Innovations in the Treatment of Substance
Addiction

MW01120591

André Luiz Monezi Andrade
Denise De Micheli
Editors

Innovations in the Treatment of Substance Addiction

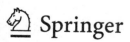 Springer

Editors
André Luiz Monezi Andrade
Departamento de Psicobiologia
Universidade Federal de São Paulo
São Paulo
Brazil

Denise De Micheli
Universidade Federal de São Paulo
São Paulo
Brazil

ISBN 978-3-319-82752-0   ISBN 978-3-319-43172-7   (eBook)
DOI 10.1007/978-3-319-43172-7

Printed on acid-free paper

This Springer imprint is published by Springer Nature
The registered company is Springer International Publishing AG Switzerland

Acknowledgments

Firstly, I would like to dedicate this book to health professionals who devote the majority of their professional lives dealing with all aspects of drug rehabilitation and to the family members of those suffering from addiction.

My deep gratitude to my parents for their love and support throughout my life.

Thanks to my wife for her constant love, encouragement, and understanding during those times I have spent researching and writing this book.

I want to thank my students, who over the years have helped me to discover the joy of teaching.

Finally, I would like to thank many people whose help and inspiration made this project possible.

André Luiz Monezi Andrade

For from Him and through Him and for Him are all things. (Romans 11:36)

To Nicolau, my love and great encourager... together we are always better and stronger!

For Nicolas and Carla, who teach me every day about unconditional love and day by day make me feel the most special person in the world.

To my parents, Regina and Gian, examples of love and perseverance.

Denise De Micheli

Contents

Editors and Contributors

About the Editors

André Luiz Monezi Andrade obtained MD and Ph.D. in psychobiology (with an emphasis on substance dependence) from the Universidade Federal de São Paulo (UNIFESP)—Escola Paulista de Medicina and graduated in psychology from the Universidade Positivo. At present, he is an associate editor of the International Journal of Psychology and Neuroscience (ISSN 2183-5829). He has experience in basic research that evaluates the effects of the dopaminergic and serotoninergic systems on the behavioral sensitization to the stimulant effects of alcohol in rodents. He has developed several works in clinical research that evaluate different models of prevention of drug use and abuse. Additionally, he was the supervisor of the courses SUPERA (System for the Abusive use of and Dependence on Psychoactive Substances: Referral, Brief Intervention, Social Reinsertion and Follow-up) and Faith in Prevention, both sponsored by the National Secretary of Policy on Drugs (SENAD), which have already qualified over 70,000 health professionals and religious leaders from all the states of the country. He is a member of an International Multicentric Study coordinated by the World Health Organization in which Brazil, India, Mexico, and Belarus participate, focused on the evaluation of the effectiveness of virtual interventions on alcohol use. He also gives classes at the Department of Psychology of Universidade Anhembi Morumbi—Laureate International Universities®.

Denise De Micheli obtained a bachelor's degree in psychology at Universidade Paulista and master's and doctoral degrees at the Universidade Federal de São Paulo. She is a professor in the Department of Psychobiology at Universidade Federal de São Paulo, also serves as chief of the Interdisciplinary Centre of Studies in Neuroscience Adolescent Health and Education, and is a member of the Association for Medical Education and Research in Substance Abuse.

Contributors

Rui Ferreira Afonso Master's degree in Psychobiology from Universidade Federal de São Paulo and doctoral student in neurosciences. Yoga and meditation's teacher.

André Bedendo Psychologist from the Universidade Federal de Juiz de Fora and Master of Sciences from the Department of Psychobiology of the Universidade Federal de São Paulo, where he is presently a doctoral student. He is a researcher at the Núcleo de Pesquisa em Saúde e Uso de Substâncias (NEPSIS) (Nucleus of Research in Health and Substance Use) and supervisor of the distance learning course SUPERA (System for the Abusive use of and Dependence on Psychoactive Substances: Referral, Brief Intervention, Social Reinsertion and Follow-up), sponsored by the National Secretary of Policy on Drugs (SENAD).

Kirk J. Brower Department of Psychiatry and Addiction Research Center, University of Michigan; 4250 Plymouth Road, Ann Arbor, MI 48109-2700.

Susan Brown is a Licensed Clinical Social Worker (LCSW), Board Certified Diplomate, has been in private practice in La Mesa, CA. since 1987, and a Certified Approved Consultant through the EMDR International Association.

Oleg Chaban Psychosomatic Medicine and Psychotherapy Department, Ukrainian Research Institute of Social and Forensic Psychiatry and Drug Abuse; Department of Psychoneurology, Railway Clinical Hospital #1, station Kyiv; 8a Kotsubinskiy str., Kyiv, Ukraine, 01030.

Deirdre A. Conroy Clinical Associate Professor, Department of Psychiatry and Addiction Research Center, University of Michigan; 4250 Plymouth Road, Ann Arbor, MI 48109-2700.

Erica Cruvinel is a psychologist, obtained master's degree in collective health, a Ph.D. student of the Post-graduation Program in Psychology at Federal University of Juiz de fora, and a researcher at Reference Center in Alcohol and Other Drugs Research, Intervention and Evaluation.

Dianne da Rocha Prado is an undergraduate student doing Bachelor of Science and Technology at Universidade Federal do ABC, and performs training in neurosciences and cognition and investigating the effect of ayahuasca in models of morphine dependence and withdrawal syndrome.

Víviam Vargas de Barros is a psychologist and has a master's in psychology from the Universidade Federal de Juiz de Fora. She is currently a doctoral student at the Department of Psychobiology of the Universidade Federal de São Paulo. She has professional training in cognitive behavioral therapy from the Núcleo de Estudo Interdisciplinar em Saúde Mental (NEISME) (Center of Interdisciplinary Study in Mental Health). She is a certified practitioner in Mindfulness-based Relapse Prevention (MBRP) from the University of California, San Diego Medical School, and advanced training for Professors in MBRP from the Centre for Addiction Treatment Studies—Warminster, England. She is currently a member of the Brazilian Center of Research and Training in Mindfulness-based Relapse Prevention (MBRP Brasil), a subgroup of the Núcleo de Pesquisa em Saúde e Uso de Substâncias (NEPSIS) (Center of Studies in Health and Substance Use), as well as of the Mente Aberta (Open Mind—Brazilian Center of Mindfulness and Health Promotion). The focus of her studies is substance use and mindfulness-based interventions.

Marco Tulio de Mello graduated in physical education from the Universidade Federal de Uberlândia (UFU), specialized in Physical Education for Persons with Special Needs from the UFU, a doctor in psychobiology from the Universidade Federal de São Paulo, and a full professor from the Universidade Estadual de Campinas. Mello is an associate professor at the Department of Sports in the College of Physical Education, Physical Therapy and Occupational Therapy at the Universidade Federal de Minas Gerais.

Lúcio Garcia de Oliveira graduated in biomedicine from the Universidade Federal de São Paulo (UNIFESP) and in psychology from the Centro Universitário Paulistano (Unipaulistana). He specialized in neuropsychology at the Center of Psychosurgical Studies (CEPSIC) of Hospital das Clínicas (HC-FMUSP) and in cognitive behavioral therapy in the Program of Anxiety (AMBAN) of the Institute of Psychiatry at the Faculdade de Medicina da Universidade de São Paulo FMUSP. He has a master's and a doctoral degree from the Department of Psychobiology at the Universidade Federal de São Paulo UNIFESP, has a post-doctoral degree from the Department and Institute of Psychiatry at Faculdade de Medicina da Universidade de São Paulo (FMUSP), and is a doctoral student at the Department of Forensic Medicine, Medical Ethics and Social and Work Medicine (FMUSP). He is currently working as a psychologist at Hospital Municipal Dr. Fernando Mauro Pires da Rocha, in the south region of the city of São Paulo, and carrying out research in epidemiology, cognitive evaluation, neuropsychology, and drug abuse and dependence.

Isabel Cristina Weiss de Souza is a clinical psychologist and a doctoral student at the Department of Psychobiology of the Universidade Federal de São Paulo (UNIFESP). She has a master's degree in public health from the Universidade Federal de Juiz de Fora (UFJF) and is a specialist in cognitive therapies from the Faculdade de Medicina da Universidade de São Paulo (USP). She had training in Mindfulness-based Relapse Prevention (MBRP) from the University of California, San Diego School of Medicine, and advanced teacher training from the Centre for Addiction Treatment Studies (UK). She worked at the Centro de Atenção Psicossocial Álcool e Drogas (CAPS-AD) (Center of Psychosocial Care—Alcohol and Drugs) between 1992 and 2008. She is currently working as a collaborator at the Centro de Pesquisa, Intervenção e Avaliação em Álcool e Outras Drogas (Crepeia/UFJF) (Center of Research, Intervention and Evaluation on Alcohol and

Other Drugs), and at the Núcleo de Pesquisa em Saúde e Uso de Substâncias (Nepsis/UNIFESP) (Center of Research in Health and Substance Use).

Fateme Dehghani-Arani Department of Psychology, University of Tehran, Dr Kardan Street, Nasr Bridge, Jalal al Ahmad Street, Chamran Highway, Tehran 1445983861, Iran

Paulo Daubian Rubini dos Santos Nosé graduated in physical exercise from the Faculdades Metropolitanas Unidas—FMU and is taking a master's degree in the post-graduation course of Sciences of Nutrition and Sports and Metabolism in the College of Applied Sciences at the Universidade Estadual de Campinas—FCA/UNICAMP.

Frederico Eckschmidt graduated in psychology at Universidade Presbiteriana Mackenzie (2004), specialized in substance dependence from the Department and Institute of Psychiatry at the Medical School at Universidade de São Paulo (2011), and is taking a master's degree at the School of Preventive Medicine at USP, with a focus on traffic hazards associated with mixing alcoholic beverages and caffeine. He has experience in the treatment and research of substance use-related disorders, with articles published in national and international journals with epidemiological data and their consequences. He works mainly on the following issues: substance use-related disorders, epidemiology, treatment, and rehabilitation.

Andrea Maculano Esteves graduated in physical education (1999) and specialized in adapted sports (2000) from the Universidade Federal de Uberlândia (2000). She holds a master's degree in psychobiology (2003), doctoral degree in sciences (2007), and postdoctoral (2011) from the Universidade Federal de São Paulo. She is presently a professor at the Universidade Estadual de Campinas (UNICAMP) in the College of Applied Sciences (FCA) and certified in the post-graduation course Sciences of Nutrition and Sports and Metabolism from the same institution. She is a coordinator of the Laboratory of Sleep and Physical Exercise (LASPE) with experience in research (basic and clinical), teaching, and extension in the area of psychobiological aspects with emphasis on physical education. Her main areas of activity are sleep, sleep disorders, adapted physical education, physical exercise, and shift work.

Maira Leon Ferreira is a psychologist, obtained a master's degree, a Ph.D. student of the Post-graduation Program in Psychology at Federal University of Juiz de Fora, and a researcher at Reference Center in Alcohol and Other Drugs Research, Intervention and Evaluation.

Iryna Frankova Psychosomatic Medicine and Psychotherapy Department, Ukrainian Research Institute of Social and Forensic Psychiatry and Drug Abuse; 8a Kotsubinskiy str., Kyiv, Ukraine, 01030.

Luis Pereira Justo is a psychiatry doctor, obtained a master's in sciences from the Universidade Federal de São Paulo, and a researcher at Association Fund of Incentive to Research (AFIP—Associação Fundo de Incentivo à Pesquisa).

Justo is a physician at the Center of Reference and Training in STD-Aids of the Secretariat of Government of the State of São Paulo (CRT-DST-Aids da Secretaria de Estado de Governo do Estado de São Paulo), 04023-062, Brazil.

Elisa Harumi Kozasa majored in biological sciences from the Universidade de São Paulo, has a postdoctoral, a doctoral, and a master's degree from the Department of Psychobiology of the Universidade Federal de São Paulo. She is a researcher and a professor in neuroscience in the post-graduation program in Health Sciences of the Instituto Israelita de Ensino e Pesquisa Albert Einstein. Her main researches address the neurophysiology and effects of mind–body interventions such as meditation, evaluated by functional neuroimaging. She is an instructor in the program Cultivating Emotional Balance.

Alexander Mazur Department of Anatomy and Cell Biology, McGill University; 3640 University Street, Montreal, Quebec, Canada H3A 0C7.

Fúlvio Rieli Mendes graduated in biomedical Sciences at Universidade Federal de São Paulo, with master's and doctorate at the same institution. He is a professor of pharmacology at the Universidade Federal do ABC (UFABC), advisor at the graduate program in Neuroscience and Cognition at UFABC, and collaborator of the Brazilian Center for Psychotropic Drug Information (CEBRID).

Ricardo Monezi holds a master's from the School of Medicine at the Faculdade de Medicina da Universidade de São Paulo; doctor from Escola Paulista de Medicina/Universidade Federal de São Paulo; a postdoctoral student at the Department of Preventive Medicine at the Escola Paulista de Medicina/Universidade Federal de São Paulo; a member of the Nucleus of Medicine and Integrative Practices (NUMEPI) of the Escola Paulista de Medicina/Universidade Federal de São Paulo; and a teacher at the Pontifícia Universidade Católica, São Paulo.

Ana Regina Noto graduated in psychology from the Faculdade Paulistana de Ciências e Letras (1997) and in biochemical pharmacy from the a Pontifícia Universidade Católica de Campinas (1988). She holds a master's degree (1995) and doctoral degree (1998) in psychobiology from the Universidade Federal de São Paulo. She is presently a professor at the Department of Psychobiology of the Universidade Federal de São Paulo and a coordinator of the Nucleus of Research in Health and Substance Use (NEPSIS) and the Centro Regional de Referência em Crack e outras Drogas—CRR-DIMESAD-UNIFESP (Regional Center of Reference on Crack and Other Drugs). Her line of research is focused on psychosocial aspects related to the use of psychotropic substances and their implications for health, both as an epidemiological and a qualitative reference. She also focuses on clinical and community trials of evaluation of preventive and therapeutic interventions from the perspective of developmental and cognitive psychology. Her main study themes are use of alcohol/drugs in socially vulnerable populations; relapse prevention based on mindfulness; and drug use, violence, and family.

Anna Oliinyk Department of Psychoneurology, Railway Clinical Hospital #1, station Kyiv; 8a Kotsubinskiy str., Kyiv, Ukraine, 01030.

Laisa Marcorela Andreoli Sartes is a psychologist and obtained master's degree and Ph.D. in sciences at the Psychobiology Program of UNIFESP. She is a psychology associate professor of Federal University of Juiz de Fora and researcher at Reference Center in Alcohol and Other Drugs Research, Intervention and Evaluation.

Adriana Scatena graduated in psychology from the Faculdade Paulistana de Ciências e Letras and specialized in Hospital Psychology from Universidade de Santo Amaro. She has experience in training and development with a focus on human resources; hospital psychology with a focus on different levels of prevention (primary, secondary, and tertiary); and in clinical psychology (brief psychotherapy) with an emphasis on childhood and adolescence. She has a master's in childhood and adolescence from the Universidade Federal de São Paulo.

Michael P. Schaub is a senior lecturer in psychology at the University of Zurich and the scientific director of the Swiss Research Institute of Public Health and Addiction ISGF, a WHO Collaborating Centre, associated with the University of Zurich. He is a trained psychotherapist with a strong clinical and scientific background in the area of substance use disorders. He completed his Ph.D. in 2005 on the topic of cannabis use, its associated personality dimensions in the general population, and co-occurring mental health problems in vulnerable persons. In 2012, he received his postdoctoral lecture qualification (Habilitation) for psychology, with the specialization for "treatment and diagnostic of substance use disorders" at the University of Zurich.

Dr. Schaub has published more than 50 peer-reviewed papers in scientific journals. He is a scientific expert in addiction research for the World Health Organization (WHO) and at the United Nations Office on Drugs and Crime UNODC. Currently, he is the PI of the effectiveness study on the new WHO Web-based self-help intervention Drink Less conducted in Belarus, Brazil, India, and Mexico.

Francine Shapiro obtained Ph.D. in clinical psychology, Professional School of Psychological Studies, San Diego, California; ABD in English Literature, New York University; California licensed psychologist (PSY12160); and executive director, EMDR Institute, Inc.

Shapiro is a executive director, EMDR Humanitarian Assistance Programs Senior Research Fellow-Mental Research Institute, Palo Alto, California and developed Eye Movement Desensitization and Reprocessing (EMDR) Method.

Julie Stowasser is a licensed Marriage and Family Therapist practicing in California. Emphasizing a strong general practice for all ages, her specialties include EMDR therapy, along with the treatment of male and female adults and children, who are or were victims or perpetrators of violence or other forms of abuse and neglect. In seeking to fulfill a goal of strengthening and enhancing the most competent and ethical administrations of EMDR therapy, Julie edits and writes, assists in the training of new EMDR clinicians and provides consultation, and offers workshops and presentations nationally and internationally.

André Wagner is a psychologist from the Universidade Federal de Juiz de Fora and has a master's in sciences from the Department of Psychobiology of the Universidade Federal de São Paulo, where he is presently a doctoral student. He is a researcher at the Núcleo de Pesquisa em Saúde e Uso de Substâncias (NEPSIS) (Nucleus of Research in Health and Substance Use) and supervisor of the distance learning course SUPERA (System for the Abusive use of and Dependence on Psychoactive Substances: Referral, Brief Intervention, Social Reinsertion and Follow-up), sponsored by the National Secretary of Policy on Drugs (SENAD).

Gabriela Arantes Wagner is an adjunct professor of epidemiology at the Department of Preventive Medicine at the Universidade Federal de São Paulo. She has a postdoctoral degree in epidemiology from the pela Faculdade de Saúde Pública at USP (2011–2014), a doctoral degree in sciences from the Program of Post-Graduation at the Department of Psychiatry at Medical School at the Faculdade de Medicina da USP (2011), Professional Development in Analytic Toxicology from the Universidade Estadual de Campinas (2003), and graduated in pharmaceutical sciences with a major in Clinical and Toxicological Analyses from the Pontifícia Universidade Católica in Campinas (2001).

Juçara Xavier Zaparoli is a bachelor of biological science at Federal University of Sao Paulo (EPM/UNIFESP), with post-graduation (master's degree—Master of Science) in psychobiology at the Psychobiology Department of the UNIFESP. She has experience on developing clinical research to investigate the effects of omega-3 fatty acid family on nicotine dependence.

Nataliya Zhabenko Department of Psychiatry and Addiction Psychiatry, State Establishment "The Lugansk State Medical University"; 50 rokiv Oborony Luganska 1, Luhansk, Ukraine, 91045.

Olena Zhabenko Psychosomatic Medicine and Psychotherapy Department, Ukrainian Research Institute of Social and Forensic Psychiatry and Drug Abuse; Department of Psychoneurology, Railway Clinical Hospital #1, station Kyiv; 8a Kotsubinskiy str., Kyiv, Ukraine, 01030.

Robert A. Zucker Department of Psychiatry and Addiction Research Center, University of Michigan; 4250 Plymouth Road, Ann Arbor, MI 48109-2700.

Part I
Introduction to Substance Abuse

Chapter 1
Characterization of Substance Dependence

**Lúcio Garcia de Oliveira, Frederico Eckschmidt
and Gabriela Arantes Wagner**

Introduction

The phenomenon of dependence has often been associated exclusively with the severe neurophysiological effects related to severe symptoms of tolerance and withdrawal from certain substances or objects as, for example, illicit drugs or gambling. In recent years, however, a new definition and comprehension appeared, indicating that the several symptoms of this disorder and its multiple expressions actually share a common biopsychosocial etiology (Shaffer et al. 2004; Sussman et al. 2011; Goodman 2008). The conventional view implicitly associates the cause of dependence with the properties of those substances or objects and encourages different treatments for that compulsive behavior (Shaffer et al. 2004). Nevertheless, a more comprehensive view of this disorder is called for, since there is a wide range of common characteristics among addictive behaviors.

In this scenario, the individual ends up wasting a lot of time thinking about or engaging in behaviors regarding the consumption of psychoactive substances (PAS) such as tobacco, alcohol, and illicit drugs, and the compulsive ingestion of food or engagement in other objects such as gambling, Internet, pathological love, sex, physical exercise, work, and shopping (Shaffer et al. 2004; Sussman et al. 2011).

L.G. de Oliveira (✉) · F. Eckschmidt
Departamento de Medicina Preventiva, Universidade de São Paulo, Av. Dr. Arnaldo, 455 - 2o. andar, São Paulo, SP 01246-903, Brazil
e-mail: lucgoliver@gmail.com; luciogoliver@usp.br

F. Eckschmidt
e-mail: fredeckschmidt@gmail.com

G.A. Wagner
Departamento de Medicina Preventiva, Universidade Federal de São Paulo, Rua Botucatu, 740 5o andar, São Paulo, SP 04023-062, Brazil
e-mail: gabriela.wagner@gmail.com

© Springer International Publishing Switzerland 2016
A.L.M. Andrade and D. De Micheli (eds.), *Innovations in the Treatment of Substance Addiction*, DOI 10.1007/978-3-319-43172-7_1

As regards substance use disorder (SUD), bulimia, pathological gambling, and compulsive sexual behavior, in addition to the suffering inflicted upon the individual, all of them share a series of clinical characteristics, namely (a) the course of the disease, since the disorders generally appear in adolescence or early adulthood, running a chronic course, with remissions and exacerbations; (b) the maintenance of the behavior in spite of the harmful consequences and the narrowing of the repertoire; (c) the subjective experience of the individuals, presenting intense desire, concern, or excitement during the preparatory activity, in addition to the feeling of loss of control; (d) progressive development; (e) tolerance, that is, reduction of strength of the reinforcing effects; (f) withdrawal, with physical or psychological discomfort by the interruption or reduction of the behavior; (g) likelihood of relapses, with the continuous return to harmful patterns after a period of withdrawal or control; (h) propensity to substitution for other addictive behaviors; (i) harm or neglect in other aspects of life (work, social activities or hobbies, insufficient social relations, criminal activities and legal problems, involvement in dangerous situations, bodily injury, financial loss or emotional trauma); and (j) recurring content in the way individuals relate with themselves and others, including low self-esteem, self-centeredness, denial, rationalization, and the conflicts between dependence and control (Sussman et al. 2011; Goodman 2008).

In the case of any dependence, we can observe that the disorder involves the loss of capacity to freely choose whether to continue or quit the behavior (loss of control), which leads to adverse consequences. At any rate, even though some substances or objects do not seem to create an obvious physical dependence, all of them produce a subjective necessity of a deeper involvement for the individual to reach satiety and, thereafter, symptoms such as depression, intense anxiety, hopelessness, helplessness, and irritability in the event of its the sudden withdrawal (Sussman et al. 2011).

Disorders Due to Substance Use (DSU)

The use of PAS involves a coevolutionary relationship that started at least 200 million years ago with the first arboreals and plants, possibly being explored by the first mammals as substitutes for the nutritionally costly neurotransmitters produced endogenously (Sullivan and Hagen 2002).

Over this period, countless genetic adaptations were necessary for our body to metabolize alkaloids and alcohol. This hypothesis is supported by the several chemical adaptations necessary for the metabolization of those substances and in the structure of the plants that evolved to mimic neurotransmitters and interfere with their functions (Sullivan and Hagen 2002; McGovern 2009).

Therefore, certain substances are endowed with a property known as psychoactivity; that is, the ingestion of those compounds might interfere with several mental processes as, for example, cognition and humor (SENAD 2006), with behaviors and awareness, in such a way that "the effects might range from a mild stimulation caused by a cup of coffee or tea to the deeply changing effects produced by hallucinogenics as LSD" (Ott 1996).

This group of compounds can be categorized according to the several effects they have on the central nervous system (CNS). In general, they are classified into three categories: (a) psycholeptic, that is, substances that inhibit the mental tonus or the functioning of the CNS; (b) psychoanaleptic, substances that stimulate the mental tonus or the functioning of the CNS; or (c) psychodysleptic, substances that disturb the mental tonus or the functioning of the CNS (Seibel 2010). The chemist A. Hoffmann later added the (d) neuroleptics, substances with anxiolytic and antipsychotic properties, of which the group of *Rauvolfia serpentina* constitutes the natural prototype (Ott 1996).

However, even though this system is didactic and simple, it draws together the action and effects of the PAS excessively, thus losing precision as a result of extreme reductionism. A more accurate description of its effects on the CNS could, therefore, include other characteristics, as suggested by the ethnobotanist Ott (1996): (a) narcotic, with sedation properties as the opioids; (b) intoxicant, as alcohol and other solvents and as chloroform, ether, and benzene; (c) hypnotic, that is, related to sleep and the hypnagogic states, as barbiturates and benzodiazepines tranquilizers; (d) stimulant, as caffeine, cocaine, and amphetamines; (e) entheogen or psychedelic (hallucinogenic), which deeply affect sense perception, mood, and behaviors, as mescaline, LSD, psilocybin, DMT, and ibogaine; and (f) sedative neuroleptic, as meprobamate and chlorpromazine.

Yet, that model does not address the presence of several substances in more than one category, as in the case of tobacco, which is a stimulant and a depressor concomitantly, or MDMA (*ecstasy*), a stimulant and psychedelic, or one of the two main cannabinoids, THC, which is stimulant, depressant, and psychedelic, and the CBD, which is antipsychotic, and countless others, as psychologist McKim (2007) suggests.

Those definitions are important, but they do not describe the addictive power of the substances, since some of them (tobacco and alcohol) are commercialized almost freely in spite of favoring the development of dependence, while others are prohibited without entailing no type of dependence or withdrawal syndrome, as entheogens, for example (Ott 1996). Consequently, although practically all PAS might be related to contexts of abuse and even cause other damaging effects, not all of them are associated with dependence, independently of being illicit or not. Accordingly, some substances are more addictive, as opiates and tobacco, and others have a lower or no addictive power, as LSD or psilocybin.

Diagnostic Criteria

Numerous terms are used to describe the full spectrum of PAS use as well as their effects and the disorders they cause. Drug use can be defined as, for each and every consumption, experimental, sporadic, or frequent. Those categories are not necessarily related to harmful use or dependence syndrome.

Disorder takes place when there is a problematic use of PAS, a maladaptive pattern. Its diagnosis can be based on two distinct systems: the ICD-10 (International Catalogue of Diseases in its 10th version) (WHO 2005) and the DSM-5 (Diagnostic and Statistical Manual of Mental Disorders in its 5th version) (APA 2014).

According to the ICD-10, this group of disorders is defined as "Mental and behavioral disorders due to psychoactive substance use" (WHO 2005). This classification system uses letter F (relative to Chapter 5, dedicated to mental and behavioral disorders), the second item typifies the disorder due to the use of PAS, which is number 1, and the third digit of the code identifies the substance used. Therefore, the system comprises the following codes:

- **F10**. – due to the use of alcohol.
- **F11**. – due to the use of opiates.
- **F12**. – due to the use of cannabinoids.
- **F13**. – due to the use of sedatives and hypnotics.
- **F14**. – due to the use of cocaine.
- **F15**. – due to the use of other stimulants, including caffeine.
- **F16**. – due to the use of hallucinogenics.

The fourth item of the classification regards the clinical condition, or its specificities, where mainly the following aspects are classified: a (.0), which is acute intoxication; a (.1), which typifies the use that is harmful to health, and a (.2), which indicates the development of dependence syndrome, among others.

Contrariwise to acute intoxication, which can happen on one single occasion, harmful use is characterized by recurrent and significant damage related to the repeated use of the substance. In order to be diagnosed, the individual should meet the following diagnostic criteria:

- Physical or psychological damage
- Identifiable nature of the damage
- Persistent use in spite of the complications
- Does not meet criteria for dependence

Dependence syndrome, on the other hand, is diagnosed only when the individual presents three or more of the behaviors listed below in the last 12 months:

- Strong craving or compulsion
- Incapacity of control
- Withdrawal
- Tolerance
- Progressive dropout of pleasant activities/interests
- Persistent use in spite of harmful consequences

Therefore, in order to meet criteria for dependence, the individual should present basically three symptoms: (a) craving, the person is unable to stop thinking about or using the drug; (b) tolerance, which makes the individual use higher and higher doses, and (c) withdrawal, characterized by a general feeling of uneasiness when it is discontinued or lacking.

An important concept here is that abstinence crisis differs from the simple craving. The latter possesses a more psychological component and manifests as a strong will to use the substance. In withdrawal, additionally to the will, there are unpleasant physical phenomena such as nausea, irritability, tremors, insomnia.

The other system of diagnostic classification is the DSM-5 (APA 2014; Dawson et al. 2013). Despite being polemic, in 2013, there was a conceptual change in the way substance use disorder (SUD) is understood. It abolished the distinction between abuse and dependence present until the 4th version. Currently, the system encompasses the two distinct manifestations under one single disorder: substance-related and addictive, now classified according to severity as mild, moderate, or severe.

This change was necessary to incorporate the old criteria of the DSM-4 for substance dependence that had already been inserted regarding severity, but also by the evidence that abuse does not necessarily precede the incidence of dependence (APA 2014). As a result, the diagnosis of substance-related and addictive disorders requires at least two or more criteria, and severity began to be classified according to the number of criteria met: two or more indicate mild disorder; four or five indicate moderate disorder; and six or more criteria indicate severe disorder (Araújo and Lotufo Neto 2014).

This alteration became polemic especially in the case of individuals who presented one single criterion as, for example, using illicit drugs or drunk driving, who are no longer considered abusers. Another aspect involves individuals who met only two dependence criteria of the old DSM-4 and now would be classified as having moderate severity according to the DSM-5 (Dawson et al. 2013). Another important conceptual change was the inclusion of gambling disorder among the substance-related and addictive disorders in the DSM-5; there is growing evidence that such behavior acts on the reward system with similar effects to those of drugs of abuse (Araújo and Lotufo Neto 2014), a fact that also corroborates the idea of a common etiology.

Etiology

However, there are different risk factors (or variables) that interfere in the development of drug dependence. Those factors are **biopsychosocial**; that is, they are related to the drug itself, the user, and the environment the user is in. Literature points that genetic factors account for 40–60 % of an individual's vulnerability to develop dependence. This estimate includes the effects caused by environmental factors on the function and expression of a person's genes, the epigenetic heritage. Factors involved in the psychological development and other medical conditions also influence the development of the disorder. In addition, adolescents and individuals with other mental disorders (comorbidities) face a higher risk of drug abuse and dependence than the general population (NIDA 2014).

Drug-Related Variables

An important pathway for the understanding of drug effects on the brain is the reward pathway. This pathway involves several parts of the brain, among which the ventral tegmental area (VTA), the nucleus accumbens, and the prefrontal cortex. When this pathway is activated by a rewarding stimulus (as, for instance, food, water, sex, and drugs), the information travels from the VTA to the nucleus accumbens and then to the prefrontal cortex. Some behavioral theories on drug dependence consider that the behavior learned or sustained by means of animal models characterizes drug dependence, since they share the common fact that those substances have a positive reinforcing capacity from use, as the activation of the serotoninergic, dopaminergic, and GAGAergic pathways. In this context, drugs might have a higher or lower abuse potential, which might be directly related to the effect of the substance itself and its capacity to activate the reward pathway in each individual, as drugs present individual variability, that is, the potential for reinforcement and abuse differ for each one (Formigoni and Abrahão 2010).

Important characteristics to be considered other than the pharmacological properties of the drugs of abuse are their pharmacokinetic characteristics. The faster the speed of arrival to the site of action of a drug, the higher the biotransformation and excretion speed, which makes its use be repeated more constantly. A classic example is the difference between smoked cocaine (crack freebase) and powder cocaine (cocaine chloridrate). Both drugs have the sympathomimetic agent, but in the smoked mode, the absorption speed and the plasmatic concentration are higher for being conferred by its absorption via the pulmonary alveoli, similarly to cocaine administered intravenously. This speeds up the onset of effects. Aspired (snorted) powder cocaine is absorbed by nasal–oropharyngeal membranes, which demands higher drug absorption time and more time for the effects to take place (Moreau and Camarini 2014).

Tolerance mechanisms and withdrawal syndrome are other characteristics of drug dependence. Those phenomena result from physiological adaptations that happen as a result of exposure to drugs. Tolerance is the decrease of the effect of the drug in spite of the dose being maintained; that is, the user needs to increase the dose to reach its desired effect. Withdrawal syndrome is a set of symptoms that happen as a consequence of the sudden absence of a dependence-inducing drug, which can be considered as a "rebound" effect of the drug withdrawal (Formigoni and Abrahão 2010; Moreau and Camarini 2014).

Epidemiology and Current Scenario

Another important characteristic for one to understand the phenomenon of dependence is the frequency and the damage caused by the excessive use of PAS. First, it is crucial to highlight the fact that recreational or social use is usually not related to problems or disorders (Seibel 2010), even in the case of illicit substances. Its frequency is usually measured by populational and statistical surveys, and the replication of those surveys from time to time allows the construction of historical series. The analysis of those series allows researchers to highlight (or not) changes in use over time as well as identify new trends of use and, finally, compare its use by the population according to the political and social–historical situation.

In this sense, the "World Drug Report" is a statistical survey carried out by the "United Nations Office on Drug and Crime—UNODC" that measured the use of psychoactive substances by individuals between 15 and 64 years old all over the world by means of three indicators: (a) *lifetime use* (use at least once in life, which then represents experimental use), *annual use* (or in the last 12 months, which then represents sporadic use), and use *in the past* 30 *days* (which represents *a present and possibly regular use*; UNODC 2014).

Currently, out of seven billion individuals the world over, approximately 240 million used illicit substances at least once in the year (UNODCCP 2013), also counting occasional users. This number drops to half when consumption in the last 30 days is assessed, hence most of the users who make a more frequent use (UNODCCP 2012). Still considering that total, only 12 % of illicit drug users, or 0.6 % of the world population between 15 and 64 years old, will develop some use-related disorder, as drug abuse or dependence (UNODCCP 2013).

Therefore, the fact that a substance is illicit does not mean it will trigger the disorder. Quite the contrary, when we compare the use of illicit substances or even the problematic use of illicit substances with that of licit substances as alcohol and tobacco, we may notice that the latter cause much more damage in terms of populational percentage (UNODCCP 2013).

In this scenario, it is important to stress the fact that alcohol is the psychotropic substance most consumed all over the world. Its harmful use is defined by the World Health Organization (WHO) as a drinking behavior that causes social and health consequences to the drinker and those in his immediate surroundings, as well as any kind of use associated with adverse effects to health (UNODC 2014). The harmful use of alcohol is responsible for 3.3 million annual deaths (5.9 % of all the deaths in the world); hence, it appears as the eighth risk factor for deaths, preceded by hypertension, tobacco use, diabetes, physical inactivity, overweight and obesity, high cholesterol, and unprotected sex, affecting especially middle-income countries (WHO 2009).

Still in this scenario, alcohol use is responsible for 5.1 % of the global burden of illnesses and injuries in the world, leading to 139 million loss regarding disability-adjusted life years (DALYs) due to premature death or incapacitating condition (World Health Organization 2014), affecting mainly middle-income countries, as mentioned for the mortality rate (WHO 2009).

Thus, the use of alcohol is associated with the occurrence of *two hundred* health conditions (ICD-10) whose incidence or progression is affected by alcohol, namely (World Health Organization 2014):

1. Neuropsychiatric conditions: alcohol harmful use and dependence;
2. Illnesses of the gastrointestinal tract: hepatic cirrhosis and pancreatitis;
3. Cancer: mouth, nasopharynx, oropharynx, larynx, colon, rectum, liver, pancreas, and breast;
4. Intentional damage: suicide and homicide;
5. Unintentional damage: the higher the blood alcohol concentration, the higher the probability of psychomotor effects, placing the individual at risk, as in the case of traffic accidents (TA);
6. Cardiovascular Diseases (CVDs): the beneficial effect of alcohol disappears as the pattern of use becomes more intense;
7. Fetal alcohol syndrome (FAS);
8. Diabetes mellitus;
9. Infectious–contagious diseases: Alcohol weakens the immune system, giving room for opportunistic diseases. In this case, a relation between the harmful use of alcohol and the incidence of HIV/AIDS and tuberculosis has been pointed.

The global burden of alcohol use-related diseases is associated mainly with neuropsychiatric diseases. Consequently, it is noteworthy that about 25 % of the years of working life lost due to incapacity (DALYs) are a result of psychiatric disorders, causing more incapacity than mortality.

According to the WHO, the world population between 15 and 64 years old consumes an average of 6.2 L of pure alcohol/year. Out of that population, 38.3 % are alcohol users, 13.7 % do not ingest alcoholic beverages anymore, and 48 % are teetotalers. The highest alcohol consumption can be observed in Europe and America. The European population between 15 and 64 years old consumes on average 10.9 L of alcohol/year, while Americans consume on average 8.4 L of pure alcohol/year. A little over 65 % of the European population (66.4 %) ingests some type of alcoholic beverage, in contrast to 61.5 % of Americans, prevalence that is higher than those observed for the world population in this age bracket. It should be mentioned that the lowest prevalence of teetotalers is observed in America, with com 18.9 %. Another remarkable fact is that 7.5 % of the world population engage in the pattern of use known as heavy episodic drinking, defined as the use of 60 g of alcohol or more of pure alcohol (6 + alcoholic doses) on one single occasion and at least once a month.

Finally, 4.1 % of the world population between 15 and 64 years old have some alcohol-related psychiatric disorder, out of which 1.8 % make harmful use of alcohol and 2.3 % can already be considered dependent. Europe is the region that presents the highest prevalence of alcohol-related psychiatric disorders, with 7.5 % of the total population (3.5 % making harmful use and 4.0 % already dependent), followed again by 6 % in the regions of America (2.6 % harmful use and 3.4 % already dependent; World Health Organization 2014).

Those data might indicate that something is wrong as regards the priority on which important financial resources of the health system and the legal system are spent, and the way this issue is handled, through a unicausal view focused exclusively on the drug consumption, an approach that ends up criminalizing several ethnic groups and individuals with higher vulnerability, creating violence, deaths and prison overcrowding.

Psychosocial Factors Involved

In particular, because not every PAS user develops some sort of disorder (quite the contrary, most of them seem to make recreational use without major problems), the need of a broader comprehension of this phenomenon is evident. For this to happen, attention should also be given to psychosocial factors that deeply influence the development of dependence.

Since only some PAS users become problematic or compulsive, researchers should evaluate etiologic mechanisms other than the substance itself in order to understand the harmful use and the development of dependence: the contexts and vulnerability associated with the history of the individuals, their environment, cultural and epigenetic characteristics, gender, possible places where PAS can be acquired, etc.

Initially, it is fundamental to reinforce that it is not only the substance that causes dependence, but rather the combination among the PAS effects, the body, and the context in which consumption takes place. For example, a stock market operator in New York might use the chloridrate (salt) to enhance his performance and cognitive capacity, while a worker in Bolivia might chew the leaves of the *Erythroxylum coca* bush to obtain the same effects and to suppress hunger.

The two modes of administration and the power of the effects are different (snorted and ingested), the meaning for both is different (in one context, it is expensive and illegal; in the other, it has a millennial and religious use), and the individuals are different. Each one has a life history, and each one has their own reaction to the substance, from an unpleasant situation of paranoia and tachycardia to an increment at some level. Therefore, if only the psychopharmacological effects of the substance were considered, both users would develop dependence, which is not observed in the clinical practice. On the contrary, cocaine was added to several tonics as Coca-Cola and Mariani wine in the beginning of the twentieth century, offered even in the form of tablets to children with a toothache, due to its "invigorating" and topic anesthetic power.

Therefore, each organism that uses a PSA generates a phenomenon known as *reinforcement*, being stimulated to continue the use or not, depending on the context or the result. In the example of the workers, perhaps both reached enhanced production and, consequently, higher income. However, what the individual sometimes searches for is self-medication or a substance that helps him cope with some difficult social or emotional situation. In that case, it is common to observe shy people who find themselves more sociable after the ingestion of alcohol, or individuals who do not have support or knowledge to deal with their own sexuality, situations of abuse, or comorbid mental disorders and resort to PAS in order to better cope with those difficulties. The higher risk for the development of dependence is present in those situations, since there are social and individual vulnerabilities that favor the onset of the disorder. In those cases, there is a neuropsychological matching of a pleasant sensation with a dopaminergic stimulation of the brain reward system along with the avoidance of an unpleasant situation or suffering.

Consequently, this distinction of context is important, since unfortunately there is still the myth that if you use marijuana, even if it is once, you will become dependent, and in the case of crack, one single use already leads the person to totally lose control of their lives and become zombies. There is nothing more fallacious than this type of argument, as the lack of information often makes the dialogue with the individual who is already suffering even more difficult and often makes him the victim of a system from which he finds no way out. One of the first experiments that evidenced this social–environmental relation was performed by psychologist Alexander et al. (1978) who, in 1978, showed the effects of social environment and gender on the self-administration of morphine in rats.

In order to determine the effects of habitat conditions on morphine self-administration, rats were isolated in two types of cages: a standard laboratory cage, and another large open box (8.8 m^2) in an environment that allowed for leisure and socialization. The study showed that on the day of choice between drinking water or the morphine solution, the isolated rats drank significantly more morphine than the rats in environments that favored social relations and entertainment, and the isolated females drank significantly more morphine than the males (Alexander et al. 1978). Their research, therefore, indicated that the isolated rats increased their morphine consumption, while the animals housed socially decreased it. This result started a broad debate, questioning the results presented in previous researches on small and isolated cages as well as the fact that those situations might happen on a daily basis.

That experiment became classic, but, later on, countless other experiments showed that PAS abuse and dependence are associated with a multitude of risk factors in different contexts of development. Several sociodemographic risk factors (e.g., poverty, geography, family, and peer groups) may influence the onset and evolution of SUD and other activities (gambling, for instance) in the same way that they can affect the development of dependence (Shaffer et al. 2004). Additionally, several researches show that the presence of psychopathology is higher among individuals who are dependent on multiple PAS than in the general population. Shaffer et al. highlight the fact that many of those who search for the treatment for SUD have higher rates of anxiety and depressive disorders. Moreover, populations with psychopathological conditions (major depression, generalized anxiety disorder, or post-traumatic stress disorder) frequently present an increased prevalence of SUD, and several studies show psychiatric comorbidity conditions often precede alcohol and cocaine abuse (Shaffer et al. 2004). Major depression, bipolar disorder, borderline personality disorder, and post-traumatic stress disorder are especially associated with suicidal behavior in individuals with addictive disorders (Yuodelis-Flores and Ries 2015).

Hence, a considerable number of prospective and longitudinal studies have found several traces of pre-morbid personality, as unconventional individuals, that demonstrate rejection of or nonconformity with social rules; those who suffer from social anxiety; searchers for sensations; pessimistic, impulsive, extrovert, and aggressive individuals; and those who have labile or irregular humor all of them have strong associations with the later development of psychoactive substance abuse (Goodman 2008).

There are also other factors as the history of the individual, with sexual abuse, for instance. The relevance of this aspect is evident when one analyzes the cases in a Spanish study. According to its author, 46 % of the patients ($n = 115$) who presented substance use disorder were victims of abuse. There was a statistically significant difference between men (37.8 %) and women (79.6 %; Fernandez-Montalvo et al. 2015).

In Brazil, the use of crack was associated with poor quality of life, worse functioning, impaired academic performance, and reduced religious involvement. Maternal presence and paternal absence were also more pronounced among crack users, who also showed more prone to search for psychologic and psychiatric treatment than the general population (Narvaez et al. 2015).

Consequently, in addition to the genetic and cognitive mechanisms, it is necessary to include other factors that interfere in the individual subjectivity, triggering the harmful use, involving the factors that the individuals establish in relation to the micro- and macro-social–cultural context in which they live, such as culture, religion, legislation, and geographical region that will determine substance offer, government system, situation of stress in childhood, psychiatric comorbidities, etc.

Conclusion

In short, dependence is a chronic non-transmissible disease characterized by three most prevalent symptoms and signs: compulsion, tolerance, and abstinence. The phenomena involved regard both the biological characteristics of the individual (e.g., genetic, physiologic, neurocognitive) and the psychological (e.g., presence of associated disorders or not) and social ones (e.g., peers, family, violence) that determine the disease. Those characteristics, however, are individual, and not all dependents will present the same risk factors for the development of the disease. As a result, scientists resort to studies that allow them to consider the important characteristics so that they can devise projects of treatment and health prevention for those individuals, in order to make them less vulnerable from the biopsychosocial perspective. In this sense, the most important tool for the non-development of the disease is prevention. It should be built based on information that also works as a model of positive identification in the practice of learning healthy behaviors. For this to actually happen, there must be favorable contextual conditions such as jobs, health, and social inclusion.

References

Alexander, B. K., Coambs, R. B., & Hadaway, P. F. (1978). The effect of housing and gender on morphine self-administration in rats. *Psychopharmacology (Berl), 58*(2), 175–179.

APA. (2014). Diagnostic and statistical manual of mental disorders: DSM-5. http://www.dsm5.org/.

Araújo, Á. C., & Lotufo Neto, F. (2014). A nova classificação Americana para os Transtornos Mentais: o DSM-5. *Revista Brasileira de Terapia Comportamental e Cognitiva, 16*, 67–82.

Dawson, D. A., Goldstein, R. B., & Grant, B. F. (2013). Differences in the profiles of DSM-IV and DSM-5 alcohol use disorders: Implications for clinicians. *Alcoholism, Clinical and Experimental Research, 37*(Suppl 1), E305–E313.

Fernandez-Montalvo, J., Lopez-Goni, J. J., & Arteaga, A. (2015). Psychological, physical, and sexual abuse in addicted patients who undergo treatment. *Journal of Interpersonal Violence, 30*(8), 1279–1298.

Formigoni, M. L. O. S., & Abrahão, K. P. (2010). Neurobiologia da Dependência de Substâncias psicoativas. In S. D. Seibel (Ed.), *Dependência de Drogas* (2ª ed.). São Paulo: Editora Atheneu.

Goodman, A. (2008). Neurobiology of addiction: An integrative review. *Biochemical Pharmacology, 75*(1), 266–322.

McGovern, P. E. (2009). *Uncorking the past: The quest for wine, beer, and other alcoholic beverages.* Berkeley: University of California Press. (xv, 330 pp).

McKim, W. A. (2007). *Drugs and behavior: an introduction to behavioral pharmacology* (6th ed.). Upper Saddle River, NJ: Pearson Education. (xvi, 416 p., 4 p. of plates p).

Moreau, R. L. M., & Camarini, R. (2014). Drogas de abuso. In S. Oga, M. M. A. Camargo, & J. A. O. Batistuzzo (Eds.), *Fundamentos de Toxicologia* (4th ed.). São Paulo: Atheneu.

Narvaez, J. C., Pechansky, F., Jansen, K., Pinheiro, R. T., Silva, R. A., Kapczinski, F., et al. (2015). Quality of life, social functioning, family structure, and treatment history associated with crack cocaine use in youth from the general population. *Revista Brasileira de Psiquiatria, 37*(3), 211–218.

NIDA. (2014). NIH Pub No. 14-5605: National Institute on Drug Abuse; 2014 [updated 13. set.2015]. http://www.drugabuse.gov/publications/drugs-brains-behavior-science-addiction/drug-abuse-addiction.

Ott, J. (1996). *Pharmacotheon: Entheogenic drugs, their plant sources and history* (2nd ed.). Kennewick, WA: Natural Products Co. (639 pp).

Seibel, S. D. (2010). Conceitos básicos e classificação geral das substâncias psicoativas. In S. D. Seibel (Ed.), *Dependência de Drogas* (2nd ed.). São Paulo: Editora Atheneu.

SENAD. (2006). *Glossário de álcool e drogas/Tradução e notas: J. M. Bertolote.* Brasília: Secretaria Nacional Antidrogas.

Shaffer, H. J., LaPlante, D. A., LaBrie, R. A., Kidman, R. C., Donato, A. N., & Stanton, M. V. (2004). Toward a syndrome model of addiction: Multiple expressions, common etiology. *Harvard Review of Psychiatry, 12*(6), 367–374.

Sullivan, R. J., & Hagen, E. H. (2002). Psychotropic substance-seeking: Evolutionary pathology or adaptation? *Addiction, 97*(4), 389–400.

Sussman, S., Lisha, N., & Griffiths, M. (2011). Prevalence of the addictions: A problem of the majority or the minority? *Evaluation and the Health Professions, 34*(1), 3–56.

UNODC. (2014). *World drug report 2014.* New York: United Nations Office on Drugs and Crime.

UNODCCP. (2012). *World Drug Report 2012.* Viena: United Nations Office for Drug Control and Crime Prevention.

UNODCCP. (2013). *World Drug Report 2013.* Viena: United Nations Office for Drug Control and Crime Prevention.

WHO. (2005). ICD-10: International statistical classification of diseases and related health problems—tenth revision. Geneva: World Health Organization. http://www.who.int/classifications/apps/icd/icd10online2003/fr-icd.htm.

WHO. (2009). *Global health risks: Mortality and burden of disease attributable to selected major risks.* Genebra: World Health Organization.

World Health Organization. (2014). *Global status report on alcohol and health 2014.* Geneva: World Health Organization.

Yuodelis-Flores, C., & Ries, R. K. (2015). Addiction and suicide: A review. *The American Journal on Addictions, 24*(2), 98–104.

Chapter 2
Neurobiology of Substance Abuse

André Bedendo, André Luiz Monezi Andrade and Ana Regina Noto

Introduction

Drug dependence is understood as a complex disorder associated with biological, emotional, and social factors. Consequently, an individual might develop dependence as a result of the interaction of those factors or even one of them alone, which favors the repetitive use that leads to dependence.

According to the Diagnostic and Statistical Manual of Mental Disorders, Fifth Edition (DSM-V), the disorders caused by substance use are characterized by a pattern of use which entails severe clinical damage that might be physical, psychological, or social, and have significant impact on the life of the users and those around them. Among the clinical diagnoses for dependence of the DSM-V are: failure to control use; social damage; recurring use even in situations that imply in physical danger, or pharmacological criteria (presence of tolerance or abstinence).

Concerning the neurobiological bases of drugs of abuse, the first fundamental hypothesis about drugs of abuse, which attempted to explain the action of drugs on the brain, was formulated in the 1980s. Supported by several previous studies, this theory has been enhanced and many efforts have been devoted, and still are, for

---

The original version of this chapter was revised: Name of two authors were excluded from Chapter 2. The erratum to this chapter is available at 10.1007/978-3-319-43172-7_15

A. Bedendo (✉) · A.L.M. Andrade · A.R. Noto
Departamento de Psicobiologia, Universidade Federal de São Paulo, Rua Botucatu, 862 – 1o Andar, Edifício de Ciências Biomédicas, São Paulo, SP 04023-062, Brazil
e-mail: andrebedendo@gmail.com

A.L.M. Andrade
e-mail: andremonezi@gmail.com

A.R. Noto
e-mail: anareginanoto@gmail.com; ana.noto@unifesp.br

© Springer International Publishing Switzerland 2016
A.L.M. Andrade and D. De Micheli (eds.), *Innovations in the Treatment of Substance Addiction*, DOI 10.1007/978-3-319-43172-7_2

researchers to understand the neurobiological effects of drugs, mainly those associated with dependence. By studying the central nervous system (CNS), neurobiology aims at understanding and identifying the areas involved in the behavior of continuous drug use. This understanding will allow therapeutic strategies to be developed, shed light on the etiology of dependence, and promote the perception of drug dependence as a health-related disorder rather than a moral issue.

Therefore, the objective of the present chapter is to describe the main neurobiological aspects involved in the dependence on drugs of abuse, hence help understand the etiology of this dependence.

Basic Concepts: Psychopharmacology and Neuroanatomy

The brain of an adult human has approximately 170 billion cells, out of which 86 billion cells are neurons (Azevedo et al. 2009). Neurons are the main cells of the CNS responsible for the transmission of information. One of their particular characteristics is their form. They comprise a *cell body*, which processes all the basic activities of a cell and the region where the nucleus of the cell lies; the *dendrites*, which are ramifications that receive most of the information from other neurons; and the *axon*, a slender projection of a nerve cell, responsible for conducting the nervous impulse to the other neurons. Once a given stimulus reaches a neuron, this can activate it and promote the transmission of the information received, forwarding it to different brain regions. For example, when an individual sees a cake or a drug, the neuron that receives this sensory information may trigger it to other neurons that in turn might evoke a memory of how tasty that cake is or how pleasant the use of a certain substance.

Additionally, most of the neurons do not touch physically; hence, the communication among them is permeated by *synapses*. A synapse is composed by a set of two neurons (pre- and post-synaptic) and a gap between them (synaptic cleft). The information is transmitted by chemical signals from the neurotransmitters (NTs) which interact with their respective receptors. Once an electrical signal reaches the end of a neuron, called axon terminal, NTs are released into the *synaptic cleft*, allowing them to bind with their *receptors*. The binding between NTs and receptors takes place through the chemical attraction among the molecules. In a specific way, an NT can only bind with a compatible receptor. The best analogy to explain the interaction between NTs and receptors is the relation between a key and its lock. A key can only open the lock it was designed for, not working for other models. In the same way, a dopamine molecule (DA), a type of neurotransmitter, can only bind with specific dopamine receptors. Once coupled to its binding site, the NT may activate or inhibit the receptors, spreading or interrupting the transmission of information to the post-synaptic neuron.

Similarly to the NTs, drugs of abuse are chemical substances that alter the functioning of the CNS directly or indirectly. Such alterations may lead to changes in the basal activity of the brain. For example, some drugs may increase the amount of NTs released into the synaptic cleft or even increase the time they are available in the cleft. There are several physiological mechanisms that allow drugs to perform their modulations in the brain. Drugs of abuse may act by hindering the *reuptake* of NTs (their removal from the synaptic cleft); binding directly to receptors and acting independently of the presence of NTs; binding to receptors in different sites from those of the NTs (allosteric sites), modulating the action of NTs; inhibiting the degradation of NTs by binding to enzymes that are specific for this function; taking the place of NTs in the *synaptic vesicles* (site where NTs are stored); or binding directly to the membrane of the pre-synaptic neuron, promoting the release of NTs.

Neurobiology and Behavioral Aspects

According to the neurobiological theory of drug dependence, the behavior of continuously seeking for the substance or its specific effects (euphoria, relaxation, motor alterations, sleepiness, etc.) results in alterations the drugs promote in the brain activity by changing, for instance, the amount of time of action of the NTs in the synaptic cleft. The study of the neurobiology of drugs of abuse is directly related to the study of behavior. From the neurobiological perspective, the behavior of continuous consumption of drugs might be understood as a learning process in which the drug acts as reinforcement. Therefore, basic concepts of behaviorism such as stimulus, response, operant conditioning, punishment, and positive and negative reinforcements are important for the understanding of the neurobiological basis of drug use. A *stimulus* might be defined as an event or something that might cause a specific reaction, known as *response*. Responses can be of biological, psychological, or behavioral nature. Using the example we already mentioned, a cake and drugs are considered *stimuli* that might trigger a *response*: The memory of how tasty the food or how pleasant the use of the drug can be. When a *stimulus* **increases** the frequency of a *response*, it is called *reinforcement* or *reinforcing stimulus*. *Punishment*, on the other hand, **decreases** the frequency of the *response*. *Reinforcement* can be of two types: *positive* or *negative*. It is considered *positive* when its **presence** increases the frequency of a response, and *negative* when its **withdrawal** or **absence** promotes the increase in the frequency of a response.

If an individual uses the drug (stimulus) and presents a sensation of well-being (response), which enhances the chances of that behavior being repeated, the drug will be considered a *positive reinforcement*. In a negative situation, when individuals are experiencing a negative state, as in the withdrawal syndrome, they will feel relaxed and well (*response*) when they use the drug (*stimulus*), the drug will be a *negative reinforcement*, since it increases the frequency of drug-using behavior in order to relieve the discomfort of a withdrawal syndrome. Therefore, a *stimulus* does not necessarily trigger a response. When that is the case, it is called a *neutral stimulus*. However, it may start to trigger a response once the person is conditioned to produce that response. This learning process is called *conditioning*. There are two basic types of conditioning: *classic and operant*. In the *classic conditioning*, a *neutral stimulus* is associated with an *unconditioned stimulus* (a stimulus that produces an innate response, such as a type of food that makes one's mouth water). After repeated pairing of the *neutral stimulus* with the *unconditioned stimulus,* a type of learning occurs in which the *neutral stimulus* begins to elicit the response. It is then called *conditioned stimulus.* The other type of conditioning, called *operant*, postulates that learning takes place through reinforcement and punishment. In that case, unlike in the *classic* conditioning, the *operant* conditioning is based on the fact that there is an **increase** or a **decrease** of the chances of a response depending on the consequences associated with the behavior. An important aspect of the *operant conditioning* is that it deals with *voluntary* behaviors, such as eating a piece of cake or using a drug. Conversely, the classic conditioning is frequently based on involuntary responses, such as physiological responses (e.g., pain, salivation, and sweating).

Common Action of Drugs of Abuse: The Brain Reward System

Considering the basic behavioral aspects associated with substance use that have been presented, now we can better understand which are the neurobiological basis of the drugs of abuse. In this section, we will discuss the similarities regarding the brain functioning when there is drug use, and how this use changes the transmission of information in the brain. Later on we will discuss some particularities of the action of each drug of abuse, better explaining how the different effects are generated by each class of drug (depressant, stimulant, and hallucinogenic). Drug use may range from one single use in life to a frequent and daily use. In other words, not every initial use of drugs will evolve into a condition of dependence. In fact, only a small proportion of individuals who have already used some type of drug develop dependence. As an example we can mention the use of alcohol by the adult Brazilian population: while 74 % drink, only, approximately 12 % fulfill the diagnostic criteria for dependence (Carlini et al. 2007). The way individuals consume a drug (sniffed/snorted, inhaled/smoked, intravenous, oral, etc.) will also interfere in the odds of their evolving to a more severe pattern of use, and the pattern itself might increase or decrease their odds of becoming dependent.

Every psychoactive drug needs to reach the brain to produce its effect. The different routes of administration have a direct effect on the time the substance takes to reach the brain. Some routes provide a fast access of the substance to the bloodstream, quickly increasing its levels in the blood. As a result, it reaches the brain almost immediately, causing faster effects. On the other hand, the faster the drug reaches the brain, the faster its effects wear off. Due to the characteristics of the lungs, the substance reaches the bloodstream very fast. Thereafter the blood, already containing the substance, reaches the heart, being directly pumped to the whole body, including the brain. A large concentration of the drug will soon be available to reach the brain quickly, causing fast yet transient effects. A study comparing equivalent doses of cocaine in different routes of administration (smoked, sniffed/snorted, and injected) concluded that the alterations resulting from some physiological reactions (increased blood pressure, increased heart rate, and mydriasis) happen in a similar way for the smoked or injected route. Cognitive-behavioral effects (euphoria, pleasure, and perception of the intensity of effect), however, are stronger in the smoked use. In the use of snorted cocaine (cocaine chlorhydrate), the cognitive-behavioral effects have a slower onset, and the physiological effects take place in a more slowly and less intense manner than in the smoked or intravenous use. Taken together, these data point to a higher potential for cocaine abuse and dependence in its smoked (crack) and injected route when compared to the snorted route (cocaine chlorhydrate) (Cone 1995).

Dependence on any drug of abuse cannot and should not be diagnosed based on one single use of the substance. As discussed before, there are diagnostic criteria that should be met, as the examples present in the DSM-V (American Psychiatric Association 2013), in order for dependence to be characterized. All of them are related to the recurring or continuous use of the drug (use for long periods; unsuccessful attempts to quit or cut down on use; continuous use even in situations that involve physical, psychological, or social damage to oneself or others; tolerance; withdrawal syndrome; and craving). Moreover, the severity of symptoms, characterized by the number of criteria met, reflects the increase or decrease in the frequency or number of doses used. Hence, independently of the route of administration of the substance, it is not possible to characterize dependence in an individual who has used drugs only once.

Since there should be a repetitive behavior of drug use to characterize dependence, the study of the neurobiological bases of drugs is strongly related to behavioral aspects. Several studies, especially those with animals, were conducted in order to determine which are the brain regions involved in dependence. Even though there are numerous animal models to study it, one of the main ones is the paradigm of *self-administration*. In this paradigm, an animal is placed in a box with access to a lever (Skinner box). By pressing the lever, the animal can receive a number of rewards as food and water, and also drugs of abuse. Animals deprived of food and water initially explore the environment and, over time, learn that they receive the reward by pressing the lever. When they are presented with two levers, one that supplies water and the other that supplies some drug, many animals choose to press the lever that provides the drug rather than the one that provides the natural rewards. Once this happens, one may assume that substance is passible of self-administration. Variations of this model include the injection of drugs directly in the circulation, in brain regions, and even the electric stimulation in specific brain regions. Using a variation of the traditional self-administration model through the use of electrodes that promoted electric stimulation of the brain, Olds and Milner (1954) published a study that aimed at detecting the reinforcing characteristics of electric stimulation of some brain areas of rats. The authors observed that when a certain region was stimulated (septal area), the animal pressed the lever several times, similarly to what happened with natural reinforcing stimuli (food and water). Therefore, they assumed they had detected a brain system responsible for the reinforcing effect of behaviors. In the following years, until the 1960s, several studies were conducted that identified other regions associated with the reinforcing effects and the data of Olds and Milner (1991). Among those regions were the *ventral tegmental area* (VTA), the *nucleus accumbens* (Nacc), regions of the do *pre-frontal cortex* (PFC), and the *amygdala* (Wise 1996). Those regions stood out initially in the study of a pathway called "*reinforcement pathway*" or "*pleasure pathway*," exactly the one that would explain the reinforcing effect of behaviors.

The reinforcement pathway consists of two pathways of dopaminergic neurons, the *mesolimbic* and the *mesocortical pathways*, known as the *mesocorticolimbic system* when taken together. The pathway of neurons that goes from the *VTA* into the *Nacc* is called *mesolimbic pathway*. Other regions of the limbic system are also part of the mesolimbic pathway, as the amygdala, which is associated with the reinforcement and pleasure generated by drugs of abuse, in addition to the memories associated with the use and conditioned responses (Koob and Bloom 1988) (see *conditioned stimuli* in the section "Neurobiology and Behavioral Aspects"). The neurons that go from the *VTA* into the *PFC* form the *mesocortical pathway*. This pathway seems to be associated with the compulsive behavior of drug use, low inhibitory control, and the emotional valence of the drug (Volkow and Fowler 2000). The reinforcement pathway is activated by natural reinforcing stimuli as food, water, and sex, as well as by artificial stimuli as drugs of abuse. Every time it is activated it promotes the release of an important component to understand the neurobiological bases of dependence: the neurotransmitter *dopamine* (*DA*). When any of the reinforcers is presented, there is the release of *DA* into the Nacc, generating a feeling of pleasure. In fact, once DA is released into the Nacc, the response to the stimulus is facilitated, giving it more salience. When this happens, the behavior tends to be repetitive, enhancing associative learning. This condition attaches excessive value to the stimulus or to the contexts associated with the use of the drug (Di Chiara and Bassareo 2007; Di Chiara et al. 1999). Dopamine is released into the PFC as well. In that case, the release is involved with cognitive processes, as the regulation of attention, memory, motivation, and executive functions (Seamans and Yang 2004).

Some substances as cocaine and amphetamines promote the release of DA directly into the Nacc as a result of their direct action in that region. Other drugs, on the other hand, promote the release of DA into the Nacc by activating the neurons of the mesolimbic pathway in the VTA (Koob and Volkow 2010). The release of DA into the Nacc seems to be important for the feeling of pleasure caused by the use of drugs, the compulsive behavior, and the motivation to search for the substance. When the *mesolimbic pathway* is stimulated, there might be release of DA into the *amygdala*, in addition to the release of that neurotransmitter into the Nacc (Weiss et al. 2000), since the amygdala is involved in the learning of memories associated with the use of drugs. An example is the pleasant memories caused by the use of the substance. Moreover, the amygdala might be activated when something associated with the drug is close, as the view of a place where the drug is usually used. Hence, the amygdala plays a fundamental role in the learning of clues associated with the drug and the evoking of some memory associated with its use (Stahl 2010).

Some regions of the PFC are believed to be involved in drug dependence, namely the portions of the *ventromedial pre-frontal cortex*, associated with emotions and affective states; *dorsolateral frontal cortex*, related to memory and decision making, and the *orbitofrontal cortex*, associated with the inhibition of responses (Noël et al. 2006). Broadly speaking, these PFC regions seem to regulate the decision making toward or away from the use of substances. In short, different information seems to be integrated into the PFC, allowing the modulation of responses by means of their efferent connections (Volkow and Fowler 2000). Another interesting point is that the *orbitofrontal cortex* is activated in individuals in different phases of dependence, as intoxication, craving, and abuse, while it is deactivated during abstinence. In that case, the activation would be associated with motivation, tracking, modulation, and updating of salience of a reinforcing stimulus, as drugs, according to context, control abilities and inhibition of associated responses (Goldstein and Volkow 2002). When this happens, stimuli associated with the use of drug might evoke pleasant memories associated with the use, hence favoring the reuse of the substance. At the same time, the PFC regions may also be activated and evoke negative memories associated with use. As the PFC is related to decision making and response inhibition, the behavior might be suppressed, preventing a future use of the drug (Bechara 2005; Noël et al. 2006).

As discussed above, both natural and artificial reinforcing stimuli can promote the release of DA into the pleasure pathway. Those reinforcers, however, seem to act differently in the brain from the natural ones (basic activities of survival, as feeding and reproduction). Such stimuli are innate and unconditioned, evoking behaviors of search or flight, depending on their characteristics (Di Chiara 2002; Glickman and Schiff 1967). After repeated exposure to a reinforcing stimulus, one might reach an adaptive stage called *habituation*, in which the responses to the stimulus are reduced or paralyzed. Conversely, behaviors associated with non-natural reinforcers, such as drugs of abuse, might get around this adaptive mechanism. This would, in turn, lead to an excessive motivation of the stimuli conditioned to the drug, favoring the onset of dependence (Di Chiara and Bassareo 2007). Another relevant aspect is that the response resulting from the use of drugs might promote a high increase in the amount of extracellular DA in the Nacc, higher than that generated by food, sex, or other reinforcers (Fibiger 1993). Moreover, even though both the natural and the non-natural stimuli promote the release of DA into the Nacc, the action of those two different types of reinforcers is different regarding the neurobiological regions affected. While natural reinforcers release DA into the portion known as *core* of the Nacc, non-natural reinforcers release DA into the portion *shell* of the Nacc (Di Chiara and Bassareo 2007).

The release of DA into the Nacc might happen both when the reinforcing stimulus is presented and when one is about to receive the reinforcer. Behaviors associated with reinforcing stimuli can be subdivided into *preparatory* (related to the anticipation of the behavior, working as encouragement that promotes approaching the reward and facilitates the production of a response) and *consummatory* (immediately after the behavior, as orgasm after intercourse, or chewing after the contact with food). Both of them promote the release of DA into the Nacc. As a result, anticipatory signals to the use of substances lead to the release of DA into the Nacc (Blackburn et al. 1989), favoring the repetition of the behavior.

Different Action of the Drugs in the Brain Reward System

Drugs of abuse share the same action in the brain, causing the release of DA into the Nacc and promoting the feeling of pleasure, which makes the body perceive this eliciting stimuli as more salient. The DA release into the Nacc might happen in different ways, be it directly, as in the case of cocaine and amphetamine, or indirectly, through its action in different brain regions (see below).

Drugs of abuse have different effects depending on their class, the main ones being *depressant, stimulant, and hallucinogenic*. Depressant drugs work by reducing the brain activity and causing slowing down of the CNS. Some examples are alcohol, opioids, and benzodiazepines. Stimulant drugs act in the opposite way, increasing the activity of the CNS. Some examples of this class of drugs are cocaine/crack, amphetamine, and tobacco. Hallucinogenic drugs are those that affect the working of the CNS in a qualitative way, changing the perception of the individual, as in the case of marijuana.

From the neurobiological viewpoint, what makes those substances cause such different effects is the type of neurotransmission system involved, its mechanisms of action, and the brain areas the substance acts on. Therefore, although cocaine and heroin cause release of DA into the Nacc, these drugs have particular effects. In the case of cocaine, the effects are clearly stimulant. In the case of heroin, however, the effects are depressors of the CNS.

Alcohol

The acute effects of alcohol on the CNS are mediated especially by the potentialization of the inhibitory action of GABA (main inhibitory neurotransmitter of the CNS) and the reduction of the stimulant action of glutamate (main excitatory neurotransmitter of the CNS). In the chronic use of alcohol, there seems to be an inversion, in which there is an increase in the activity of glutamate receptors and a reduction in the function of the GABA receptors (Samson and Harris 1992). The use of alcohol increases the concentration of DA in the Nacc through the activation of neurons in the VTA. This release seems to be associated with both the action of alcohol on GABA receptors and of glutamate receptors. The activation of GABA inhibits the GABAergic interneurons that communicate with the VTA. As GABA is the main inhibitory neurotransmitter of the CNS, this reaction causes the disinhibition of the DA neurons of the VTA, releasing DA in the Nacc. At the same time, alcohol might inhibit glutamatergic receptors, decreasing its stimulant action on the same GABAergic interneurons, which will once again reduce the inhibitory effect of GABA on the VTA (Gilpin and Koob 2008; Tabakoff and Hoffman 2013). The reinforcing actions of alcohol also seem to affect the endogenous opioid system. As discussed above, GABA interneurons in the VTA keep the release of dopamine into the Nacc inhibited. Opioid receptors inhibit GABA interneurons, disinhibiting the release of DA into the Nacc (Herz 1997). The activation of opioid receptors might occur by the action of both β-endorphins and enkephalins (released by neurons from the arcuate nucleus, for example). Alcohol seems to act stimulating the release of those substances (Gianoulakis 1996; Stahl 2010).

Cocaine and Crack

Cocaine and crack are the same substances concerning their action on the CNS. Their main differences lie in the process of production of the drug and their most common routes of administration. Their action on the CNS is stimulant and happens through the blockade of monoamine transporters (dopamine, serotonin, and noradrenaline), especially by blocking DA transporters. Hence, the blockade of the latter, responsible for removing the neurotransmitter from the synaptic cleft, causes an increase in the amount and length of time in which DA is available in the synaptic cleft. As a result, there are higher chances that DA binds with post-synaptic receptors, potentializing the normal effects of DA. This increased DA availability favors the learning of associations among the subjective and physiologic effects of the use of cocaine/crack and environmental and behavioral stimuli (Kalivas 2007).

The stimulant effects of cocaine/crack, as euphoria, are a consequence of their effects on different brain regions, as the VTA, the Nacc, the amygdala, the hippocampus, and the frontal cortex. Particularly the Nacc seems to be of utmost importance in the repetitive behavior of cocaine/crack use, since the amount of DA released into that region is very large, outweighing the physiological levels associated with natural activities as sex (Nestler 2005). Consequently, greater salience is conferred to the drug when compared with other natural reinforcements (Kalivas 2007). Another significant aspect is that cocaine/crack, due to their mechanism of action, might stimulate the release of DA directly into the dopaminergic terminals of the Nacc (Koob and Le Moal 2005a).

Amphetamines

The group of drugs classified as amphetamines includes substances as ephedrine, methamphetamine, and methylphenidate, among others. Those substances might be of natural or synthetic origin, licit, or illicit. They share the characteristic of stimulating the CNS, just as cocaine/crack. Amphetamines are similar to cocaine/crack not only in relation to their effects on the CNS, but also regarding the blockade of noradrenaline, DA, and serotonin (Koob and Le Moal 2005a). Nevertheless, they use other mechanisms, acting as inhibitors of monoamine oxidase (enzyme responsible for the degradation of monoamines), to promote a greater availability of DA (Robinson 1985) and the displacement of DA to outside the synaptic vesicles, taking its place inside the vesicle. As a result, the intracellular concentration of DA increases, releasing it into the synaptic cleft (Stahl 2010). The action of amphetamine is mediated by mesolimbic and mesocortical dopaminergic pathways, and the release of DA might happen into both the Nacc and the amygdala (Koob and Le Moal 2005a).

Opioids

This class of substances includes heroin, codeine, morphine, and opium, among many others. Some opioid drugs can be obtained directly from the poppy flower (*Papaver somniferum*) or be produced in laboratories. Their main effects are depressor and include analgesia, sedation, respiratory depression, and sensation of euphoria. The same way as amphetamines, the class of opioids includes both licit (morphine and codeine) and illicit (heroin) drugs.

The action of opioids on the CNS is mediated by different types of opioid receptors. Their main effect on the CNS is the dopaminergic stimulation in the VTA and the increase of DA release into the Nacc. Those receptors are involved in the effects of exogenous opioids (drugs) as well as the endogenous opioids (substances naturally present in the CNS, with similar action to that of drugs of abuse; World Health Organization 2004). Hence, opioids activate their receptors in the VTA, Nacc, and amygdala, and promote the release of DA into the Nacc by means of the action of the VTA or the Nacc itself (Koob and Le Moal 2005a).

Benzodiazepines

Benzodiazepines (BZD) are medications used in the treatment of anxiety, convulsions, and sleep induction. They appeared as an alternative to the use of barbiturates for being safer from the therapeutic point of view. The main mechanism of action of BZDs happens through their binding to GABA receptors. By binding to the receptor, BZDs modulate the functioning of the neuron, potentializing and prolonging the GABA effects, activating the chloride channels, increasing the GABA capacity of allowing chloride ions to enter the neuron, and inhibiting the neuron. BZD actions require less GABA to open the ion channel (World Health Organization 2004; Petursson and Lader 1981).

The potential of BZDs to cause dependence is extensively discussed in the literature. Among the clear clinical aspects, we can mention the fast development of tolerance to some of their effects and the withdrawal syndrome (Ashton 2005; World

Health Organization 2004; Owen and Tyrer 1983; Petursson and Lader 1981). However, few studies point to the capacity of BZDs to bring about the sensation of pleasure associated with the use of drugs as amphetamines and cocaine.

Marijuana

Marijuana is a natural drug of abuse that produces hallucinogenic effects on the CNS. There are other synthetic compounds, as the synthetic marijuana, that produce similar effects to those of that plant. Even though marijuana contains dozens of psychoactive substances known as cannabinoids, its main hallucinogenic effects result from the delta-9-tetrahydrocannabinol. The compounds of this class are not found exclusively in plants. The endogenous version (produced in our body) of cannabinoids is called endocannabinoids, and their main example is the anandamide. Cannabinoids and endocannabinoids bind to specific receptors, the two main ones being CB1, present predominantly in the CNS, and CB2, present in peripheral tissues and the immune system (Gong et al. 2006; Wang and Ueda 2008). Cannabinoid receptors are present in several regions associated with the reinforcement of drugs of abuse, including the PFC, the Nacc, and the VTA. The reinforcing action of cannabinoids seems to happen through the increase in the activity of dopaminergic neurons of the mesolimbic pathway, even though cannabinoid receptors are not directly present in those neurons. The action happens by means of their activity on GABA and glutamate neurons (Fattore et al. 2008; Maldonado et al. 2006).

The activation of cannabinoid receptors in the VTA seems to promote the release of DA through the inhibition of GABA neurons. In the Nacc, the cannabinoid receptors present in the glutamate neurons (from the PFC) inhibit the release of glutamate. Such inhibition makes the GABA neurons that project from the Nacc to the VTA be inhibited as well, which will result in the release of DA into the Nacc through the mesolimbic pathway (Maldonado et al. 2006).

Tobacco

The action of tobacco in any of its forms (cigarettes, cigars, snuff, etc.) is mediated in the CNS by nicotine. This activity happens in a series of receptors spread over several brain regions. Nicotine is a stimulant of the CNS and reaches the brain very quickly when smoked in the form of cigarettes (see route of administration in the section "Common action of drugs of abuse: the brain reward system"). Moreover, large amounts of nicotine are made available in the body after each cigarette puff.

Nicotine acts in acetylcholine nicotine receptors. Nicotine dependence seems to be primarily associated with its reinforcing properties that result from the action in the receptors of dopaminergic neurons in the VTA. Therefore, its action promotes the direct or indirect release of DA into the Nacc, a crucial aspect for the behavioral effects associated with reinforcing properties (World Health Organization 2004). In a direct way, nicotine acts on dopaminergic receptors present in the post-synaptic neurons in the VTA; in an indirect way, the action happens by means of the desensitization of the GABAergic interneurons in the VTA, reducing the release of GABA that acts inhibiting the dopaminergic neurons.

Main Neurobiological Theories on Drug Dependence

Even though several studies raise the hypothesis that the use of drugs of abuse activates brain regions related to the reward system (mesolimbic and mesocortical pathways), there is no complete definition of all the mechanisms of action of drugs on the human brain. This is so especially because of methodological restrictions or techniques that limit the studies. Consequently, the assertions are based on scientific information that was tested and replicated over decades, and corroborate the hypotheses formulated.

Below we present two important neurobiological theories on drug dependence.

Dependence, Dopamine, and the Mesolimbic Pathway

The first significant neurobiological theory about drugs of abuse was presented in 1980 by Roy Wise, researcher in the Department of Psychology at Concordia University in Montreal, Canada (Wise 1980). His hypothesis was that several types of reinforcement, including drugs of abuse, would activate the reinforcement pathway (related to the dopaminergic system) at least partially. This system would be directly activated by drugs as cocaine and amphetamine (the direct action of opioids was still uncertain then). Other drugs, on the other hand, would act not by the direct activation of the dopaminergic fibers of the reinforcement pathway, but rather by the excitation or inhibition of the dopaminergic system by means of its afferences. Such drugs would include opioids, benzodiazepines, ethanol, and barbiturates (Wise 1980). In 1987, in another work in which he shared the authorship with Michael Bozarth, Wise further suggested that all the drugs with a potential to cause dependence had the ability of psychomotor stimulation (Wise and Bozarth 1987). According to this theory, every positive reinforcement would share the same biological mechanism involving dopaminergic pathways. This time Wise stated that opioids would have a common action with cocaine and amphetamine, that is, promoting the psychomotor activity directly in the reinforcement pathway. The psychostimulant action of nicotine, caffeine, barbiturates, benzodiazepines, marijuana, and phencyclidine, on the other hand, would result from the direct stimulation of the dopaminergic fibers of the reinforcement pathway or by means of circuits associated with it (Wise and Bozarth 1987). In short, in this new phase of their theory, Wise and Bozarth declare that all drugs of abuse have a stimulant action on the psychomotor activity, mediated by dopaminergic neurons of the reinforcement pathway and its connections with other systems.

Over 20 years later, another study was published with much information added to the original theory of 1980 and enlarged in 1987. In that version, more recent and complete, Wise points the dopaminergic mesolimbic pathway as the key point of the brain circuitry in the reinforcement of drugs of abuse (Wise 2002). Cocaine and amphetamine would be reinforcers for releasing dopamine into the Nacc. The action of nicotine would be a result of actions in the cholinergic receptors present mainly in the VTA, and its activation would also promote the release of DA into the Nacc. Heroin and morphine, both opioids, would act in two ways: one by inhibiting the GABA neurons, which normally keep the mesolimbic pathway inhibited, disinhibiting it; the other by inhibiting the neurons that come out of the Nacc. Marijuana and alcohol seem to act by unknown mechanisms, increasing the triggering of the mesolimbic dopaminergic neurons. Caffeine seems to have a reinforcing effect by means of an independent circuit. Finally, benzodiazepines and barbiturates seem to activate one or more circuits of GABAergic neurons, not necessarily associated with the dopaminergic system, thus activating their habit-generating effects (Wise 2002). A noteworthy point in this new version of Wise's theory is that the mesolimbic system could be activated both by the direct message of the reinforcement that is present and by sensory stimuli that pointed to the closeness of a reinforcer. Consequently, the drug does not necessarily have to be present for the mesolimbic pathway to be activated, and it only takes signals that the drug is near.

Dependence as a Disorder Associated with Stress

George Koob is another eminent researcher who proposed a theory to explain the common action of drugs on the brain. His theory was based on the perspective of the reinforcement and the pleasure produced by drugs on the brain. He suggests that the brain reinforcing pathway is associated with several neuropharmacological elements that have neuroanatomic elements in common (Koob 1992). Three key neurotransmission systems are thought to be involved in the reinforcing capacity of drugs: the opioid, the GABAergic, and the dopaminergic systems. Initially, Koob's theory addressed opioids, hypnotic/sedative substances, cocaine, and amphetamine. All those drugs would have a significant action on the mesocorticolimbic system (mesolimbic and mesocortical pathways).

DA appears to be critical in the reinforcing properties of cocaine and amphetamine, though not so strong in the case of opioids and hypnotic/sedative substances. In those situations, DA would contribute to the reinforcing properties, but not in an essential way. As for opioids, Koob suggests that their receptors in the Nacc and VTA would be critical for reinforcement. In the case of hypnotic/sedative substances, mainly alcohol, the GABA receptors would be the initial sites of the reinforcing action, especially those present in the Nacc and amygdala (Koob 1992).

The hypothesis Koob proposes differs considerably from the theory proposed by Wise (1980), since for Koob DA does not play a critical role in the reinforcing action of all the drugs, as suggested by Wise.

In 1997, Koob and Le Moal (1997) published a review on the use of drugs in which they proposed that the vulnerability to dependence would not only involve a spiraling sequence triggered by the acute use of drugs (binge/intoxication pattern), but also involve stages of withdrawal/negative feelings and concern/anticipation. Consequently, the authors concluded that the cycle of dependence cannot be explained only by the association to responses that result from the initial drug use (Koob and Le Moal 1997). Therefore, according to the theory proposed by Koob as regards drug dependence, that condition is characterized by a chronic disorder that involves relapse and comprises three specific stages: (1) compulsion for the search and use of the drug; (2) loss of control in limiting the use; and (3) presence of negative emotional states such as dysphoria, anxiety, and irritability when the access to the drug is limited (Koob and Volkow 2010). This view places particular importance on strategies of *negative* reinforcement in the maintenance of dependence, not limiting it only to *positive reinforcement* (pleasure generated by the use of the substance). Even if the first use is promoted by the pleasure generated by the substance (positive reinforcement), the maintenance of use would happen as an attempt to relieve the negative consequences (physical and emotional) of the lack of drug (negative reinforcement; Kreek and Koob 1998). This leads to another important point in the difference between the theories of Wise and Koob, since the hypothesis of Wise is based mainly on the positive reinforcement aspect of the drug, while to Koob it may act as a negative reinforcement as well, especially in the cases of drug dependence.

During the intoxication phase (acute), the reinforcing effects of drugs make the reward system favor the creation of habits through the activation of the reinforcement systems, which would involve both the action of dopamine and the opioid system in the Nacc and the dorsal striatum (related to the learning process and habit formation; Koob and Volkow 2010). However, due to the excessive stimulation of the reward system (by means of positive reinforcements that would lead to the release of opioid peptides), there would be the activation of dynorphin (an endogenous opioid) in the Nacc and VTA, suppressing the release of DA. As a consequence, this decrease in the release of DA would favor negative states after the withdrawal of the drug (Koob et al. 2014).

Several studies by Koob and other researchers give consideration to the role of the regulatory system of stress in the pathway of reinforcement and maintenance of dependence (Koob and Le Moal 1997; Kreek and Koob 1998; Piazza and Le Moal 1996, 1998). According to George Koob, drug use activates the brain system of stress (Koob et al. 2014; Kreek and Koob 1998). He believes that both the system of stress and that of dependence are associated with a series of neuroadaptations that result from the prolonged use of drugs. The use of drugs, initially motivated by social reasons and the search for reinforcement in an acute way, might lead to the development of a compulsive pattern of use in some individuals, and eventually to dependence (Koob and Le Moal 2005a). During this process of transition from social use to dependence, there would be excessive and prolonged stimulation of the mechanisms of stress regulation (Koob et al. 2014). In that way, the use of drugs in the long term would promote alterations in the pleasure pathway and in the brain system of stress, connected to important changes in the motivation to use. In the view of Koob and Le Moal, this would be the "dark side" of drug use, known as the antireinforcement system (Koob and Le Moal 2005b, 2008). In the second phase of the spiral proposed by Koob, the stress mechanism seems to act promoting negative emotional states. His hypothesis is that by the activation of the brain system of stress during drug withdrawal there would be a sensitization through the release of corticotropin, noradrenaline, and dynorphin that would promote such negative states. One of the associated regions would be the amygdala (Koob et al. 2014; Koob and Volkow 2010).

Finally, the phase of concern/anticipation, or the craving stage, has been pointed out as a key element in relapse. This stage would involve the processing of conditioned reinforcement in the amygdala, of contextual information in the hippocampus, and the executive control dependent on the PFC, which would include the representation of contingencies and outcomes associated with the drug, in addition to the value attributed to the drug and the subjective states related to it (Koob and Volkow 2010).

Final Considerations

The study of the neurobiology of drugs allowed the identification of several brain regions associated with substance use and, consequently, considered as possible therapeutic targets. Moreover, the neurobiological view of dependence is fundamental for a better understanding of this process as a health disorder rather than a moral issue. The main drugs of abuse have already been pointed as important in the mediation of the response to a given stimulus, giving it special value and providing higher chances for the behavior to be repeated. From the neurobiological view, this is possible through the release of dopamine into the Nacc. On the other hand, the way through which the drugs promote the release of that neurotransmitter is highly variable- that is, it might take place in a direct way or through associated pathways, as the mesolimbic and the mesocortical pathways. The different ways drugs act on the brain allow the understanding of their different cognitive, behavioral and physiological effects.

As important as the study of the neurobiological bases of dependence, it is noteworthy that substance use should always be considered a multifactor disorder of biopsychosocial nature. This means that once any of those aspects is neglected, the attention to the substance-dependent individual will be faulty or at least incomplete. Even though neurobiological factors might be determining in the development of dependence in certain individuals, this alone should not be considered the factor responsible for the whole dependence process.

References

American Psychiatric Association. (2013). *Diagnostic and statistical manual of mental disorders* (5th ed.). Washington, DC.

Ashton, H. (2005). The diagnosis and management of benzodiazepine dependence. *Current Opinion in Psychiatry, 18*(3), 249–255. doi:10.1097/01.yco.0000165594.60434.84.

Azevedo, F. A., Carvalho, L. R., Grinberg, L. T., Farfel, J. M., Ferretti, R. E., Leite, R. E., et al. (2009). Equal numbers of neuronal and nonneuronal cells make the human brain an isometrically scaled-up primate brain. *Journal of Comparative Neurology, 513*(5), 532–541. doi:10.1002/cne.21974.

Bechara, A. (2005). Decision making, impulse control and loss of willpower to resist drugs: A neurocognitive perspective. *Nature Neuroscience, 8*(11), 1458–1463. doi:10.1038/nn1584.

Blackburn, J. R., Phillips, A. G., Jakubovic, A., & Fibiger, H. C. (1989). Dopamine and preparatory behavior: II. A neurochemical analysis. *Behavioral Neuroscience, 103*(1), 15–23.

Carlini, E. A., Galduróz, J. C., Noto, A. R., Carlini, C. M., Oliveira, L. G., & Nappo, S. A. (2007). *II Levantamento domiciliar sobre o uso de drogas psicotrópicas no Brasil: Estudo envolvendo as 108 maiores cidades do país—2005.* São Paulo: Páginas & Letras.

Cone, E. J. (1995). Pharmacokinetics and pharmacodynamics of cocaine. *Journal of Analytical Toxicology, 19*(6), 459–478.

Di Chiara, G. (2002). Nucleus accumbens shell and core dopamine: Differential role in behavior and addiction. *Behavioural Brain Research, 137*(1–2), 75–114.

Di Chiara, G., & Bassareo, V. (2007). Reward system and addiction: What dopamine does and doesn't do. *Current Opinion in Pharmacology, 7*(1), 69–76. doi:10.1016/j.coph.2006.11.003.

Di Chiara, G., Tanda, G., Bassareo, V., Pontieri, F., Acquas, E., Fenu, S., et al. (1999). Drug addiction as a disorder of associative learning. Role of nucleus accumbens shell/extended amygdala dopamine. *Annals of the New York Academy of Sciences, 877*, 461–485.

Fattore, L., Fadda, P., Spano, M. S., Pistis, M., & Fratta, W. (2008). Neurobiological mechanisms of cannabinoid addiction. *Molecular and Cellular Endocrinology, 286*(1–2 Suppl 1), S97–S107. doi:10.1016/j.mce.2008.02.006.

Fibiger, H.C. (1993). *Mesolimbic dopamine: An analysis of its role in motivated behavior.* Paper presentd at the Seminars in Neuroscience.

Gianoulakis, C. (1996). Implications of endogenous opioids and dopamine in alcoholism: Human and basic science studies. *Alcohol and Alcoholism, 31*(Suppl 1), 33–42.

Gilpin, N. W., & Koob, G. F. (2008). Neurobiology of alcohol dependence: Focus on motivational mechanisms. *Alcohol Research and Health, 31*(3), 185–195.

Glickman, S. E., & Schiff, B. B. (1967). A biological theory of reinforcement. *Psychological Review, 74*(2), 81–109.

Goldstein, R. Z., & Volkow, N. D. (2002). Drug addiction and its underlying neurobiological basis: Neuroimaging evidence for the involvement of the frontal cortex. *The American Journal of Psychiatry, 159*(10), 1642–1652.

Gong, J. P., Onaivi, E. S., Ishiguro, H., Liu, Q. R., Tagliaferro, P. A., Brusco, A., et al. (2006). Cannabinoid CB2 receptors: Immunohistochemical localization in rat brain. *Brain Research, 1071*(1), 10–23. doi:10.1016/j.brainres.2005.11.035.

Herz, A. (1997). Endogenous opioid systems and alcohol addiction. *Psychopharmacology (Berlin), 129*(2), 99–111.

Kalivas, P. W. (2007). Neurobiology of cocaine addiction: Implications for new pharmacotherapy. *American Journal on Addictions, 16*(2), 71–78. doi:10.1080/10550490601184142.

Koob, G. F. (1992). Drugs of abuse: Anatomy, pharmacology and function of reward pathways. *Trends in Pharmacological Sciences, 13*(5), 177–184.

Koob, G. F., & Bloom, F. E. (1988). Cellular and molecular mechanisms of drug dependence. *Science, 242*(4879), 715–723.

Koob, G. F., Buck, C. L., Cohen, A., Edwards, S., Park, P. E., Schlosburg, J. E., et al. (2014). Addiction as a stress surfeit disorder. *Neuropharmacology, 76*, 370–382. doi:10.1016/j. neuropharm.2013.05.024.

Koob, G. F., & Le Moal, M. (1997). Drug abuse: Hedonic homeostatic dysregulation. *Science, 278* (5335), 52–58.

Koob, G. F., & Le Moal, M. (2005a). *Neurobiology of addiction.* Cambridge: Academic Press.

Koob, G. F., & Le Moal, M. (2005b). Plasticity of reward neurocircuitry and the 'dark side' of drug addiction. *Nature Neuroscience, 8*(11), 1442–1444. doi:10.1038/nn1105-1442.

Koob, G. F., & Le Moal, M. (2008). Addiction and the brain antireward system. *Annual Review of Psychology, 59*, 29–53. doi:10.1146/annurev.psych.59.103006.093548.

Koob, G. F., & Volkow, N. D. (2010). Neurocircuitry of addiction. *Neuropsychopharmacology, 35*(1), 217–238. doi:10.1038/npp.2009.110.

Kreek, M. J., & Koob, G. F. (1998). Drug dependence: Stress and dysregulation of brain reward pathways. *Drug and Alcohol Dependence, 51*(1–2), 23–47.

Maldonado, R., Valverde, O., & Berrendero, F. (2006). Involvement of the endocannabinoid system in drug addiction. *Trends in Neurosciences, 29*(4), 225–232. doi:10.1016/j.tins.2006. 01.008.

Milner, P. M. (1991). Brain-stimulation reward: A review. *Canadian Journal of Psychology, 45* (1), 1–36.

Nestler, E. J. (2005). The neurobiology of cocaine addiction. *Science and Practice Perspectives, 3* (1), 4–10.

Noël, X., Van Der Linden, M., & Bechara, A. (2006). The neurocognitive mechanisms of decision-making, impulse control, and loss of willpower to resist drugs. *Psychiatry (Edgmont), 3*(5), 30–41.

Olds, J., & Milner, P. (1954). Positive reinforcement produced by electrical stimulation of septal area and other regions of rat brain. *Journal of Comparative and Physiological Psychology, 47* (6), 419–427.

Owen, R. T., & Tyrer, P. (1983). Benzodiazepine dependence: A review of the evidence. *Drugs, 25*(4), 385–398.

Petursson, H., & Lader, M. H. (1981). Benzodiazepine dependence. *British Journal of Addiction, 76*(2), 133–145.

Piazza, P. V., & Le Moal, M. (1998). The role of stress in drug self-administration. *Trends in Pharmacological Sciences, 19*(2), 67–74.

Piazza, P. V., & Le Moal, M. L. (1996). Pathophysiological basis of vulnerability to drug abuse: Role of an interaction between stress, glucocorticoids, and dopaminergic neurons. *Annual Review of Pharmacology and Toxicology, 36*, 359–378. doi:10.1146/annurev.pa.36.040196. 002043.

Robinson, J. B. (1985). Stereoselectivity and isoenzyme selectivity of monoamine oxidase inhibitors. Enantiomers of amphetamine, N-methylamphetamine and deprenyl. *Biochemical Pharmacology, 34*(23), 4105–4108.

Samson, H. H., & Harris, R. A. (1992). Neurobiology of alcohol abuse. *Trends in Pharmacological Sciences, 13*(5), 206–211.

Seamans, J. K., & Yang, C. R. (2004). The principal features and mechanisms of dopamine modulation in the prefrontal cortex. *Progress in Neurobiology, 74*(1), 1–58. doi:10.1016/j. pneurobio.2004.05.006.

Stahl, S.M. (2010). *Psicofarmacologia: Base neurocientífica e aplicações práticas* (3 ed.). Guanabara Koogan.

Tabakoff, B., & Hoffman, P. L. (2013). The neurobiology of alcohol consumption and alcoholism: An integrative history. *Pharmacology, Biochemistry and Behavior, 113*, 20–37. doi:10.1016/j. pbb.2013.10.009.

Volkow, N. D., & Fowler, J. S. (2000). Addiction, a disease of compulsion and drive: Involvement of the orbitofrontal cortex. *Cerebral Cortex, 10*(3), 318–325.

Wang, J., & Ueda, N. (2008). Role of the endocannabinoid system in metabolic control. *Current Opinion in Nephrology and Hypertension, 17*(1), 1–10. doi:10.1097/MNH.0b013e3282f29071.

Weiss, F., Maldonado-Vlaar, C. S., Parsons, L. H., Kerr, T. M., Smith, D. L., & Ben-Shahar, O. (2000). Control of cocaine-seeking behavior by drug-associated stimuli in rats: Effects on recovery of extinguished operant-responding and extracellular dopamine levels in amygdala and nucleus accumbens. *Proceedings of the National Academy of Sciences of the United States of America, 97*(8), 4321–4326.

Wise, R. A. (1980). Action of drugs of abuse on brain reward systems. *Pharmacology, Biochemistry and Behavior, 13*(Suppl 1), 213–223.

Wise, R. A. (1996). Addictive drugs and brain stimulation reward. *Annual Review of Neuroscience, 19*, 319–340. doi:10.1146/annurev.ne.19.030196.001535.

Wise, R. A. (2002). Brain reward circuitry: Insights from unsensed incentives. *Neuron, 36*(2), 229–240.

Wise, R. A., & Bozarth, M. A. (1987). A psychomotor stimulant theory of addiction. *Psychological Review, 94*(4), 469–492.

World Health Organization. (2004). *Neuroscience of psychoactive substance use and dependence*. Geneva: World Health Organization.

Part II
Innovations in The Treatment of Substance Addiction

Chapter 3
What Can We Expect from the Pharmacological Treatments for Dependences Presently Available?

Luis Pereira Justo

Introduction

The problematic use of substances such as alcohol, marijuana, cocaine, tobacco, and others imposes a major destabilization as regards the well-being of individuals and societies in several countries, including Brazil. In addition to the risk of dependence, those substances might entail various types of aggression to the human body and contribute to a significant increase in the onset of diseases, incapacitation, and mortality (Saitz 2007). The damage caused by the use of alcohol and tobacco, substances whose use is permitted, that is, licit drugs, is certainly more prevalent and costly all over the world than that resulting from the use of illicit drugs, such as marijuana, cocaine, and crack. We should also mention that some medications prescribed by physicians may become drugs of abuse, as in the case of benzodiazepines and opioid analgesics, with extremely harmful consequences to their users. The problems associated with all those substances are disseminated in populations around the world, reaching the various strata that compose society, with no restriction as to socioeconomical power. The damage inherent to the use of drugs (here we include alcohol, tobacco, and any other substances classified in the patterns of abuse) can be detected in both the users and those close to them. Even those who do not have direct contact with the users and are often not aware of the extension of the damage caused by those substances can be affected. An American study demonstrated that 63 % of the society reported, by the time the study was being carried out, suffering the negative impact of alcohol, tobacco, or illicit drug use, independently of having direct contact with the user (Jupp and Lawrence 2010). Therefore, one should not be surprised at the great concern of multiple sectors of society, such as health professionals who work directly with users, public

L.P. Justo (✉)

Departamento de Psicobiologia, Universidade Federal de São Paulo, Rua Botucatu, 862 - 1º Andar, Edifício de Ciências Biomédicas, São Paulo, SP 04023-062, Brazil

e-mail: lpjusto@gmail.com

© Springer International Publishing Switzerland 2016

A.L.M. Andrade and D. De Micheli (eds.), *Innovations in the Treatment of Substance Addiction*, DOI 10.1007/978-3-319-43172-7_3

37

health managers in charge of creating policies targeted to the collectivity, policy makers, religious leaders, and the general population, as they understand the severity of the problem.

When actions that address drug-related problems are devised, there are always more questions than satisfactory answers, since the complexity of the theme is actually considerable. The use of alcohol, marijuana, and some other drugs is a very old fact in the history of civilization, dating back to thousands of years. Over time, the man has dealt in different ways with their peers who are affected by problems that might arise from the use. Understanding the reason or reasons why the use of those substances might produce such serious problems is a challenge, especially as regards the loss of control over behaviors that lead to this consumption and end up characterizing dependence. In this scenario, moral judgements have great weight and, we must say, hinder the struggle in the appeasement of difficulties.

A careful look should be directed to alcohol or drug users or dependent individuals. This care implies in one not starting off from prejudicial premises, but rather searching for a comprehensive and humanized understanding of the dependent individual and the circumstances surrounding dependence. Moreover, researchers must look for really viable solutions for the treatment. Additionally, and perhaps the most difficult and at the same time fundamental aspect, dependent individuals should not be segregated from their immediate environment and the rest of society. Finally, those are tasks that require much effort from all the people involved.

What we call treatment of dependence should more adequately be called treatment of the dependent, with the possible inclusion of those who comprise their closest relationship network, which implies in some sophistication of the approach. People are different, and so are the conditions in which the problems exist. Consequently, it is necessary to recognize the particularities of each case before using resources that are standardized for large groups. Those resources, however, should not be discarded, since they may be effective along with other therapeutic measures. In other words, we should add elements of treatment that can be effective to many individuals, and the knowledge we have of the singularity of each case or individual.

The therapeutic possibilities are varied, and it is desirable that different modalities be combined in one single treatment in order for the chances of success to be increased. In this sense, we can resort to several forms of psychotherapy with therapists well prepared for that: self-help groups (as the Alcoholics Anonymous); psychoeducation methods; activities of various nature with therapeutic objectives as, for example, a job that fits the individual's condition in that particular moment; participation in group tasks; artistic expression; physical exercises; meditation; and many more. Those resources include several medications, known as pharmacotherapy. They may help both in the treatment of withdrawal syndrome and detoxification, and in the maintenance of abstinence from the substance(s) one is addicted to. Moreover, they may help preserve general aspects of well-being and mental health. An aspect worth mentioning is that, when we try to treat dependent individuals, we often find out they have other health problems, not as a result of drug use but associated with it. Those problems are called comorbidities. In those cases, the use of medication other than that used to treat the dependence may also be necessary.

Reinforcing what we exposed above, the best therapeutic approaches should be multidisciplinary, involving various professionals from distinct areas. Physicians should be among those professionals, since their evaluation and the medications they may prescribe are fundamental in the process. The knowledge of the neurobiology associated with drug dependence allows us to believe it is a phenomenon with a strong biological basis, whether it is regarding the vulnerability one has to become dependent when exposed to a given substance, or the behavioral characteristics one begins to have after they become dependent. However, one cannot assert that the environmental factors and the psychological functioning of each person are less important in this process. Those factors are painful for those who experience it directly as well as those who have direct or indirect contact with the individuals involved in dependence. Even though researchers still need to find a way to optimize the action of medication, their use may represent a crucial component in the treatments. Unfortunately, there are no medications yet whose significant effectiveness has been demonstrated to treat each kind of substance dependence. Therefore, even though the pharmacological approach may help, medication should not be the only treatment modality. There is great variability from person to person in response to medications. None of them is universally efficacious and effective.

Another point worth mentioning is that it is the physician who prescribes the medications. This professional detains the necessary knowledge on the normal and the pathological functioning of the body, and the potential action of medications on it. Experts in the field of dependence are usually better prepared to treat morbid conditions associated with dependence, since they had specific training and usually have more experience than general practitioners or physicians in other specialties. Most of those specialists are psychiatrists. They should also be alert and able to neutralize the manifestations of intolerance and prejudicial attitudes often targeted to alcohol and other drug users. The mission of physicians is not to impose their own moral values or be the messengers of social and family norms of the individual under treatment. Their first duty is to help human beings relieve their suffering. This is the commitment that should guide pharmacological treatments.

A diagnosis should be established before the beginning of any treatments. In order to do so, physicians should have general knowledge of the problems at stake. They should know the history of the individuals concerning its multiple aspects: their route until they reached the drug, the type of drug, how often and under which circumstances it is used, and whether other drugs are used concomitantly and whether there are other health or psychiatric diagnoses. The physician is also expected to be updated as regards new researches on drugs, related problems, and their treatments, therefore becoming knowledgeable of the most recent and valid scientific evidence. By doing so, they will be able to apply the most general knowledge to each particular case, since the singularity of each patient is too important for physicians to decide on the set of information that will determine the medical approach. Hence, no pharmacological scheme is invariably good to all individuals, and according to this line of thought, physicians have no ready solution to any individual who needs their services. Treatments work, at least partially, as therapeutic trials that should be periodically evaluated as to their effectiveness.

When dependence sets in, that means the body will be chronically affected in most cases. Even though the use of medication does not necessarily have to be chronic, other kinds of care should. For example, the individual should not use any amount of the substance anymore and should avoid situations that were previously associated with use. There must be special attention to psychiatric comorbidities, that is, disorders such as depression, anxiety, and psychotic syndromes, among others, as they may work as risk factors for the individual to return to the substance use.

In this chapter, we will discuss some medications used in the treatment of dependences, and the situations in which they are prescribed to users of alcohol, drugs, and even prescription drugs.

Short-term Treatments: Detoxification

When someone dependent on a substance discontinues or substantially reduces its use, they may start having extremely uncomfortable and even threatening symptoms for the maintenance of good health conditions. Those manifestations are commonly described as withdrawal syndrome. They comprise a set of symptoms that are often characteristic of certain substances. In the mildest cases, they may represent anxiety, irritability, discouragement, lack of pleasure in things that are usually significant, physical agitation, insomnia and appetite alterations, among others. Those symptoms, for being transient and disappearing spontaneously, may not require pharmacological treatment. In the most severe cases (for some substances, the severity of dependence is more evident and striking), the capacity of the body to remain physiologically balanced might be compromised, and there might be severe symptoms as lowered level of consciousness with loss of contact with reality and alterations in the cardiovascular and hydroelectrolytic functioning. Those cases of homeostasis breakdown must be quickly treated, both for the safety of the individual in the immediate moment, and so that they are not followed by the restart of drug consumption, once the symptoms might act as a "negative reinforcement," that is, highlighting the need to ingest the substance in order to stop the discomfort. The ingestion of the substance once again actually makes the symptoms disappear, which generates the notion that the individual cannot go without it. It is in this stage that detoxification treatments are important, for they not only guarantee the safety and comfort of the user at the moment, but also make the way for the later therapeutic work of abstinence promotion in a lasting way.

When we talk about detoxification of an individual who is dependent on alcohol or other drugs, we may be talking about different things according to the substances, the frequency of use, the amount ingested, the conditions of use, and what the word means to the individual. As a consequence, we must define what detoxification is. In this context, it is the process of substance withdrawal in a safe way for the global health and also with the least suffering possible for the individual (Diaper et al. 2013). It is also a way to start approaches of relapse prevention in the periods immediately after the discontinuation of the substance one is dependent on (Kattimani and Bharadwaj 2013). Detoxification treatments vary according to the case. Sometimes they are carried out by the gradual removal of the substance, while other times it implies in its total removal, but with the administration of medications that have a substitution action. Still in other cases, it involves the complete cessation of substance use, without any medication of substitution action, but with the treatment of symptoms that might appear in the initial withdrawal phase. The approach will be determined by the type of substance the individual is dependent on, their life conditions, global health, where and who they live with, their motivation for treatment, etc.

As we mentioned before, acute detoxification treatments should be considered the initial phase of treatment for dependence rather than an objective in themselves. Relapses soon after a detoxification period are quite frequent; hence, it is desirable that health professionals already start introducing strategies that aim at long-term treatments, mainly with a view to preventing the individual from returning to the behavior of substance use (Diaper et al. 2013).

It is a common notion that dependence on any substance requires a detoxification phase. That is not entirely precise. Detoxification may be a significant phase in the treatment for certain substances as alcohol, opioids, benzodiazepines, and cocaine/crack. Those substances can cause such intense withdrawal syndromes that they may be life threatening or force the individual to return to the substance use. Other drugs such as marijuana, LSD, and amphetamines, to mention a few, do not produce significantly intense withdrawal syndromes in most cases and hence do not require a specific detoxification treatment, that is, the abrupt discontinuation of use does not demand acute therapeutic interventions. Evidently, there are exceptions as regards dependence on these latter drugs that might need therapeutic detoxification interventions. Withdrawal syndrome is a set of signs and symptoms that are characteristic of each substance and may occur when there is abrupt discontinuation or substantial decrease in drug intake, or even when there is an intercurrent acute disease. Those signs and symptoms vary from case to case as to intensity and quality. One should bear in mind that withdrawal syndromes are self-limited, that is, they last for a limited period of time even if there is no pharmacological treatment.

The consumption of ethanol, the type of alcohol most frequently found in drinks, is part of the dietary habits of most human societies. The majority of people do not get to the point of having major drinking problems, but some do. The problems can be acute, as in drinking and driving, without necessarily implying in dependence, or chronic, as in the case of dependence, a condition that is quite difficult to manage.

Perhaps, the best known withdrawal syndrome is that of alcohol. It may follow a milder course, with only anxiety, some agitation, light sweating, insomnia, and craving, or it might be a severe occurrence, to the point of causing deep consciousness alterations such as motor agitation, thought and behavioral confusion, illusions, delirium, and hallucination (frequently with the view of animals that are not in the same environment the person is), in addition to intense sweating and tremor; changes in the sleep/wake cycle, and other physical signs such as alterations of blood pressure, heart beat, and body temperature. In the most severe cases, there might also be seizures (Kattimani and Bharadwaj 2013). Those cases are called delirium tremens, and it is adamant that the individual be hospitalized for detoxification. For the milder cases mentioned above, if acute treatment is required, it can take place in an outpatient setting. Without the use of adequate medication, it is difficult and even risky to go through a more severe case of alcohol withdrawal syndrome. The medications most commonly used in alcohol detoxification are benzodiazepines, such as diazepam and chlordiazepoxide, as well as others less frequently used. The treatment in this acute phase also involves the vitamins of the B complex, in particular thiamine, vitamin C, and correction of the hydroelectrolytic balance, with attention to magnesium (Kattimani and Bharadwaj 2013; Perry 2014; Manasco et al. 2012). Data from clinical research point to the usefulness of acamprosate already in the treatment phase of alcohol withdrawal syndrome, since that component controls the excessive brain excitability of this period, and consequently has a protective action against neuronal damage and prevents seizures (Grant et al. 1990; Kampman et al. 2009). There are physicians who use anticonvulsants such as topiramate, carbamazepine, gabapentin, or sodium valproate from the beginning of treatment on, since they believe this way they can work around the neural toxicity, and more occasionally with antipsychotics and antihypertensives as adjuvants (Perry 2014; Kenna et al. 2009; Krupitsky et al. 2007). The use of anticonvulsants for alcohol detoxification is still controversial, considering that the evidence yielded by clinical research does not provide a solid basis for their prescription. Moreover, they might have the potential to alleviate certain symptoms and prevent some brain damage, but they do not seem to be effective candidates to replace benzodiazepines in the initial treatment phase (Minozzi et al. 2010).

Opioids are a group of substances derived from herbal opium in its natural form, or also synthetic drugs that have chemical structure and action similar to those of natural opium and its derivates. Among the examples of opioids, we can mention morphine, heroin, and a large variety of synthetic ones. In Brazil, those drugs have little penetration for recreational use. On the other hand, we can find individuals who are addicted to opioids used as analgesic. The treatment for opioid dependence is difficult, as it is usually severe. In that case, too, detoxification is important. It is done by the gradual reduction of the substance the individual is dependent on, or by the substitution for another opioid with a biochemical profile that is more favorable as regards dependence and risks to the user. In general, treatment for these cases is administered in specialized clinics.

Benzodiazepines are widely used medications, mainly to control anxiety and for sleep induction, even though they may have several other uses in medicine. They are good medications when used correctly, but might constitute a problem otherwise. There are many different types in the market, such as diazepam, clonazepam, lorazepam, bromazepam, midazolam, oxazolam, and flurazepam, with several trade names. Sometimes they are prescribed for long periods (over three consecutive months and at relatively high dosages), which may lead to dependence. Therefore, they should not be prescribed for long-term use, except in very special cases when it is clearly justifiable. When an individual becomes dependent on a benzodiazepine, the treatment itself implies in detoxification, since it should be withdrawn gradually or substituted by another that will also be gradually withdrawn thereafter. The greatest problems with benzodiazepines tend to happen when people use them to sleep, for they end up fearing insomnia and resist its withdrawal. In that case, an alternative is to try a temporary substitution for substances that help sleep but are less likely to cause dependence, for instance, zolpidem, melatonin, trazodone, amitriptyline, and quetiapine (at low doses). Nevertheless, the prolonged use of benzodiazepines is undesirable in most cases and, should insomnia persist, other types of treatment would be advisable. The withdrawal of benzodiazepines should not be abrupt due to the possible onset of anxiety and insomnia symptoms, in particular.

When health professionals discuss detoxification treatment for powder cocaine and especially for its smoked form (crack), what they want is the change of the environment and the way of life of the dependent individuals, as their removal from the environment where they have access to the drug (which greatly facilitates its purchase), rather than the administration of pharmacological treatments that might inhibit the craving for the drug. The medications often prescribed during the period of detoxification serve various purposes as, for example, calming the individual down; inducing sleep; reducing irritability, agitation and aggressiveness, when they occur. We are not talking about detoxification that implies in a gradual withdrawal of cocaine or crack. Those drugs must be withdrawn at once. The withdrawal symptoms do not work the same way as in the dependence of alcohol, opioids, and benzodiazepines. The medications used in those cases are unspecific, that is, they are not exclusive for the treatment of dependence per se, and might be of different types, usually the class of benzodiazepines and sedative antipsychotics. Much has been researched to find medications that act on the craving for cocaine/crack, but so far none of them has shown a robust enough result to be considered effective (Diaper et al. 2013). Among the substances already tried and studied, we have topiramate, amantadine, tiagabine, gabapentin, modafinil, bupropion, and disulfiram, to mention a few (Diaper et al. 2013). The same is true for other stimulants of the central nervous system, such as amphetamines, which were used for a long time to reduce appetite and facilitate weight loss diets.

Marijuana can also cause withdrawal syndrome when it is used for a long time and in large amounts. The symptoms usually arise 48 h after the last use and disappear from 2 weeks to 3 months without a new use (Greydanus et al. 2013). In that case as well, the detoxification treatment aims at controlling symptoms such as irritability, anxiety, insomnia, and subjective discomfort, and there are no specific medications to control the craving to use marijuana. Studies suggest that dronabinol, a derivative of the plant *Cannabis sativa*, source of marijuana, could relieve the symptoms of marijuana withdrawal (which result from another component of Cannabis, the delta-9-THC) (Greydanus et al. 2013). Sodium valproate, bupropion, fluoxetine, nefazodone, and mirtazapine have already been studied for that purpose. They had a small effect on craving that seemed, in any case, better than that of placebos (Diaper et al. 2013). Individuals who use small amounts or make infrequent use do not present withdrawal syndrome when they interrupt the use of marijuana. There are now synthetic forms of delta-9-THC in the market. They are more potent than the herbal marijuana and receive the street names "spice" and "K2," among others. Those drugs have been little studied yet, but they might cause a more severe dependence, with a stronger withdrawal syndrome.

In the case of tobacco, the treatment for dependence is also strongly associated with detoxification. Behavioral and pharmacological techniques have been studied. As regards the pharmacological ones, a very common treatment is the administration of bupropion or nortriptyline, both are antidepressants, which in some cases reduce the craving for smoking. Another common treatment is the administration of the above-mentioned medications along with a program of progressive reduction of the number of cigarettes smoked daily until complete cessation (Jupp and Lawrence 2010). When those combined techniques are not successful, health professionals resort to nicotine replacement administered by a route other than smoked (for example, transdermal or adhesive patches applied to the skin). The concentrations of the patches are gradually reduced, with their complete withdrawal within about 3 months. It is essential that individuals do not make use of tobacco while they are receiving nicotine by oral or transdermal route or spray. It is possible not to make use of the antidepressants mentioned above, only replace the smoked nicotine by its compatible dose by means of an alternative route, and proceed to the gradual reduction until complete withdrawal. There are oral nicotine preparations or sprays, but these are more used in maintenance treatments, when necessary. Another therapeutic modality for smoking is the use of varenicline, commercialized specifically for this treatment (Garrison and Dugan 2009). Clonidine (Gourlay et al. 2004) is mentioned in some studies as well. According to some authors, clonidine is considered a second-line treatment (Diaper et al. 2013). People who stop smoking sometimes present depressive symptoms that should be treated even if mild, especially as a way to reduce the chances of relapse. Several types of antidepressants can be used for that purpose, as the class of selective serotonin re-uptake inhibitors (fluoxetine, citalopram, escitalopram, sertraline, for instance), but it is worth considering the use of nortriptyline which, in spite of entailing more side effects, acts on the craving to smoke.

Other drugs, among the many existing ones, such as ecstasy, methamphetamine, LSD, and psilocybin, do not have the characteristic of producing withdrawal syndrome, and therefore do not require detoxification treatments for most users.

Long-Term Treatments: Relapse Prevention, Damage Reduction, and Control of Psychiatric Comorbidities

It is a lot more an exception than a rule that someone dependent on alcohol or other drugs has their problems solved by detoxification treatments alone. Considering dependence brings about changes in the brain that are not corrected in the short term, and may never be overcome, the problem should be understood as chronic. Consequently, there will always be the risk of relapse, even if the dependent person is determined not to return to the use of the substance. This condition certainly requires long-lasting treatments.

Long-term treatments for dependence might have two distinct objectives. The first is relapse prevention, whose objective is the complete cessation of alcohol or other drug use. The second would be therapeutic actions that aim at helping dependent individuals to reduce and have some control over their consumption, thus reducing the damage caused by the substance. The latter approach is known as damage reduction treatment. Concomitantly, researchers should investigate psychiatric comorbidities that work as risk factors for substance use and treat them accordingly. These long-term therapeutic interventions will vary according to the drug: the severity of dependence, the possible existence of one or more comorbidities, and the general conditions of the dependent person.

Below we will address some pharmacological treatments that show better efficacy for the dependence on some substances.

With the objective of preventing relapse of alcohol ingestion, disulfiram was approved for this kind of treatment in the United States of America in 1948, being the first medication used for that purpose (Zindel and Kranzler 2014). Someone under treatment with disulfiram will have very unpleasant physical reactions in the event of alcohol ingestion. Whenever this happens, the result is the same. It happens because disulfiram prevents alcohol from being metabolized in a physiologically normal way, and one of the intermediate metabolites, acetaldehyde, accumulates in the body in toxic amounts, causing discomfort. As a result, it is expected that the person develops some kind of aversion to alcohol consumption. Therefore, this type of treatment is called aversive. For ethical reasons, disulfiram should not be administered without the person's knowledge. Its usefulness seems to be stronger in those individuals who are intent on quitting drinking and count on the supervision of someone close, for it is difficult for them to agree to take the medication or actually take it if they are not supervised (Laaksonen et al. 2008).

A medication that has been increasingly used to control the craving for alcohol is an antagonist of opioid receptors (involved in the neurobiological mechanisms of dependence) called naltrexone (Jupp and Lawrence 2010). It seems to reduce the "positive reinforcement" associated with alcohol by reducing the subjective feeling of reward connected to the ingestion of alcohol, increasing the chances of people reducing their drinking behavior (Sinclair et al. 2002). Another substance that has been tested with some success and similar mechanisms of action to reduce long-term alcohol craving is nalmefene (Gual et al. 2014).

Acamprosate has been used in the struggle against relapse, so common in alcohol-dependent individuals. It acts through the inhibition of one of the receptors in the neurotransmitter system called glutamatergic, which seems to have a strong relation with the physiological brain alterations that favor relapse, even in those individuals who have been abstinent for a relatively long time (De Witte et al. 2005; Kennedy et al. 2010). A possible adverse effect of acamprosate over time is the development of a phenomenon known as tolerance, by which the medication starts having little therapeutic effect or no effect at all; thus, researchers have questioned its usefulness (Jupp and Lawrence 2010).

Topiramate, initially commercialized as an anticonvulsant, has been studied and used both in the short- and in the long-term treatment for alcohol-dependent individuals. It seems to inhibit the reward effects acutely produced by the consumption of alcoholic beverages, reducing or suppressing its ingestion, and reducing the deleterious brain reactions caused by long exposure (Blodgett et al. 2014; Johnson et al. 2008). Topiramate has the additional advantage of not being extensively metabolized by the liver, except at high doses; hence, it is safer for use by alcohol-dependent individuals, who often present hepatic impairment (De Sousa 2010). A meta-analysis, the analysis of a number of studies to obtain a synthesis of estimates, detected that topiramate seems to have higher effectiveness in the treatment of alcoholism than some other medications used (Blodgett et al. 2014). At least one recent study shows advantages in the association of topiramate and naltrexone, considering it is possible to use smaller doses of both with good results (Moore et al. 2014). Other anticonvulsants are used in the treatment for alcohol dependence, namely carbamazepine and gabapentin (Jupp and Lawrence 2010).

Baclofen, a substance that has been studied in the treatment of alcoholism, seems to induce some reduction in alcohol craving, but it has the adverse effect of being significantly sedative, especially if the individual ingests alcohol concomitantly. The results of the studies so far do not provide enough data for its indication as a first-choice treatment (Brennan et al. 2013).

The antidepressants in the class of the selective serotonin re-uptake inhibitors seem useful in some cases of alcohol dependence, as long as they do not have a genetic variable as a causal component that classifies them as a distinct subtype of alcohol dependence (Johnson 2008).

The long-term treatment for opioids dependence is usually difficult due to the tendency to relapse the users display. Various therapeutic modalities are tried, including the maintenance with more controllable opioids such as methadone for long periods of time, but always under strict medical supervision (Jupp and Lawrence 2010). Ideally, the dependent person should remain completely abstinent from all sort of consumption, an achievement that can be rather difficult, especially for the users of heroin and morphine.

The treatments for dependence on psychostimulants such as cocaine/crack and amphetamines and its derivates do not have medications with robust efficacy or clear specificity for that purpose yet. As the consumption of cocaine and crack is becoming almost epidemic in several countries, researchers spare no efforts to find therapeutic solutions. Several substances that act as enhancers of dopaminergic neurotransmission (which those stimulants also do) were tested, but most of the studies did not show their efficacy in the reduction of craving for cocaine/crack and amphetamines in humans. Bupropion, another antidepressant with dopaminergic action, yielded some benefits in methamphetamine-dependent individuals (Heinzerling et al. 2014). Some positive results seem possible with anticonvulsants such as topiramate (mainly at higher doses), tiagabine, vigabatrin, gabapentin, and even valproic acid (Jupp and Lawrence 2010). Dissulfiram, best known for its use in the treatment for alcoholism, seems effective in the treatment for cocaine dependence, even though the evidence available is not enough to guarantee the safety of its use neither explain its mechanism of action (Shorter and Kosten 2011). Further studies are needed to clarify the efficacy of those agents, and the specific circumstances under which they may adequately fulfill their role of therapeutic agents.

Since the serotonergic system is implied in the brain actions of psychostimulants, some agents that act predominantly on this system are potential pharmacological therapeutic instruments in the treatment for the craving for cocaine, crack, and amphetamines. The studies carried out with sertraline, venlafaxine, fluoxetine imipramine, and paroxetine did not show favorable results (Jupp and Lawrence 2010). Citalopram, a serotonergic agent, on the other hand, showed some effectiveness (Moeller et al. 2007).

Some atypical antipsychotics such as risperidone and quetiapine have been used to cocaine and crack dependence, even though there are reports of abusive use of the latter (Jupp and Lawrence 2010). Biperiden, an anticholinergic agent, was recently studied to treat this dependence with positive results, mainly as regards control of craving, with consumption reduction (Dieckmann et al. 2014). Here again, further studies are required to confirm and broaden these results.

Vaccines have been created to try and control the effects of cocaine and crack, but studies on them are not easily feasible for researchers to know whether they would be a useful treatment. In the case of amphetamines, however, vaccines have shown more promising results in some studies (Jupp and Lawrence 2010). Laboratories have tried to create vaccines to treat smoking, but at least so far the results have not been satisfactory (Havermans et al. 2014), therefore not representing a clinical modality to be used.

Herbal marijuana is still the most used illicit drug all over the world. Until some years ago, there were no good-quality scientific information that could reveal the potential benefits it may bring and the harm it may cause to users. Nowadays, there is enough information to know that *Cannabis sativa* as a whole is a plant that produces a large amount of cannabinoid substances, among which a psychoactive drug that can be extremely harmful to humans (delta-9-THC). Nevertheless, it also contains cannabinoids that can be transformed into possible medications with some therapeutic indications. The heavy and frequent use of marijuana might lead to dependence and cause withdrawal syndrome when interrupted. There are no medications approved by the regulatory health organizations for the specific long-term treatment of this dependence. In any case, some alternatives have been tested, but the results are still frail. Among the medications under study, we can mention gabapentin, dronabinol, sodium valproate, lithium, buspirone, and lofexidine (Jupp and Lawrence 2010).

Conclusion

Even though pharmacological treatments show some efficacy and effectiveness and are imperative in the present scenario of therapies for substance dependence, the prevalence of consumption and the alcohol-/other drugs-related problems are still high, with a heavy burden to society. Consequently, substantial investment is necessary both on research of new medications that might be effective and other psychosocial interventions that produce more tangible results and might be useful to expressive populations of users. Even if we consider the socioeconomic deficient conditions that caracterizes some countries and the possible involvement of this in the management of drug addiction, it is worth pointing out that in more developed societies problems with substance abuse is very difficult to deal either.

References

Blodgett, J. C., Del Re, A. C., Maisel, N. C., & Finney, J. W. (2014). A meta-analysis of topiramate's effects for individuals with alcohol use disorders. *Alcoholism Clinical and Experimental Research, 38*(6), 1481–1488.

Brennan, J. L., Leung, J. G., Gagliardi, J. P., Rivelli, S. K., & Muzyk, A. J. (2013). Clinical effectiveness of baclofen for the treatment of alcohol dependence: A review. *Clinical Pharmacology: Advances and Applications, 5*, 99–107.

De Sousa, A. (2010). The role of topiramate and other anticonvulsants in the treatment of alcohol dependence: A clinical review. *CNS & Neurological Disorders Drug Targets, 9*(1), 45–49.

De Witte, P., Littleton, J., Parot, P., & Koob, G. (2005). Neuroprotective and abstinence-promoting effects of acamprosate: Elucidating the mechanism of action. *CNS Drugs, 19*(6), 517–537.

Diaper, A. M., Law, F. D., & Melichar, J. K. (2013). Pharmacological strategies for detoxification. *British Journal of Clinical Pharmacology, 77*(2), 302–314.

Dieckmann, L. H., Ramos, A. C., Silva, E. A., Justo, L. P., Sabioni, P., Frade, I. F., et al. (2014). Effects of biperiden on the treatment of cocaine/crack addiction: A randomised, double-blind, placebo-controlled trial. *European Neuropsychopharcology, 24*(8), 1196–1202.

Garrison, G. D., & Dugan, S. E. (2009). Varenicline: A first-line treatment option for smoking cessation. *Clinical Therapeutics, 31*(3), 463–491.

Gourlay, S. G., Stead, L. F., & Benowitz, N. L. (2004). Clonidine for smoking cessation. *Cochrane Database of Systematic Reviews, 3*, CD000058.

Grant, K. A., Valverius, P., Hudspith, M., & Tabakoff, B. (1990). Alcohol withdrawal seizures and the NMDA receptor complex. *European Journal of Pharmacology, 176*, 289–296.

Greydanus, D. E., Hawver, E. K., Greydanus, M. M., & Merrick, J. (2013). Marijuana: Current concepts. *Frontiers in Public Health, 1*, 42.

Gual, A., Bruguera, P., & López-Pelayo, H. (2014). Nalmefene and its use in alcohol dependence. *Drugs of Today, 50*(5), 347–355.

Havermans, A., Vuurman, E. F., van den Hurk, J., Hoogsteder, P., & van Schayck, O. C. (2014). Treatment with a nicotine vaccine does not lead to changes in brain activity during smoking cue exposure or a working memory task. *Addiction, 109*(8), 1260–1267.

Heinzerling, K. G., Swanson, A. N., Hall, T. M., Yi, Y., Wu, Y., & Shoptaw, S. J. (2014). Randomized, placebo-controlled trial of bupropion in methamphetamine-dependent participants with less than daily methamphetamine use. *Addiction*. doi:10.1111/add.12636.

Johnson, B. A. (2008). Update on neuropharmacological treatments for alcoholism: Scientific basis and clinical findings. *Biochemical Pharmacology, 75*(1), 34–56.

Johnson, B. A., Rosenthal, N., Capece, J. A., Wiegand, F., Mao, L., Beyers, K., et al. (2008). Topiramate for Alcoholism Advisory Board; Topiramate for Alcoholism Study Group. Improvement of physical health and quality of life of alcohol-dependent individuals with topiramate treatment: US multisite randomized controlled trial. *Archives of Internal Medicine, 168*(11), 1188–1199.

Jupp, B., & Lawrence, A. J. (2010). New horizons for therapeutics in drug and alcohol abuse. *Pharmacology & Therapeutics, 125*, 138–168.

Kampman, K. M., Pettinati, H. M., Lynch, K. G., Xie, H., Dackis, C., Oslin, D. W., et al. (2009). Initiating acamprosate within-detoxification versus post-detoxification in the treatment of alcohol dependence. *Addictive Behaviors, 34*, 581–586.

Kattimani, S., & Bharadwaj, B. (2013). Clinical management of alcohol withdrawal: A systematic review. *Industrial Psychiatry Journal, 22*(2), 100–108.

Kenna, G. A., Lomastro, T. L., Schiesl, A., Leggio, L., & Swift, R. M. (2009). Review of topiramate: An antiepileptic for the treatment for the alcohol dependence. *Current Drug Abuse Reviews, 2*(2), 135–142.

Kennedy, W. K., Leloux, M., Kutscher, E. C., Price, P. L., Morstad, A. E., & Carnahan, R. M. (2010). Acamprosate. *Expert Opinion on Drug Metabolism & Toxicology, 6*(3), 363–380.

Krupitsky, E. M., Rudenko, A. A., Burakov, A. M., Slavina, T. Y., Grinenko, A. A., Pittman, B., et al. (2007). Antiglutamatergic strategies for ethanol detoxification: Comparison with placebo and diazepam. *Alcoholism, Clinical and Experimental Research, 31*(4), 604–611.

Laaksonen, E., Koski-Jännes, A., Salaspuro, M., Ahtinen, H., & Alho, H. (2008). A randomized, multicentre, open-label, comparative trial of disulfiram, naltrexone and acamprosate in the treatment of alcohol dependence. *Alcohol and Alcoholism, 43*(1), 53–61.

Manasco, A., Chang, S., Larriviere, J., Hamm, L. L., & Glass, M. (2012). Alcohol withdrawal. *Southern Medical Journal, 105*(11), 607–612.

Minozzi, S., Amato, L., Vechi, S., & Davoli, M. (2010). Anticonvulsants for alcohol withdrawal. *Cochrane Database Systematic Review, 3*, CD005064.

Moeller, F. G., Schmitz, J. M., Steinberg, J. L., Green, C. M., Reist, C., Lai, L. Y., et al. (2007). Citalopram combined with behavioral therapy reduces cocaine use: A double-blind, placebo-controlled trial. *The American Journal of Drug and Alcohol Abuse, 33*(3), 367–378.

Moore, C. F., Protzuk, O. A., Johnson, B. A., & Lynch, W. J. (2014). The efficacy of a low dose combination of topiramate and naltrexone on ethanol reinforcement and consumption in rat models. *Pharmacology, Biochemistry and Behavior, 116*, 107–115.

Perry, E. C. (2014). Inpatient management of acute alcohol withdrawal syndrome. *CNS Drugs, 28*(5), 401–410.

Saitz, R. (2007). Treatment of alcohol and other drug dependence. *Liver Transplantation, 11*(suppl 2), S59–S64.

Shorter, D., & Kosten, T. R. (2011). Novel pharmacotherapeutic treatments for cocaine addiction. *BCM Medicine, 9*, 119. doi:10.1186/1741-7015-9-119.

Sinclair, J. D., Alho, H., & Shinderman, M. (2002). Naltrexone for alcohol dependence. *New England Journal of Medicine, 346*(17), 1329–1331.

Zindel, L. R., & Kranzler, H. R. (2014). Pharmacotherapy for alcohol use disorders: Seventy years of progress. *Journal of Studies on Alcohol and Drugs, 75*(suppl17), 79–88.

Chapter 4
Use of Herbal Medicine to Treat Drug Addiction

Fúlvio Rieli Mendes and Dianne da Rocha Prado

Initial Considerations

The treatment of drug addiction is complicated, and most of the available approaches are ineffective, either pharmacological or no pharmacological (behavioral). The main approaches to the treatment of drug addiction are to reduce the craving (desire for drugs), decrease or prevent its reinforcing power (pleasant feeling obtained with the use of the substance), and minimize or abolish the unpleasant symptoms caused by the drug withdrawal, i.e., symptoms that occur upon the abrupt discontinuation of drug use (Kreek et al. 2002). Another approach is the replacement therapy, in which a medicine produces similar effects to the drug, but less potentially harmful, especially in cases where it is difficult to stop using the drug because it can generate a very intense withdrawal syndrome. An example is the replacement of heroin or morphine (obtained illegally) by methadone, a drug administered orally and which requires lower doses and induces weaker withdrawal symptoms. Another approach less currently used is the aversion therapy, in which the use of a therapeutic substance makes a person feel very badly while taking the drug, and the best-known example is disulfiram, which accentuates the negative symptoms of alcoholic intoxication.

The use of alternative therapies is an option as a primary or complementary treatment and has grown as a result of the failure of classical pharmacological approaches using synthetic drugs. Among the alternative therapy options, the use of herbal medicine is considered a promising approach, though not widely used, as will be seen throughout this chapter.

The use of plants for medicinal purposes is an ancient practice. At the same time, humans began to use various plants or plant preparations to experience pleasurable

F.R. Mendes (✉) · D.R. Prado
Centro de Ciências Naturais e Humanas, Universidade Federal do ABC, Rua Arcturus, 03, São Bernardo do Campo, SP 09606-070, Brazil
e-mail: fulvio.mendes@ufabc.edu.br; fulviorm@hotmail.com

© Springer International Publishing Switzerland 2016
A.L.M. Andrade and D. De Micheli (eds.), *Innovations in the Treatment of Substance Addiction*, DOI 10.1007/978-3-319-43172-7_4

51

feelings, or as part of rituals and habits of certain societies; therefore, it is clear that the use of mind-altering plants has always fascinated human beings (Carlini 2003). Some examples are the use of hallucinogenic plants and mushrooms and also the preparation of fermented and distilled beverages from various plants for the production of alcoholic beverages. However, the use of certain plants or derivatives can cause addiction, such as tobacco and alcohol, or substances isolated from plants such as cocaine from coca leaves, morphine from opium, and its synthetic analogue heroin.

Among the drugs of abuse, there are synthetic and natural substances or preparations derived from them. On the other hand, the nature also appears to be source of plants and active principles useful in treating chemical dependence. The main known plants and their active principles with this utility are discussed in this chapter.

Medicinal Plant Versus Herbal Medicines

First of all, it is important to discern a medicinal plant and a herbal medicine or phytotherapic. Any plant which is commonly used for the treatment of a disease or its symptoms, or even prophylactically is considered a medicinal plant. In folk medicine, several plants or their parts may be employed and the preparation form can be very different. The preparation of peppermint tea by infusing its leaves in boiling water, the guaco honey syrup, or a aloe vera gel are examples of specific forms of preparations with different uses. In all these cases, the preparation is homemade, with recipes passed from generation to generation, spread through popular culture. While some of these uses are widely disseminated, they have not been validated by the scientific medical community, that is, there is no scientific evidence attesting to their effectiveness.

On the other hand, the herbal medicine or phytotherapic is produced by a pharmaceutical laboratory, usually presented in the form of typical pharmaceutical preparations, such as tablets, pills, capsules, syrups, ointments, and sprays with defined dosage. The legislation concerning the registration of phytotherapics is different in some countries. In Europe, the herbal medicine must be registered by regulatory agencies like other synthetic drugs, but in the USA, they are sold as supplement food (not under FDA registration). Usually, a new herbal medicine must present proof of safety and efficacy to be registered, although a special group called "traditional phytotherapic" can be registered based on the tradition, if well documented by the scientific literature, as is the case in Brazil (Anvisa 2014). The herbal medicine must present a label drug with description of its chemical composition, indications, and expiration date. As we will see in this chapter, several plants are popularly used for the treatment of drug addiction, but few have actually been studied and generated a medically approved herbal medicine for this purpose.

Plants Used for the Treatment of Drug Addiction

The interest about the use and research of plants for drug addiction treatment has increased in recent years, reflected by the increasing number of publications evaluating the effects of crude extracts, active principles, and plant associations on the treatment of addiction. Although there are a considerable number of plants mentioned as useful in the treatment of drug addiction, only few species have been consistently studied and only a minority has been evaluated in clinical trials. In fact, most of the experimental evidences on plants capable of decreasing the drug abuse and reducing the withdrawal syndrome and drug relapse were obtained from laboratory animals (Rezvani et al. 2003; Abenavoli et al. 2009; Mendes et al. 2012). It is not the goal of this chapter to discuss in depth the mechanisms of action of these plants, but show an overview of the main studies and their possible indications. The main plants with scientific support for the treatment of drugs are described on the next pages.

Iboga (*Tabernanthe iboga*) and Ibogaine

Ibogaine is a psychoactive indole alkaloid obtained from the roots of iboga (*Tabernanthe iboga*), an African plant with hallucinogenic property used for centuries in rituals of certain tribes (Fig. 4.1). Scrapings of iboga root bark are used in small doses to combat fatigue, hunger, and thirst, and in high doses as a sacrament in the Bwiti religion in Gabon and West-Central Africa for spiritual experiences (Alper et al. 2008). There are other similar alkaloids, but ibogaine is the most studied and seems to be the most potent (Mačiulaitis et al. 2008). The scientific literature indicates that ibogaine is effective in the treatment of different drugs of abuse such as morphine, heroin, cocaine, and nicotine (Rezvani et al. 2003; Overstreet et al. 2003; Abenavoli et al. 2009).

The first reported use of ibogaine was a study conducted in 1962 where several hallucinogens were experienced in controlled situation and the individuals who have made the use of ibogaine reported no symptoms of heroin withdrawal syndrome (Alper et al. 2008). Since then, several animal and clinical studies have been conducted with iboga preparations, ibogaine alone, and also using synthetic analogues. The iboga alkaloids do not induce self-administration in animals, and the repeated treatment does not lead to a withdrawal syndrome when discontinued, suggesting that ibogaine does not produce addiction. Most animal studies indicated attenuation of the opioid withdrawal syndrome with the use of iboga or ibogaine. Other studies also showed decreased self-administration of morphine, cocaine, alcohol, amphetamine, methamphetamine, and nicotine after the iboga/ibogaine treatment (Dworkin et al. 1995; Glick and Maisonneuve 1998; Carai et al. 2000; Jupp and Lawrence 2010), and it is believed that the effect is due to its metabolite noribogaine (Mačiulaitis et al. 2008). The mechanism of action of ibogaine remains

Fig. 4.1 *Tabernanthe iboga*
bush with fruits. The ibogaine
is extracted from its roots.
Source: http://upload.
wikimedia.org/wikipedia/
commons/e/e4/Tabernanthe_
iboga_MS_4098.jpg

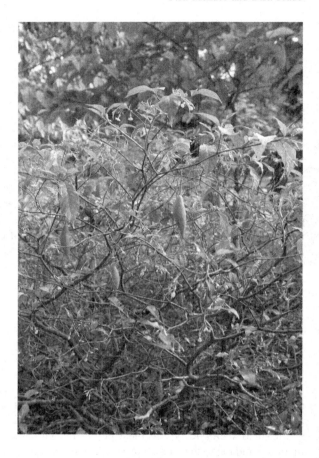

unclear, and the literature is somewhat controversial (Mačiulaitis et al. 2008; Brown 2013). Ibogaine and its metabolite noribogaine bind with a different potency to several receptors (such as dopamine and serotonin receptors), interfering with the secretion of some hormones and intracellular pathways (Mačiulaitis et al. 2008; Abenavoli et al. 2009). It is believed that the introspection experienced during the effect of ibogaine, which often includes a certain degree of self analysis and reevaluation of the life style, is an important psychological factor in the decision of stop using drugs (Brown 2013).

Some clinical studies have been conducted with ibogaine in drug dependents and showed satisfactory results in the reduction of opioid withdrawal syndrome. Many reports are case studies that describe the absence or an alleviation of the withdrawal syndrome and craving after the drug abstinence (detoxification period), and many individuals stopped using drug or had a long period of abstinence, but there are also cases of relapse (Brown 2013). A retrospective study of alcohol, marijuana, cocaine, and crack users that had been subjected to treatment with ibogaine associated with psychotherapy showed that 61 % of participants were abstinent at the time of the interview, that is, they had stopped using drugs. Patients that received a single dose of ibogaine had an average abstinence time of 5.5 months, while the treatment with multiple doses led to an average abstinence over 8 months (Schenberg et al. 2014). No serious adverse events were observed, suggesting that the treatment with ibogaine is safe and effective for the dependence of other drugs in addition to morphine and heroin.

Ibogaine-based treatment for drug addiction may be found in the clinics of Europe and North/Central America, particularly in Mexico, but the treatment cost is very high. In addition, the use of ibogaine in many of these clinics is unofficial, with advertisements published on the Internet, since the trade and clinical use of ibogaine are not regulated in most countries. The treatment with ibogaine is mainly sought by the dependents of heroin and other opioids, but is also used by the dependents of alcohol, crack, and other drugs. The treatment is done with a single dose or optionally repeated doses of 10–25 mg/kg (Brown 2013). A survey that aimed to assess the ibogaine culture of use has shown that among the ibogaine provider groups are licensed physician, providers without an official medical credential, activists and self-help groups, and also groups where the ibogaine use occurs in a religious context (Alper et al. 2008). As previously reported, in many of these cases, the use of ibogaine for drug treatment occurs in an unofficial basis, what increases the risk of health issues because ibogaine is a potentially toxic psychoactive substance. By this reason, we need more clinical studies and policies to control the use of the substance in the treatment of drug addiction.

Kudzu (*Pueraria lobata*)

The kudzu (Fig. 4.2) is an Asian plant, and its roots and aerial parts are used in traditional Chinese medicine for over 2000 years. The use of tea from the roots is described in the Chinese materia medica Shen Nong (200 years BC) as a drug with antipyretic, antidiarrheal, diaphoretic, and antiemetic properties (Keung and Vallee 1998). The use of roots and leaves against alcohol abuse and intoxication was described centuries later, between 600 and 1200 AD. A mixture containing kudzu and other plants is used in China to prepare a cup of tea known as tea of sobriety. Besides kudzu, traditional Chinese medicine describes numerous drugs to stop drinking (Lu et al. 2009), most of them acting based on psychological aversion, but these plants have fallen into disuse because of their ineffectiveness or occurrence of undesirable side effects (Keung and Vallee 1998). Instead, the kudzu gained international status of antialcohol plant and is currently extensively studied.

The original study investigating the antialcohol property of kudzu was carried out with a species of hamster that has a natural preference to alcohol (i.e., when alcohol and water are offered simultaneously, these animals consume more alcohol). The alcohol intake by these hamsters is equivalent to the consumption of a heavy drinker. The administration of kudzu extract at a dose of 1.5 g/kg intraperitoneally (i.p.) over 6 days decreased the alcohol intake by hamster in a

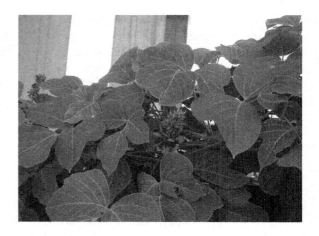

Fig. 4.2 Flowery branch of kudzu (*Pueraria lobata*). The part used in the treatment of alcoholism is the root, while the flowers have been used to alleviate alcohol hangover. *Source*: http://upload. wikimedia.org/wikipedia/ commons/e/ea/Pueraria_ lobata_ja02.jpg

model of ethanol–water-free choice. After the end of the treatment, the animals gradually increased the alcohol intake, suggesting that the effect of kudzu is reversible and occurs only during the treatment (Keung and Vallee 1998). The main plant isoflavones—puerarin, daidzin, and daidzein—were also evaluated. The daidzin at a dose of 150 mg/kg (i.p.) decreased alcohol consumption by more than 50 %. The puerarin, which is the most abundant plant isoflavone, also appears to be important for the reduction of alcohol consumption (Rezvani et al. 2003).

In a very extensive study were tested three concentrations (0.5, 0.75, and 1 g/kg) of kudzu from a commercial product (Benlhabib et al. 2004). In this study, rats were subjected to a protocol of 30 days of alcohol intake before the treatment with kudzu (to mimic the development of dependence and tolerance). Ethanol continued to be available until day 70, but was unavailable during the next 10 days to induce a withdrawal syndrome, being offered again from the 80th to the 90th day. There was a reduction in the ethanol consumption during the whole period that the animals received kudzu, and the best results were obtained with the dose of 0.5 g/kg, which reduced in 50–60 % of the alcohol intake and prevented the withdrawal signs without significantly affecting the weight of the animals.

The daidzin inhibits potently and selectively the mitochondrial aldehyde dehydrogenase (ALDH-2), an enzyme involved in the metabolism of acetaldehyde (metabolite of ethanol) and also with the metabolism of monoamines, while the daidzein and puerarin have high affinity for the benzodiazepine site of GABA receptor (Rezvani et al. 2003; Lu et al. 2009). These different mechanisms may contribute to the antialcohol effect of kudzu through an effect similar to that of disulfiram, associated with a reduction in anxiety and compulsion due to its GABAergic action. However, McGregor (2007) explain that there are two traditional kudzu preparations, a root-based extract and a flower-based extract, and advert for the risk of taking kudzu root as hangover medicine. According to the author, the flower extract is used to relieve the symptoms of the alcohol hangover and it seems to accelerate the removal of acetaldehyde, while the root extract has the opposite effect, it inhibits the ALDH-2 and should not be taken together with alcohol or under alcohol intoxication.

Despite the large number of studies with kudzu conducted on animals, there are few clinical studies. In a first study, the treatment with kudzu was not able to reduce the craving for alcohol and to help keeping sobriety of the participants (Shebek and Rindone 2000), but subsequent studies demonstrated the efficacy of the extract in moderately reducing the consumption of alcohol. The use of the extract for 1 week reduced the intake of alcohol in men and women (Lukas et al. 2005). A further study involving men with high alcohol consumption, diagnosis of abuse/dependence on alcohol, and who were not previously treated evaluated the effect of treatment for 4 weeks with a standardized extract of kudzu (250 mg of isoflavones, 3 times a day) compared to placebo. The treatment did not reduce the craving for alcohol, but reduced its consumption by 34–37 %, reduced the number of heavy drinking days, and increased the percentage of days abstinent without inducing serious adverse effects or changes in liver and renal function (Lukas et al. 2013). The administration of puerarin (1200 mg) for 1 week decreased beer consumption by heavy drinkers in a controlled condition and changed the way of drinking by the participants, who took smaller sips and took longer time to finish each beer (Penetar et al. 2012). These results suggest that kudzu and their active ingredients have moderate effectiveness in the treatment of alcohol dependence, but more studies are still needed.

St. John's Wort or Hypericum (*Hypericum perforatum*)

The European plant known as St. John's wort or hypericum (Fig. 4.3) has been extensively studied for the treatment of mild-to-moderate depression (Whiskey et al. 2001), and there are various herbal products available on the market. The St. John's wort contains flavonoids, hypericin, and hyperforin as active principles, which are involved with its antidepressant and anxiolytic activity (Mendes et al. 2012), but the substances with antiaddictive effect and their mechanisms of action are not well known.

The first studies evaluating the capability of hypericum in addiction treatment are based on the knowledge that there is a high comorbidity between depression and alcoholism (Rezvani et al. 2003). The initial study was performed with rats of genetic strains which have a natural preference to alcohol or consume large amounts of alcohol when it is freely offered. The authors evaluated the effect of the acute oral administration of doses of 100–800 mg/kg and the administration for 15 days of 400 mg/kg of hypericum extract (Rezvani et al. 1999). The doses of 200–800 mg/kg (acutely) decreased the acute alcohol intake, and the effect was maintained for 24 h with the higher doses. The chronic administration reduced the alcohol intake throughout the observation period and did not affect the food and water intake.

Fig. 4.3 Flowery branch of hypericum (*Hypericum perforatum*), known in Europe as St John's wort and used primarily for the treatment of depression. *Source*: http://upload. wikimedia.org/wikipedia/ commons/5/59/Hypericum_ perforatum_003.JPG

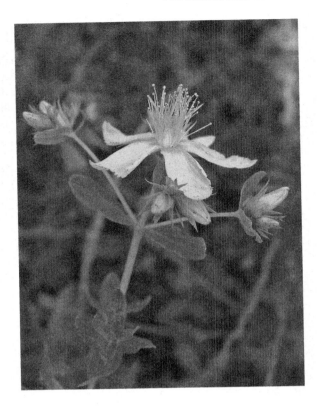

In another study, the effects of the intragastric administration of hypericum and naltrexone alone or in combination were evaluated over 7 days in rats with free access to alcohol 2 h per day (Perfumi et al. 2005). Naltrexone is an opioid receptor antagonist clinically used in the treatment of alcoholism and opiate dependence. The efficacy of two doses of each treatment was assessed; hypericum was proved to be active in reducing the ethanol intake at a dose of 125 mg/kg but not at a dose of 7 mg/kg, while naltrexone was active at a dose of 3 mg/kg and inactive at 0.5 mg/kg. However, the association between inactive doses of both treatments (hypericum 7 mg/kg and naltrexone 0.5 mg/kg) was effective in reducing the ethanol intake during the 12 days of evaluation, and there was no tolerance to the antialcohol effect (Perfumi et al. 2005). The discontinuation of the treatment led the animals to resume the alcohol consumption, suggesting that the effect was not due to a conditioned aversion to ethanol. These data indicate that the use of St. John's wort may be promising, especially in the treatment of alcoholism in patients suffering from depression, as well as an adjunct therapy acting synergistically with other medicines.

Other authors also evaluated the role of St. John's wort in morphine and heroin dependence and their withdrawal syndrome. To evaluate these outcomes, they used an experimental model in which rats were repeatedly treated with the drug (morphine or heroin) in increasing doses twice a day over 7–8 days. After the last administration of the drug, the animals received a dose of naloxone, an opioid receptor blocker, leading to an immediate precipitation of the withdrawal syndrome characterized by tremors, diarrhea, jumping behavior, etc. In one study, the oral administration of hypericum concomitant to morphine injections led to a reduction in the intensity of the signals evaluated in the withdrawal syndrome (Feily and Abbasi 2009). In the other study, different extracts prepared with hypericum reduced the physical signs of the heroin withdrawal syndrome, such as diarrhea and writhes (abdominal contractions indicative of painful sensation) (Subhan et al. 2009).

Although some animal studies support the use of hypericum in the treatment of alcoholism (Uzbay 2008), we did not find clinical studies with alcohol dependents. Instead, the effectiveness of hypericum was evaluated in the nicotine addiction in a double-blind study. Hypericum at doses of 300 or 600 mg three times a day was supplied to smokers, but the treatment with the extract did not increase the number of individuals who stopped smoking nor decreased the symptoms of withdrawal syndrome during the study period (Sood et al. 2010).

Ayahuasca (*Banisteriopsis caapi* and *Psychotria viridis*)

Ayahuasca is a psychoactive beverage originally used by indigenous people in shamanic rituals and generally prepared by decoction of two native plants of the Amazon basin region, the bark and stems of *Banisteriopsis caapi* and the leaves of *Psychotria viridis* (Fig. 4.4). The *Psychotria viridis* presents in its composition the indole alkaloid dimethyltryptamine (DMT) acting on serotonin receptors, while the *B. caapi* has alkaloids with beta-carboline structure (harmine, harmaline, and tetrahydroharmaline) which present monoamine oxidase (MAO) inhibitory action (McKenna 2004). The hallucinogenic effect of ayahuasca occurs due to the synergism of the substances in the two plants, i.e., the inhibition of the intestinal MAO facilitates the absorption of DMT which is responsible for the hallucinogenic effects of the beverage (Callaway et al. 1999; Carlini 2003; McKenna 2004). The impact of the repeated use of ayahuasca brew was evaluated in a longitudinal study with 127 users and 115 controls, and it was not found evidence of psychological maladjustment, deterioration of mental health, or cognitive dysfunction in the ayahuasca user group (Bouso et al. 2012).

The syncretic religious use of ayahuasca is accepted and regulated in several countries, but studies in animal models and in humans are still needed to assess whether its use is effective and safe as therapeutic agent against drug addiction. It is well known that many individuals seek these religious groups as alternative to help in treating disorders such as depression and addiction (Topping 1998; McKenna 2004; Labate and Cavnar 2013).

The oral pretreatment with ayahuasca (500 mg/kg) was able to block the reinforcing effect of ethanol (1.8 g/kg) in mice (Gianfratti 2009) on conditioned place

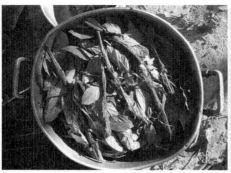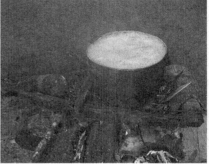

Fig. 4.4 **a** Chopped parts of the plants used in the preparation of ayahuasca: liana known as jagube or mariri (*Banisteriopsis caapi*) and leaves of chacrona or rainha (*Psychotria viridis*). Other species can be used in the beverage preparation. **b** Cooking of two plants for the preparation of ayahuasca. *Sources*: http://upload.wikimedia.org/wikipedia/commons/c/c9/Ayahuasca_and_chacruna_cocinando.jpg. http://upload.wikimedia.org/wikipedia/commons/6/60/Aya-cooking.jpg

preference, a model that simulates the influence of the environment or context on the drug craving. However, the ayahuasca alone induced place conditioning, suggesting that the preparation has reinforcing effect itself (Gianfratti 2009). This would suggest that the use of ayahuasca by addicted people works as replacement therapy, but this hypothesis has yet to be investigated. A recently published study showed that the treatment with ayahuasca was able to block the ethanol sensitization in mice (Oliveira-Lima et al. 2015), supporting the previous data that the tea may be useful in the treatment of alcohol addiction.

Most clinical studies available about ayahuasca use are observational and retrospective, where participants of the ayahuasca religions are interviewed and evaluated. Grob et al. (1996) evaluated a group of fifteen users of ayahuasca and eleven reported a history of moderate-to-severe use of alcohol and other drugs before entering the "União do Vegetal" (one of the syncretic religious groups that use ayahuasca in its ceremonies). These individuals stopped the use of drugs (without relapse reports) after starting the recurrent use of ayahuasca. Labigalini Jr (1998) evaluated a group of four individuals who were drug dependent and also stopped using drugs after they begin attending the ayahuasca rituals. In another study, teenagers from an ayahuasca religion showed lower use of alcohol and other drugs compared to the young people of the same age who have never made use of ayahuasca (Doering-Silveira et al. 2005).

The effect of the attendance in two sessions of assisted therapy with ayahuasca combined with four sessions in counseling groups was assessed on the use of substance abuse and psychological and behavioral factors in a recent observational study. It was self-reported decreased use of alcohol, tobacco, and cocaine, but not marijuana and opiate among the participants (Thomas et al. 2013). It was also observed improvement in scales of mood and quality of life, and it was suggested that the therapy used induced positive psychological and behavioral changes in the participants.

Mercante (2013) conducted a study on communities that use ayahuasca to treat addiction in Brazil and Peru. The author reports that the treatment with ayahuasca differs from a replacement therapy, such as methadone therapy for heroin addicts, because in the treatment using ayahuasca, the social issues are also considered. Therefore, this treatment provides a social and personal transformation, which reduces the chances of relapse.

The therapeutic potential of ayahuasca in the treatment of drug addiction was also evaluated in a qualitative study with health professionals and indigenous healers, and it showed evidence of the effectiveness of ayahuasca (Loizaga-Velder and Verres 2014). The data presented suggest that ayahuasca can be a strong aid in the treatment of drug addiction; however, controlled clinical studies are needed to prove the efficacy and safety of this beverage for the treatment of addiction, and it is critical to assess the importance of religion and context of use in the addiction treatment. The possible mechanisms of action of ayahuasca on drug dependence, considering both their biochemical and their psychological effects, are discussed by Liester and Prickett (2012).

Danshen or Chinese Sage (*Salvia miltiorrhiza*)

The danshen, also known as red sage or Chinese sage, is a plant widely used in traditional Chinese medicine for heart disease, insomnia, hepatitis, hemorrhages, menstrual disorders, etc., with recent data suggesting their usefulness against drug addiction (Lu et al. 2009). A standardized extract prepared with danshen roots inhibited the acquisition, maintenance, and reinstatement of alcohol consumption in rats with preference to ethanol (Lu et al. 2009).

Studies suggest that the effect of danshen is due to the active principle miltirone, but it is likely that other substances in the plant contribute to this activity (Abenavoli et al. 2009). An extract containing 4.3 % of miltirone in doses of 50–200 mg/kg decreased self-administration of ethanol by rats in two models: one that measures the reinforcing power and another motivation for alcohol use (Maccioni et al. 2014). The administration of the pure substance or extracts with different concentrations of miltirone in animals decreased alcohol intake proportionally to the concentration of the active ingredient (Colombo et al. 2006). Moreover, the extract of danshen and the miltirone decreased the blood alcohol levels of the animals, but only when administered intragastrically (not by i.p. route), suggesting that they act by decreasing the ethanol absorption. Despite the positive data in laboratory animals, we did not find controlled clinical studies confirming the antialcohol effect of the plant. The potential effect against other drugs of abuse has not been studied.

Ginseng or Korean Ginseng (*Panax ginseng*)

Korean ginseng has been used for thousands of years in China, where it is considered a real plant. The ginseng roots are used in various Asian countries as a tonic, antistress, rejuvenating, and many other purposes, and the plant is considered a typical adaptogen (Attele et al. 1999). The ginseng's active substances are saponins with a structure similar to the steroidal hormones known as ginsenosides. The ginseng roots are also used for the treatment of alcoholic intoxication what led to the investigation of this property.

Studies using the extracts of ginseng and their ginsenosides showed decrease in cocaine- and methamphetamine-induced conditioned place preference, as well as attenuation of morphine withdrawal syndrome (Takahashi and Tokuyama 1998; Lu et al. 2009). Some studies indicate that the ginseng may alter the absorption of ethanol, while others suggest that it accelerates alcohol metabolism (Abenavoli et al. 2009).

Studies in humans showed that ginseng decreased the plasma alcohol concentrations and reduced the symptoms of intoxication and hangover in healthy volunteers (Lee et al. 2014), suggesting that the ginsenosides can stimulate the enzymatic system of ethanol oxidation by increasing its metabolism and elimination. It was also hypothesized that the ginseng effect on drug addiction occurs by modulating the dopaminergic system, but there is no confirmation of this mechanism. Considering its characteristic as adaptogenic drug, able to increase the resistance to stress and improve cognition, the use of ginseng could be especially useful in the treatment of certain alcohol-related problems such as fatigue, memory loss, and irritability.

Indian Ginseng or Ashwagandha (*Withania somnifera*)

Indian ginseng is a plant used in ayurvedic medicine (traditional Indian medicine) where it is known as ashwagandha. It is used as a tonic, aphrodisiac, against stress, to improve memory, for geriatric problems, among many other uses (Kulkarni and Dhir 2008). Similar to Korean ginseng (*Panax ginseng*), it is classified as an adaptogen plant and it is believed that its antistress effect may be useful in the treatment of addiction, reducing the number of relapses.

Few studies have evaluated the effect of Indian ginseng in drug addiction models. It was reported that the plant decreased the development of tolerance to the analgesic effects of morphine and abolished the jumping behavior in mice, an effect characteristic in the withdrawal syndrome precipitated by naloxone (Kulkarni and Ninan 1997). Doses of 50 and 100 mg/kg of a standardized ashwagandha extract inhibited the acquisition and expression of the morphine-induced conditioned place preference in mice (Ruiu et al. 2013). Using the model of self-administration in rats Peana et al. (2014) showed that the treatment with the extract of Indian ginseng roots reduced the acquisition and maintenance of ethanol self-administration and also reduced the reinstatement of use after a period of forced ethanol deprivation.

The authors suggested that the effect occurs by GABAergic mechanism. Despite these recent studies indicating satisfactory results in the treatment of ethanol and morphine addiction, we did not find clinical studies with the plant.

Hallucinogens and Addiction Treatment

An increasing interest in the therapeutic use of hallucinogens has been observed recently. Among the possible therapeutic applications of natural hallucinogen, we highlight its use against drug addiction (Sessa and Johnson 2015). Some examples include ibogaine (Iboga component) and DMT (from ayahuasca) already discussed in this chapter, mescaline (from peyote) and psilocybin (from the mushroom *Psilocybe mexicana*) (Bogenschutz and Johnson 2016; Winkelman 2015). Although these substances alter the perception of reality and being illicitly used as drug of abuse, their use is often sporadic and these drugs do not induce a typical dependence as other psychotropics do.

Peyote (*Lophophora williamsii*) is a small Mexican cactus considered a gift from the gods by the native peoples of America. It has mescaline as active principle, a hallucinogenic substance that causes visual and perceptual changes. The peyote is mainly used in ritual contexts, including practices for the treatment of alcoholism (Tylš et al. 2014). Another hallucinogenic substance with possible antidrug effect is psilocybin. A study recently published showed that alcoholics under treatment with psilocybin showed a decrease in alcohol consumption, longer periods of abstinence, and decreased craving (Bogenschutz et al. 2015). According to Sessa and Johnson (2015), other clinical trials are underway evaluating the potential of psilocybin against alcohol and also ibogaine and ayahuasca for drug addiction.

Other Potentially Useful Plants for the Treatment of Drug Addiction

Animal studies have suggested that the rhodiola or golden root (*Rhodiola rosea*) may be helpful in reducing the craving and vulnerability of drug use. Rhodiola root extract prevented the development of morphine-induced conditioned place preference in mice and facilitated the extinction (loss) of preference in a situation where the drug administration was stopped, but the animals continued to be exposed to the same context (Mattioli et al. 2012). Using a similar model, it was demonstrated that rhodiola and its active principle salidroside inhibited the conditioned place preference to nicotine and prevented the relapse in mice (Titomanlio et al. 2014), but the plant produced only moderate results in the cocaine-induced conditioned place preference (Titomanlio et al. 2013).

Kava kava or kava (*Piper methysticum*) is a plant used as anxiolytic and for the treatment of insomnia, for which it has been extensively studied and there are herbal medicines already approved (Sarris and Kavanagh 2009). Kava is popularly used in some Pacific islands to help stop smoking and drinking (Lu et al. 2009), and it is believed that this effect may be related to its anxiolytic property, reducing the desire for the drug. Their anxiolytic effect is due to kavalactones which interact with various neurotransmitters. Suspected hepatotoxic effect due to the use of kava-based drugs have led many countries to ban the herbal product in their market, but the correlation of hepatotoxicity cases after the use of kava kava was not completely established and this is still a debate subject (Teschke et al. 2011).

A plant that could be useful to treat liver damage from chronic alcoholism is *Schizandra chinensis*. A plant extract was given to animals receiving a large dose of ethanol (1 g/kg, ig) for 5 weeks and promoted hepatoprotective effect (Park et al. 2014). Several other plants, including kudzu, have been reported to be beneficial for the prevention and treatment of alcoholic cirrhosis (Ding et al. 2012).

Jupp and Lawrence (2010) reported the use of reserpine (active principle of *Rauvolfia serpentina*) to reduce the cocaine use. Shi et al. (2006) cite several species and plant mixtures used in traditional Chinese medicine for the treatment of opioid addiction and report that ten formulations are already approved for clinical use in the country and clinical trials were being conducted with six of these formulations. Other species with traditional use or some studies that support their use against drug dependence or withdrawal syndrome are as follows: *Thunbergia laurifolia, Carydolis yanhusuo* (Lu et al. 2009), *Oenothera biennis, Scutellaria lateriflolia* (Abenavoli et al. 2009), *Hovenia dulcis, Thymus vulgaris, Trigonella foenum-graecum* (Tomczyk et al. 2012), *Paullinia cupana, Turnera diffusa, Passiflora quadrangularis* (Carlini et al. 2006), among others.

Final Considerations

The treatment of drug addiction is complex, and many of the approaches used today have low effectiveness, particularly when used alone. The pharmaceutical industry is still looking for more effective drugs and with less side effects, and among the possible alternatives are the herbal products. Many plants and active ingredients have been evaluated as potential for addiction treatment in preclinical studies, but few clinical studies have been conducted and just few herbal medicines were approved. This situation indicates that more clinical trials are needed to allow the development and use of herbal products in the treatment of drug dependence.

References

Abenavoli, L., Capasso, F., & Addolorato, G. (2009). Phytotherapeutic approach to alcohol dependence: New old way? *Phytomedicine, 16*(6), 638–644.

Alper, K. R., Lotsof, H. S., & Kaplan, C. D. (2008). The ibogaine medical subculture. *Journal of Ethnopharmacology, 115*(1), 9–24.

ANVISA—Agência Nacional de Vigilância Sanitária. (2014). *Instrução normativa no 4, de 18 de junho de 2014*. http://portal.anvisa.gov.br/wps/wcm/connect/10f7288044703a8bbbf8fffe3a642 e80/Guia+final+dicol+180614.pdf?MOD=AJPERES

Attele, A. S., Wu, J. A., & Yuan, C. S. (1999). Ginseng pharmacology: Multiple constituents and multiple actions. *Biochemical Pharmacology, 58*, 1685–1693.

Benlhabib, E., Baker, J. I., Keyler, D. E., & Singh, A. K. (2004). Kudzu root extract suppresses voluntary alcohol intake and alcohol withdrawal symptoms in P rats receiving free access to water and alcohol. *Journal of Medicinal Food, 7*(2), 168–179.

Bogenschutz, M. P., Forcehimes, A. A., Pommy, J. A., Wilcox, C. E., Barbosa, P., & Strassman, R. J. (2015). Psilocybin-assisted treatment for alcohol dependence: A proof-of-concept study. *Journal of Psychopharmacology, 29*(3), 289–299.

Bogenschutz, M. P., & Johnson, M. W. (2016). Classic hallucinogens in the treatment of addictions. *Progress in Neuro-Psychopharmacology and Biological Psychiatry, 64*, 250–258.

Bouso, J. C., González, D., Fondevila, S., Cutchet, M., Fernández, X., Barbosa, P. C. R., et al. (2012). Personality, psychopathology, life attitudes and neuropsychological performance among ritual users of ayahuasca: A longitudinal study. *PLoS ONE, 7*(8), e42421.

Brown, T. K. (2013). Ibogaine in the treatment of substance dependence. *Current Drug Abuse Reviews, 6*(1), 3–16.

Callaway, J., McKenna, D., Grob, C., Brito, G. S., Raymon, L., Poland, R., et al. (1999). Pharmacokinetics of Hoasca alkaloids in healthy humans. *Journal of Ethnopharmacology, 65* (3), 243–256.

Carai, M. A., Agabio, R., Bombardelli, E., Bourov, I., Gessa, G. L., Lobina, C., et al. (2000). Potential use of medicinal plants in the treatment of alcoholism. *Fitoterapia, 71*, S38–S42.

Carlini, E. A. (2003). Plants and the central nervous system. *Pharmacology, Biochemistry and Behavior, 75*(3), 501–512.

Carlini, E. A., Rodrigues, E., Mendes, F. R., Tabach, R., & Gianfratti, B. (2006). Treatment of drug dependence with Brazilian herbal medicines. *Revista Brasileira de Farmacognosia, 16*, 690–695.

Colombo, G., Serra, S., Vacca, G., Orrù, A., Maccioni, P., Morazzoni, P., et al. (2006). Identification of miltirone as active ingredient of *Salvia miltiorrhiza* responsible for the reducing effect of root extracts on alcohol intake in rats. *Alcoholism, Clinical and Experimental Research, 30*(5), 754–762.

Ding, R.-B., Tian, K., He, C.-W., Jiang, Y., Wang, Y.-T., & Wan, J.-B. (2012). Herbal medicines for the prevention of alcoholic liver disease: A review. *Journal of Ethnopharmacology, 144*(3), 457–465.

Doering-Silveira, E., Grob, C. S., De Rios, M. D., Lopez, E., Alonso, L. K., Tacla, C., et al. (2005). Report on psychoactive drug use among adolescents using ayahuasca within a religious context. *Journal of Psychoactive Drugs, 37*(2), 141–144.

Dworkin, S. I., Gleeson, S., Meloni, D., Koves, T. R., & Martin, T. J. (1995). Effects of ibogaine on responding maintained by food, cocaine and heroin reinforcement in rats. *Psychopharmacology (Berl), 117*(3), 257–261.

Feily, A., & Abbasi, N. (2009). The inhibitory effect of *Hypericum perforatum* extract on morphine withdrawal syndrome in rat and comparison with clonidine. *Phytotherapy Research, 23*(11), 1549–1552.

Gianfratti, B. (2009). *Avaliação Farmacológica do chá de Ayahuasca em modelos pré-clínicos de dependência do etanol*. Master's thesis, Universidade Federal de São Paulo, São Paulo, Brasil.

Glick, S. D., & Maisonneuve, I. M. (1998). Mechanisms of antiaddictive actions of ibogaine. *Annals of the New York Academy of Sciences, 844*(1), 214–226.

Grob, C. S., Mckenna, D. J., Callaway, J. C., Brito, G. S., Neves, E. S., Oberlaender, G., et al. (1996). Human psychopharmacology of hoasca, a plant hallucinogen used in ritual context in Brazil. *The Journal of Nervous and Mental Disease, 184*(2), 86–94.

Jupp, B., & Lawrence, A. J. (2010). New horizons for therapeutics in drug and alcohol abuse. *Pharmacology & Therapeutics, 125*(1), 138–168.

Keung, W. M., & Vallee, B. L. (1998). Kudzu root: An ancient Chinese source of modern antidipsotropic agents. *Phytochemistry, 47*(4), 499–506.

Kreek, M. J., LaForge, K. S., & Butelman, E. (2002). Pharmacotherapy of addictions. *Nature Reviews Drug Discovery, 1*(9), 710–726.

Kulkarni, S., & Dhir, A. (2008). *Withania somnifera*: an Indian ginseng. *Progress in Neuro-Psychopharmacology and Biological Psychiatry, 32*(5), 1093–1105.

Kulkarni, S. K., & Ninan, I. (1997). Inhibition of morphine tolerance and dependence by *Withania somnifera* in mice. *Journal of Ethnopharmacology, 57*(3), 213–217.

Labate, B. C., & Cavnar, C. (2013). *The therapeutic use of ayahuasca*. Berlin: Springer.

Labigalini Jr, E. (1998). *O uso de ayahuasca em um contexto religioso por ex dependentes de álcool—um estudo qualitativo*. Master's thesis, Universidade Federal de São Paulo, São Paulo, Brasil.

Lee, M.-H., Kwak, J. H., Jeon, G., Lee, J.-W., Seo, J.-H., Lee, H.-S., et al. (2014). Red ginseng relieves the effects of alcohol consumption and hangover symptoms in healthy men: A randomized crossover study. *Food & Function, 5*(3), 528–534.

Liester, M. B., & Prickett, J. I. (2012). Hypotheses regarding the mechanisms of ayahuasca in the treatment of addictions. *Journal of Psychoactive Drugs, 44*(3), 200–208.

Loizaga-Velder, A., & Verres, R. (2014). Therapeutic effect of ritual ayahuasca use in the treatment of substance dependence—Qualitative results. *Journal of Psychoactive Drugs, 46*(1), 63–72.

Lu, L., Liu, Y., Zhu, W., Shi, J., Liu, Y., Ling, W., et al. (2009). Traditional medicine in the treatment of drug addiction. *The American Journal of Drug and Alcohol Abuse, 35*(1), 1–11.

Lukas, S. E., Penetar, D., Berko, J., Vicens, L., Palmer, C., Mallya, G., et al. (2005). An extract of the Chinese herbal root kudzu reduces alcohol drinking by heavy drinkers in a naturalistic setting. *Alcoholism, Clinical and Experimental Research, 29*, 756–762.

Lukas, S. E., Penetar, D., Su, Z., Geaghan, T., Maywalt, M., Tracy, M., et al. (2013). A standardized kudzu extract (NPI-031) reduces alcohol consumption in nontreatment-seeking male heavy drinkers. *Psychopharmacology (Berl), 226*(1), 65–73.

Maccioni, P., Vargiolu, D., Falchi, M., Morazzoni, P., Riva, A., Cabri, W., et al. (2014). Reducing effect of the Chinese medicinal herb, *Salvia miltiorrhiza*, on alcohol self-administration in Sardinian alcohol-preferring rats. *Alcohol, 48*(6), 587–593.

Mačiulaitis, R., Kontrimaviciute, V., Bressolle, F., & Briedis, V. (2008). Ibogaine, an anti-addictive drug: pharmacology and time to go further in development. A narrative review. *Human and Experimental Toxicology, 27*(3), 181–194.

Mattioli, L., Titomanlio, F., & Perfumi, M. (2012). Effects of a *Rhodiola rosea* L. extract on the acquisition, expression, extinction, and reinstatement of morphine-induced conditioned place preference in mice. *Psychopharmacology (Berl), 221*(2), 183–193.

McGregor, N. R. (2007). *Pueraria lobata* (Kudzu root) hangover remedies and acetaldehyde-associated neoplasm risk. *Alcohol, 41*(7), 469–478.

McKenna, D. J. (2004). Clinical investigations of the therapeutic potential of ayahuasca: Rationale and regulatory challenges. *Pharmacology & Therapeutics, 102*(2), 111–129.

Mendes, F. R., Negri, G., Duarte-Almeida, J. M., Tabach, R., & Carlini, E. A. (2012). The action of plants and their constituents on the central nervous system. *Plant Bioactives and Drug Discovery: Principles, Practice, and Perspectives, 17*, 161.

Mercante, M. S. (2013). A ayahuasca e o tratamento da dependência. *Mana, 19*(3), 529–558.

Oliveira-Lima, A., Santos, R., Hollais, A., Gerardi-Junior, C., Baldaia, M., Wuo-Silva, R., et al. (2015). Effects of ayahuasca on the development of ethanol-induced behavioral sensitization and on a post-sensitization treatment in mice. *Physiology & Behavior, 142*, 28–36.

Overstreet, D. H., Keung, W. M., Rezvani, A. H., Massi, M., & Lee, D. Y. (2003). Herbal remedies for alcoholism: promises and possible pitfalls. *Alcoholism, Clinical and Experimental Research, 27*(2), 177–185.

Park, H. J., Lee, S.-J., Song, Y., Jang, S.-H., Ko, Y.-G., Kang, S. N., et al. (2014). *Schisandra chinensis* prevents alcohol-induced fatty liver disease in rats. *Journal of Medicinal Food, 17*(1), 103–110.

Peana, A. T., Muggironi, G., Spina, L., Rosas, M., Kasture, S. B., Cotti, E., et al. (2014). Effects of *Withania somnifera* on oral ethanol self-administration in rats. *Behavioural Pharmacology, 25* (7), 618–628.

Penetar, D. M., Toto, L. H., Farmer, S. L., Lee, D. Y.-W., Ma, Z., Liu, Y., et al. (2012). The isoflavone puerarin reduces alcohol intake in heavy drinkers: A pilot study. *Drug and Alcohol Dependence, 126*(1), 251–256.

Perfumi, M., Mattioli, L., Cucculelli, M., & Massi, M. (2005). Reduction of ethanol intake by chronic treatment with *Hypericum perforatum*, alone or combined with naltrexone in rats. *Journal of Psychopharmacology, 19*(5), 448–454.

Rezvani, A. H., Overstreet, D. H., Perfumi, M., & Massi, M. (2003). Plant derivatives in the treatment of alcohol dependency. *Pharmacology, Biochemistry and Behavior, 75*(3), 593–606.

Rezvani, A. H., Overstreet, D., Yang, Y., & Clark, E., Jr. (1999). Attenuation of alcohol intake by extract of *Hypericum perforatum* (St John's Wort) in two different strains of alcohol-preferring rats. *Alcohol and Alcoholism, 34*(5), 699–705.

Ruiu, S., Longoni, R., Spina, L., Orrù, A., Cottiglia, F., Collu, M., et al. (2013). *Withania somnifera* prevents acquisition and expression of morphine-elicited conditioned place preference. *Behavioural Pharmacology, 24*(2), 133–143.

Sarris, J., & Kavanagh, D. J. (2009). Kava and St. John's Wort: Current evidence for use in mood and anxiety disorders. *Journal of Alternative and Complementary Medicine, 15*(8), 827–836.

Schenberg, E. E., de Castro Comis, M. A., Chaves, B. R., & da Silveira, D. X. (2014). Treating drug dependence with the aid of ibogaine: A retrospective study. *Journal of Psychopharmacology, 28*(11), 993–1000.

Sessa, B., & Johnson, M. W. (2015). Can psychedelic compounds play a part in drug dependence therapy? *The British Journal of Psychiatry, 206*(1), 1–3.

Shebek, J., & Rindone, J. P. (2000). A pilot study exploring the effect of kudzu root on the drinking habits of patients with chronic alcoholism. *Journal of Alternative and Complementary Medicine, 6*, 45–48.

Shi, J., Liu, Y. L., Fang, Y. X., Xu, G. Z., Zhai, H. F., & Lu, L. (2006). Traditional Chinese medicine in treatment of opiate addiction. *Acta Pharmacologica Sinica, 27*(10), 1303–1308.

Sood, A., Ebbert, J. O., Prasad, K., Croghan, I. T., Bauer, B., & Schroeder, D. R. (2010). A randomized clinical trial of St. John's wort for smoking cessation. *The Journal of Alternative and Complementary Medicine, 16*(7), 761–767.

Subhan, F., Khan, N., & Sewell, R. D. (2009). Adulterant profile of illicit street heroin and reduction of its precipitated physical dependence withdrawal syndrome by extracts of St John's wort (*Hypericum perforatum*). *Phytotherapy Research, 23*(4), 564–571.

Takahashi, M., & Tokuyama, S. (1998). Pharmacological and physiological effects of ginseng on actions induced by opioids and psychostimulants. *Methods and Findings in Experimental and Clinical Pharmacology, 20*(1), 77–84.

Teschke, R., Qiu, S. X., Xuan, T. D., & Lebot, V. (2011). Kava and kava hepatotoxicity: Requirements for novel experimental, ethnobotanical and clinical studies based on a review of the evidence. *Phytotherapy Research, 25*(9), 1263–1274.

Thomas, G., Lucas, P., Capler, N. R., Tupper, K. W., & Martin, G. (2013). Ayahuasca-assisted therapy for addiction: Results from a preliminary observational study in Canada. *Current Drug Abuse Review, 6*(1), 30–42.

Titomanlio, F., Manzanedo, C., Rodríguez-Arias, M., Mattioli, L., Perfumi, M., Miñarro, J., et al. (2013). *Rhodiola rosea* impairs acquisition and expression of conditioned place preference induced by cocaine. *Evidence-Based Complementary and Alternative Medicine.* doi:10.1155/2013/697632.

Titomanlio, F., Perfumi, M., & Mattioli, L. (2014). *Rhodiola rosea* L. extract and its active compound salidroside antagonized both induction and reinstatement of nicotine place preference in mice. *Psychopharmacology (Berl), 231*(10), 2077–2086.

Tomczyk, M., Zovko-Koncic, M., & Chrostek, L. (2012). Phytotherapy of alcoholism. *Natural Product Communications, 7*(2), 273–280.

Topping, D. M. (1998). Ayahuasca and cancer: One man's experience. *Bulletin of the Multidisciplinary Association of Psychedelic Studies, 8*, 22–26.

Tylš, F., Páleníček, T., & Horáček, J. (2014). Psilocybin—Summary of knowledge and new perspectives. *European Neuropsychopharmacology, 24*(3), 342–356.

Uzbay, T. I. (2008). *Hypericum perforatum* and substance dependence: A review. *Phytotherapy Research, 22*(5), 578–582.

Whiskey, E., Wernecke, U., & Taylor, D. (2001). A systematic review and meta-analysis of *Hypericum perforatum* in depression: A comprehensive clinical review. *International Clinical Psychopharmacology, 16*, 239–252.

Winkelman, M. (2015). Psychedelics as medicines for substance abuse rehabilitation: Evaluating treatments with LSD, peyote, ibogaine and ayahuasca. *Current Drug Abuse Reviews, 7*(2), 101–116.

Author Biographies

Fúlvio Rieli Mendes (Mendes, FR) Graduated in Biomedical Sciences at Universidade Federal de São Paulo, with master's and doctorate at the same institution. Professor of pharmacology at the Universidade Federal do ABC (UFABC), advisor at the Graduate program in Neuroscience and Cognition at UFABC and collaborator of the Brazilian Center for Psychotropic Drug Information (CEBRID).

Dianne da Rocha Prado (Prado, DR) Undergraduate student of the Bachelor in Science and Technology at Universidade Federal do ABC. Performs training in Neurosciences and Cognition investigating the effect of ayahuasca in models of morphine dependence and withdrawal syndrome.

Chapter 5
EMDR Therapy and the Treatment of Substance Abuse and Addiction

Susan Brown, Julie Stowasser and Francine Shapiro

Introduction

Most experts today agree, as do the authors of this chapter, that substance abuse arises from complex interactions between genetics, environment, and experience. "Substance dependence is not a failure of will or of strength of character, but a medical disorder that could affect any human being. Dependence is a chronic and relapsing disorder, often co-occurring with other physical and mental conditions" (World Health Organization 2004).

The question remains, however, "Why has it been that over the course of human history, where people and cultures have had access to alcohol and potent mind-altering substances, that only some become addicted while the rest are able to regulate their use?"

We are closer to answering this question based upon current research that has demonstrated a clear relationship between early adverse life experiences and later addiction—please see Felitti et al. (1998), Felitti (2004) and Shapiro (2005).

Further, the drugs that individuals select are not chosen randomly, but result from an interaction between the psychopharmacologic action of the drug and the dominant painful feelings with which they struggle. Edward Khantzian, M.D., professor of Clinical Psychiatry at the Harvard University, observed that opiates are often preferred because of their powerful numbing action on the affects of rage and

S. Brown (✉)
4700 Spring Street, Suite 204, La Mesa, CA 91942, USA
e-mail: sbrownlcsw@gmail.com

J. Stowasser
Post Office Box 15101, San Luis Obispo, CA 93406, USA
e-mail: julie@juliestowasser.com

F. Shapiro
Mental Research Institute, Palo Alto, CA, USA
e-mail: fshapiro@mcn.org

© Springer International Publishing Switzerland 2016
A.L.M. Andrade and D. De Micheli (eds.), *Innovations in the Treatment of Substance Addiction*, DOI 10.1007/978-3-319-43172-7_5

aggression. Cocaine has its appeal because of its ability to relieve distress associated with depression. Although ill fated, "addicts discover that the short-term effects of their drugs of choice help them cope with distressful subjective states and an external reality otherwise experienced as unmanageable or overwhelming" (Khantzian 1985, p. 1263). Thus emerges a compelling hypothesis, which proposes that people use psychoactive substances in an attempt to control painful symptoms resulting from psychological trauma. This is referred to as "self-medication" (Ibid.).

Some studies in the USA show that more than 50 percent of people with mental disorders also suffer from substance dependence compared to 6 percent of the general population (World Health Organization 2004). It is from our interest in providing integrated treatment for the complex interaction of genes, environment, trauma, and psychological pain as a driving force behind co-existing disorders, that this chapter is written.

Co-occurring Mental Health and Substance Abuse

"No one ever died from their feelings, but millions of people have died from taking drugs, alcohol, and other toxic substances to help them avoid their feelings..." Weinhold & Weinhold

The co-existing problems of Mental Health (MH) and Substance Abuse (SA) disorders ignore age, gender, intellect, marital status, economic, social class, race, and nationality, leaving no one immune from their impact. The prevalence of co-occurring psychiatric and substance use disorders and the dearth of effective treatment interventions leaves individuals in a state of suffering, accompanied by impressive personal, familial, social, and economic consequences.

The correlation between trauma and other adverse experiences, especially when first experienced in childhood, and co-occurring mental health and substance abuse, is strongly established in the literature (Felitti et al. 1998; Kessler et al. 1995; Najavits et al. 1999; National Child Traumatic Stress Network (NCSTN) 2008; Ouimette and Brown 2003). A strict definition of *co-occurring disorders* (COD) states that one or more psychiatric or medical conditions co-exist with one or more addictive disorders. CODs do not simply have overlapping symptoms, but are distinct, and can be independently diagnosed from one another (American Psychiatric Association 2013).

Examples of diagnoses frequently co-occurring with addictive disorders include posttraumatic stress disorder (PTSD) and other anxiety disorders, bipolar disorder, borderline personality disorder (BPD), attention deficit disorder (ADD/ADHD), and major depression. The many possible permutations of addictions and co-existing psychiatric conditions often lead to a complicated clinical picture that is challenging to untangle and treat effectively, particularly when the contributing role of trauma is overlooked.

Co-occurring disorders are also associated with

- Poorer motivation, retention, and treatment outcomes compared to individuals with a single psychiatric disorder
- Faster relapse and greater amounts of substances used
- Less social support
- Under-employment
- Failure at work or school
- Poorer overall health conditions
- Impaired family relations
- Abuse and violence
- Legal difficulties

(Brady et al. 1994; Brown et al. 1996; Felitti et al. 1998; Najavits et al. 1999).

Historically, these areas of mental health have separate treatment, education, training, and funding avenues, creating significant barriers to receiving integrated treatment services. Currently, the development and implementation of effective, integrated treatment services is a public health challenge worldwide.

The purpose of this chapter is to

- Illustrate the relationships between trauma and other adverse life experiences, mental disorders, and the development of substance abuse and behavioral, or process, addictions (Felitti et al. 1998).
- Describe the connections between substance and behavioral addictions (Grant et al. 2006).
- Describe the Adaptive Information Processing (AIP) model as the theoretical framework for case conceptualization in EMDR therapy (Shapiro 1995, 2001, 2007; Solomon and Shapiro 2008).
- Provide a basic understanding of the principles, protocols, and procedures that define EMDR therapy (Shapiro 1995, 2001).
- Illustrate when and how to use EMDR therapy as an integrated treatment approach for co-occurring mental health and addiction disorders.

The Relationship Between Trauma, Mental Health, and Substance Abuse

"Nothing is predestined: The obstacles of your past can become the gateways that lead to new beginnings." Ralph Blum

Trauma is often the crucible from which psychiatric symptoms and addictions emerge. With trauma, *the past is present.* The Adverse Childhood Experiences (ACE) Study provides retrospective and prospective analysis of over 17,000 individuals, primarily middle-class Americans from Kaiser Permanente's Department of Preventive Medicine in San Diego, California (Felitti et al. 1998). The study examined the effect of traumatic life experiences during the first 18 years on later well-being, social function, health risks, disease burden, healthcare costs, and life expectancy.

The ten reference categories experienced during childhood are listed in Table 5.1 below, with their prevalence in parentheses.

Scoring the ACE survey is simple: Exposure to any one category above is scored as one point. Thus, an individual reporting sexual molest by one person would score the same as someone who experienced multiple sexual assaults by several individuals. As a result, these findings tend to be under, rather than over, stated. Nevertheless, the study revealed several surprising outcomes regarding the significance of early trauma and other adverse childhood experiences and the development of later substance addiction or troubling behavioral patterns. The study found "strong, proportionate relationships between the number of categories of adverse childhood experiences (ACE score) and the use of various psychoactive materials or behaviors including alcoholism and intravenous drug abuse" (op. cit.). The relationship is evident in the exponential increase in likelihood of a person having a maladaptive response to his ACEs. For example, any person with 4 or more childhood ACEs experienced a 500 % increase in potential that they will become alcoholic, while males with ACE scores of 6 or more showed a step-wise probability increase of 4600 % of becoming an intravenous drug user (Felitti 2004).

Not surprisingly, childhood trauma and neglect disrupts and can dysregulate the brain's information processing systems (Perry 1999; Schore 2002; Siegel 1999;

Table 5.1 Adverse Childhood Experiences Study (adapted from op. cit.)

	Category	Behavior	Prevalence (%)
Abuse			
1.	Emotional	Recurrent humiliation	11
2.	Physical	Beating, not spanking	28
3.	Sexual abuse	Contact sexual abuse	
	Women		28
	Men		16
	Overall		22
Household dysfunction			
4.	Mother	Treated violently	13
5.	Household member	Alcoholic or drug user	27
6.	Household member	Imprisoned	6
7.	Household member	Chronically depressed, suicidal mentally ill, in psychiatric hospital	17
8.	Household member	Not raised by both biological parents	23
Neglect			
9.	Physical	Lack of proper food, clothing, shelter	10
10.	Emotional	Isolation, lack of interaction	15

Van der Kolk et al. 1996). Lesser-known risk factors in the development of a child's brain and quest for mastery over emotional regulation are the significant roles played by the quality of parental attunement and attention (Siegel 1999). Those who are unable to manage emotional responses to everyday stressors are compelled to seek ways to control or numb their affect (Khantzian 1985).

Addictions and other compulsive behaviors temporarily change the experience of painful emotions and body sensations, thereby providing a transitory sense of relief. Often referred to as self-medication, this may be seen by the user as effectively managing distress, thereby promoting a vicious cycle of addictive coping strategies (Brown et al. 1996; Grant et al. 2006; Ouimette and Brown 2003; Volkow 2007). One study (Hien et al. 2010) found that reductions in the severity of PTSD symptoms were likely to be associated with reduced substance use in those with severe symptomotology. Results support the self-medication model and provide empirical support for integrated interventions for PTSD and substance abuse. An illustration of how this works is shown in Fig. 5.1.

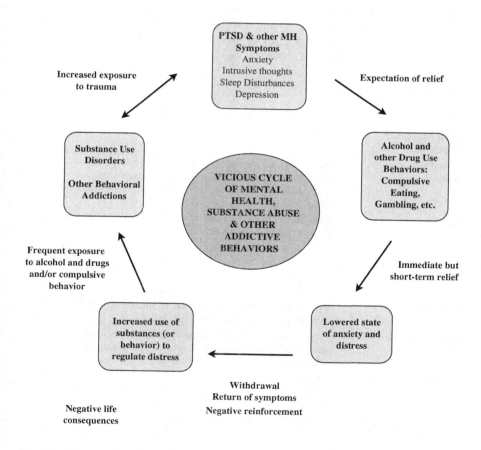

Fig. 5.1 Vicious cycle of mental health, substance abuse, and other compulsive behaviors for emotional regulation. Illustration Copyright 2009 Brown, S. (Adapted from Steward & Conrad, 2002)

The Link Between Substance and Behavioral Addictions

*"Drunkenness–that fierce rage for the slow, sure poison, that oversteps every other con-
sideration; that casts aside wife, children, friends, happiness, and station; and hurries its
victims madly on to degradation and death."* Charles Dickens

Research suggests a strong neurobiological link between chemical and behavioral,
or process, addictions. Perhaps that is because the neurochemistry associated with
"reward" or "pleasure pathways" (Grant et al. 2006; Pallanti 2006; Volkow 2007)
in the brain lead to the same loss of control and negative consequences, whether it is
a drug or a behavior to which the person becomes addicted. Therefore, it is not the
substance itself that is addictive, but rather, the individual's response to it. Not all
people who use substances become addicted, nor to common behaviors such as
gambling, yet they can both lead to similar patterns of misuse.

Research over the past decade has stressed the substantial co-morbidity of
impulse control disorders with mood disorders, anxiety disorders, eating disorders,
substance disorders, personality disorders, and with other specific impulse control
disorders (Hucker 2004). Addictions and compulsions, despite the planning aspects
involved, are also associated with a lack of impulse control and often follow similar
symptomatic cycles (Grant et al. 2006) as shown in Table 5.2

Table 5.2 Addictions, compulsions, and the similarities between them

Addictions and compulsions	Symptoms and cycles
Alcohol and other substance abuses	Preoccupation (obsession), anticipation (craving), mood modification (regulation), continued use despite adverse consequences, relapse, and potentially life-threatening medical complications
Gambling	Preoccupation, anticipation, mood modification, continued use despite adverse consequences, and relapse
Shopping	Preoccupation, anticipation, mood modification, continued use despite adverse consequences, and relapse
Sex	Preoccupation, anticipation, mood modification, continued use despite adverse consequences, and relapse
Pornography	Preoccupation, anticipation, mood modification, continued use despite adverse consequences, and relapse
Binge-eating and food restriction	Preoccupation, anticipation, mood modification, continued use despite adverse consequences, relapse, and potentially life-threatening medical complications
Compulsive exercising	Preoccupation, anticipation, mood modification, continued use despite adverse consequences, relapse, and potential medical complications
Cutting, Skin picking and hair pulling	Preoccupation, anticipation, mood modification, continued use despite adverse consequences, relapse, and potential serious medical complications

The EMDR Therapy Approach—Treatment of PTSD and Trauma

EMDR therapy is a comprehensive, integrative, A-rated and empirically validated treatment for PTSD (American Psychiatric Association 2004; Department of Veterans Affairs & Department of Defense 2004; National Institute for Clinical Excellence 2005). Twenty-three clinical trials in peer-reviewed journals attest to EMDR's efficacy with PTSD and trauma (see Shapiro, 2014 for a review).

The recent World Health Organization (WHO) practice guidelines (2013) state that EMDR therapy and trauma-focused cognitive behavioral therapy are the only psychotherapies recommended for children, adolescents, and adults with PTSD. As noted in the WHO (2013) practice guidelines, "[EMDR therapy] is based on the idea that negative thoughts, feelings and behaviors are the result of unprocessed memories. The treatment involves standardized procedures that include focusing simultaneously on (a) spontaneous associations of traumatic images, thoughts, emotions and bodily sensations and (b) bilateral stimulation that is most commonly administered in the form of repeated eye movements. Like CBT with a trauma focus, EMDR aims to reduce subjective distress and strengthen adaptive cognitions related to the traumatic event. Unlike CBT with a trauma focus, EMDR therapy does not involve (a) detailed descriptions of the event, (b) direct challenging of beliefs, (c) extended exposure, or (d) homework" (p.1).

EMDR therapy has been found equivalent to prolonged exposure (PE) therapy (Foa et al. 2007) and other cognitive behavioral therapies (CBT) in reducing PTSD symptoms (e.g., Bisson and Andrew 2007). However, EMDR therapy has also been found to be more efficient and more widely tolerated (has a lesser drop-out rate) without the client's need for 1-2 hours of daily homework as in prolonged exposure (e.g., de Roos and De Jongh 2008; Ironson et al. 2002; Jaberghaderi et al. 2004; Lee et al. 2002; Power et al. 2002).

As is true for all psychotherapies, the mechanism of action responsible for EMDR therapy's effectiveness is still unknown. A recent meta-analysis by Lee and Cuijpers (2013) examined 26 randomized controlled trials (RCTs) comparing the eye movement component of EMDR therapy to an exposure condition while participants concentrated on a disturbing memory. Pre/post-differences for both conditions demonstrated significant declines in standardized outcome measures, negative emotions, and imagery vividness. Additional studies have examined the effect of the eye movements in EMDR therapy and found that eye movements enhance retrieval of episodic memories and increase recognition of true information (Christman et al. 2003; Ricci 2006). One hypothesis regarding the development of PTSD is the failure to process episodic memory, thereby leaving upsetting memories "stuck" in the past instead of being integrated into semantic networks (Bergmann 2000, 2008; Stickgold 2002). For a more complete review of the hypothesized mechanisms of action involved in EMDR therapy, see Solomon and Shapiro (2008).

The EMDR model of psychotherapy includes an 8-phase structured protocol that integrates elements of psychodynamic, cognitive behavioral, experiential, interpersonal, and body-oriented therapies (Shapiro 2001). EMDR therapy's theoretical orientation is based on the Adaptive Information Processing model described below (op. cit.).

Theoretical Basis of EMDR Therapy: The Adaptive Information Processing Model (AIP; Shapiro 2001)

"A long habit of not thinking a thing wrong, gives it a superficial appearance of being right." Thomas Paine

The Adaptive Information Processing (AIP) model explains clinical phenomena, predicts successful treatment effects, and guides the overall practice of EMDR therapy across its wide range of therapeutic applications (Shapiro 2001). It asserts that the brain possesses an intrinsic ability to process information in the moment, interpreting and integrating current perceptions within the existing memory networks. The brain also processes distressing memories to an adaptive resolution. However, high levels of disturbance can interfere with the brain's natural information processing capabilities not only in the moment but also later when cues or triggers reactivate the disturbance.

According to the AIP, symptoms are a result of dysfunctional, physiologically stored, unprocessed memories. Some, or all, parts of the memory (imagery, emotions, body sensations, thoughts, beliefs, attitudes, and perceptions) remain fragmented in present time, distorted, and unassimilated into the more adaptive memory networks. These distortions can negatively influence an individual's thoughts, feelings, and behaviors until reprocessed and integrated into a more adaptive state.

Current situations can trigger these memories causing the individual to experience the disturbing stored affects and perspectives. This in turn influences their perceptions of the present. Externally, a trigger can be a sight, sound, smell, person, or event. Internally, a trigger can be an emotion, body sensation, mood, or dream. The purpose of EMDR therapy is to *access* the traumatic material, *activate* the information processing system, and allow the brain to *move* the dysfunctionally stored material into a more adaptive, present-oriented state.

EMDR therapy distinguishes between "Big-T" and "small-t" traumas. When diagnosing PTSD, Big-T traumas are those designated as Criterion A events (American Psychiatric Association 2013). Examples that might cause intense fear, helplessness, or horror include: experiencing, witnessing, or hearing about something that is an immediate threat to one's own or a loved one's life or safety. Physical and emotional abuse, or sexual assault or abuse, domestic violence, vehicular accident, combat, terrorism, and natural disasters are commonly identified Big-T events. However, a person can also be severely affected by more ubiquitous, adverse life experiences (small-t life events) such as attachment or attunement problems with parents, and/or siblings, bullying in school, peer problems, the death of a pet, parent's divorce, or the breakup of a romance. In EMDR therapy, unprocessed memories of trauma and other adverse life experiences are viewed as foundational to a wide range of pathology.

In support of this concept, 832 surveyed people (Mol et al. 2005) reported that their PTSD symptoms were more related to common distressing life events than to Criterion A events. The conclusion of the researchers was that the more everyday disturbing life events can generate at least as many PTSD symptoms as events designated as "traumatic" according to Criterion A (op. cit.). In EMDR therapy, these adverse experiences may be referred to as small-t traumas not because they are less traumatic, but because they are so common in our experience that they are frequently overlooked as a cause of later problems (Shapiro 1995, 2001, 2007b). Small-t traumas include some of the adverse childhood experiences previously described by Felitti et al. (1998). EMDR therapy entails identifying, accessing, and reprocessing Big-T and small-t memories that are identified as the foundation of the dysfunction.

Mental Health and Substance Abuse Through the Lens of the AIP

Case Conceptualization

Most of the current randomized controlled research on EMDR therapy focuses on the treatment of PTSD (Lee et al. 2002). However, a growing body of case studies using EMDR therapy for other mental disorders and addictions reveals a history of trauma and other adverse life experiences as contributing factors.

Examples of diagnoses and disorders other than PTSD that were treated with EMDR therapy include:

- Body dysmorphic disorder (Brown et al. 1997)
- Borderline personality disorder (Brown and Shapiro 2006)
- Choking phobia (de Roos and de Jongh 2008; Schurmans 2007)
- Deliberate self-harm (McLaughlin et al. 2008)
- Domestic violence perpetration and victimization (Stowasser 2007)
- Eating disorders (Beer 2005; Bloomgarden and Calogero 2008)

- Obsessive compulsive disorder (Whisman 1997; Whisman and Keller 1999)
- Phobias (de Jongh 2003; de Jongh and ten Broeke 2007)
- Panic disorder (Fernandez and Faretta 2007; Feske and Goldstein 1997; Whisman 1997)
- Pathological gambling (Henry 1996)
- Phantom limb pain (Russell 2008; Schneider et al. 2007; Tinker and Wilson 2005; Wilensky 2006)
- Sex offender treatment (Ricci 2006; Ricci et al. 2006).
- Social phobia (Sun and Chiu 2006)
- Substance use disorder (Brown et al. 2015; Hase et al. 2008; Marich 2009, 2010; Popky 2005; Shapiro et al. 1994; Vogelmann-Sinn et al. 1998; Zweben and Yeary 2006)

Controlled research is needed in all these areas to further determine the efficacy of EMDR therapy with these diagnoses that are implicated as causal or related to substance abuse and compulsive behaviors. However, based on this emerging literature, it does not seem to be a question of whether to consider using EMDR therapy to treat complex disorders with a basis in trauma and other adverse life experiences, but rather when, how, and with whom.

Eye Movement Desensitization and Reprocessing (EMDR): Principles, Protocols, and Procedures

"Man is made by his belief. As he believes, so he is." Goethe

EMDR therapy is taught worldwide to licensed clinicians through, for example, Eye Movement Desensitization and Reprocessing International Association (EMDRIA), EMDR Ibero-America, and EMDR-Europe approved Basic Training providers. These trainings tend to be a minimum of 6 full days of instruction and practicum with an additional 10 hours of consultation.

EMDR therapy uses a 3-prong approach within an 8-phase model to sequentially target:

(1) *past* experiential contributors that laid the groundwork for the current symptoms;
(2) *present* triggers that activate current cognitive, affective, and/or somatic symptoms; and
(3) *future* desired states and behaviors. (see Table 5.3).

Following the principles of the AIP, EMDR therapy is a treatment that recognizes that false negative beliefs or Negative Cognitions (NCs) about oneself result from dysfunctionally stored, unprocessed memories and the attendant emotions,

Table 5.3 Overview of EMDR therapy phases (Shapiro 2005)

Phase	Purpose	Procedures
1. Client history	Collect background information Assess suitability for EMDR Identify-specific treatment targets from history	Standard history taking keeping the AIP in mind Review EMDR inclusions/exclusions/client resources Elicit: (1) past events related to symptoms, (2) present-day triggers, and (3) future desired outcomes
2. Preparation	Prepare clients for EMDR processing Stabilize and increase access to positive affects	Educate about symptom development Teach stabilization techniques such as a "safe/calm place"
3. Assessment	Activate the chosen targets for reprocessing	Elicit the following: Distressing image Negative belief currently held (assess SUD 0–10) Desired positive belief (assess VOC 1–7) Current emotions Current physical sensations
4. Desensitization	Process past experiences and current triggers to an adaptive resolution (SUD of 0) Fully desensitize all channels Incorporate positive future templates	Process past, present, future Standardized EMDR protocols, including sets of bilateral stimulation, allow for spontaneous emergence of insights, emotions, sensations, and other memories If processing becomes blocked, use Cognitive Interweave to activate more adaptive information "Stay out of the way" of client's natural processing
5. Installation	Increase connections to positive cognitive networks Increase generalization effects within associated memories	Have client identify the best positive cognition (initial or emergent) Continue processing until positive cognition is a 7 on the VOC scale
6. Body scan	Complete processing of any residual distress associated with target	Concentration on physical sensations and processing any residual distress
7. Closure	Ensure client stability at the end of an EMDR session whether completely reprocessed or not	Use relaxation or guided imagery to leave client in comfortable state to leave office Ask client to monitor what happens between sessions
8. Reassessment	Evaluation of treatment effects to ensure comprehensive reprocessing	Explore what has emerged since last session by re-accessing the previous target Evaluate integration after all targets processed

body sensations, and behavioral patterns they can generate. NCs are clustered under the headings of Responsibility, Safety, and Choices. These negative beliefs are not the cause of the dysfunction; they are a symptom of the unprocessed memories at the root of pathology. Rather than directly challenging the beliefs, as in cognitive behavioral therapy (CBT) for example, EMDR therapy identifies these core, irrational, negative beliefs along with the memories that give rise to them. The desired Positive Cognitions (PCs) that the client would prefer to believe and feel are true are also identified and are measured at a "gut level" by the Validity of Cognition (VOC) scale. For genuine change to occur, the memories generating for example, the incorrect belief, "I am not good enough" must be fully reprocessed at cognitive, affective, and somatic levels such that the correct belief, "I am fine the way I am" or "I am good enough" is integrated into the nervous system until experienced as true at a "felt-sense" level.

The Use of Bilateral Stimulation in EMDR Therapy

EMDR therapy's Standard Protocol incorporates alternating bilateral stimulation (BLS) of the senses using preferably eye movements, or tactile taps or audio tones. BLS is used during the preparation Phase 2 to install and/or strengthen and enhance any needed client resources and positive affective states, such as in the Safe/Calm Place exercise. Short and slow sets of BLS are used to strengthen and enhance positive resources, rather than access and activate potentially associated negative material, which may occur naturally when faster and longer sets BLS are conducted.

EMDR therapy is organized around the principles of a client-centered model, meaning the client's internal pathways for healing override the interpretations and directives of the therapist. In EMDR therapy, clinicians do not assume they know the precise way the client needs to heal because the client's memories are linked in ways that are not always evident to the clinician or the client. Within the desensitization and reprocessing Phases 4–6, the clinician utilizes standardized protocols that encourage and support the client's internal associations regarding their targeted memories.

During desensitization and reprocessing (phases 4–6), longer and faster sets of BLS are used to access, activate, desensitize, and reprocess the distressing elements of the target. This type of purposeful activating, accessing, and moving of material liberates a person's previously painful or disturbing reactions and behaviors. Reprocessing continues until the material is integrated and a coherent narrative emerges in present time. This resolution allows the person's own intrinsic drives toward mental, physical, and spiritual health to emerge and take the place of addictive patterns.

The Treatment of Co-occurring Disorders with EMDR Therapy

The concept of a tri-stage model for treating complex trauma was first introduced by Pierre Janet in 1907 and then again by Judith Herman in 1992. The tasks of this type of model are (1) safety and stabilization; (2) trauma processing and mourning; and (3) reconnection and reintegration (Herman 1992; Janet 1907). Relapse prevention for addiction is an essential part of Janet's and Herman's 3rd stage, and EMDR therapy's 2nd and 6th phases, primarily. Please note that with complex treatment populations, neither the phases of EMDR therapy's 8-phase Standard Protocol nor the stages of the 3-stage complex trauma model are rigid or discrete, but continually intertwine and overlap as needed throughout treatment.

EMDR therapy is highly effective and efficient. However, it is also emotionally evocative in the initial phases and potentially poses an additional, though temporary, risk of relapse with addiction. Therefore, initial and concurrent attention to safety, support, and resources is paramount. Clients and family members need thorough education about the relationship between trauma and addiction. The therapist explains that EMDR therapy conceptualizes cravings and the use of substances or other behaviors as symptoms resulting from unresolved trauma. Nightmares, flashbacks, and hyper-arousal, for example, can trigger the desire to medicate with drugs and/or alcohol (National Child Traumatic Stress Network (NCSTN) 2008; Steward and Conrod 2003). It is proposed that once EMDR therapy reprocesses disturbing traumatic memories they will no longer hold any physical, emotional, or cognitive distress, and there will be less interest in and need for self-medication, thereby ultimately reducing the risk of relapse. Not all psychiatric disorders are life threatening, but because substance use and abuse can be, it is recommended that EMDR therapy is conceptualized and administered as a tri-stage model within its established 8-phase Standard Protocol.

Tasks of a Phased, Integrated Model of EMDR Therapy

STAGE ONE (Phases 1 and 2 in EMDR Therapy)

History, assessment, motivation, safety, and stabilization

- Safety and stabilization skills (Najavits 2002; Shapiro 2001)
- Motivation (Miller and Rollnick 1991; Prochaska and DiClemente 1983)
- History gathering and diagnostic assessment

Phase 1 of EMDR Therapy: History

Client history is gathered with the AIP in mind, using the designated 3-prong approach to identify (i) the past experiences causing the dysfunction, (ii) the current situations triggering disturbance, and (iii) skills needed for adaptive future functioning. It is just as important to identify, strengthen, and enhance internal and external resources to which the client has access, as it is to uncover adverse experiences. This ensures that the client will be prepared for the reprocessing phases of memory work. Reprocessing is defined as unlinking maladaptive connections and forging positive neurophysiological connections between the targeted memory and more adaptive networks. If the client does not have access to positive memory networks, there may be little to connect their dysfunctionally stored material to and reprocessing would not be expected to go smoothly or speedily (Shapiro 2001).

Clinicians are cautioned to gather history slowly when presented with lifelong, complex trauma cases in order to minimize the potential triggering of highly charged emotional material. Gradual, paced history taking is preferred, as "too much too soon" can increase the risk of relapse. The following guidelines are recommended:

- Assess for and provide any needed self-control or affect management techniques
- Gather the client's bio/psycho/social history including mental status, strengths, chronological trauma history, PTSD, anxiety, and depressive symptoms
- Assess for the presence of co-occurring disorders
- Initially screen for dissociative disorders using the Dissociative Experiences Scale (DES; Bernstein and Putnam 1986) and if indicated, seek a more formal diagnostic assessment for dissociation such as the Structured Clinical Interview for Dissociative Disorders (SCID-D; Steinberg et al. 1990). It is important to note that the presence of a dissociative disorder is contraindicated for treatment using EMDR therapy without both the specialized expertise of the clinician and readiness of the client (Forgash and Copeley 2008; Shapiro 2001)
- Elicit a detailed history of substance use/abuse/dependency/addiction and behavioral compulsion

  - Note all substances used and pattern of use, e.g., binge, regular use, increasing amounts, and maintenance
  - First use: "What was happening at the time client first started using?"
  - Assess current triggers and urges to use substances or other addictive behaviors
  - Assess relapse patterns

- Evaluate past treatment attempts and outcomes
- Assess level of readiness for treatment: precontemplation, contemplation, preparation, and action (Miller and Rollnick 1991; Prochaska and DiClemente 1983)

- Educate the family about the nature of addiction as a brain disorder and untreated trauma's contributing role—this is considered a key to successful treatment
- Assess level of support from family, friends, and co-workers—each family member's role in either supporting or undermining the treatment process should be assessed, addressed, and treated, whenever possible (Shapiro 2007)

Case Example: PTSD, Bipolar Disorder, Marijuana and Alcohol Abuse, and Compulsive Use of Pornography

Sheila referred her 33-year-old husband John (not their real names) for EMDR therapy because she had become fearful about his "rapidly deteriorating emotional state." She reported that during the last 6 months he had become increasingly more depressed, anxious, withdrawn, physically and emotionally abusive, and expressed occasional suicidal ideation and intent. His marriage was at risk of failure.

John reported that 1 year ago he had attended a family gathering where he unexpectedly saw an older cousin who had molested him between the ages of 11 and 13. He had not seen that cousin in 10 years and thought he had "already dealt with the molestation." He was upset to find he was still powerless over his reactions. His parents dismissed his distress by asking him why something from "such a long time ago" would bother him now. Admittedly attempting to "deal with" the symptoms listed below, John self-medicated with alcohol and marijuana and pornography on and off since the sexual offenses made against him during his early adolescence. These behaviors and moods again escalated after encountering his cousin and were now threatening his job and marriage.

John's History

Presenting Symptoms

- *Sleep disturbances*
- *Severe marital discord with emotional and physical rage outbursts*
- *Mood swings*
- *Self-injurious impulses*
- *Compulsive use of pornography*
- *Marijuana and alcohol abuse*

Past: To be reprocessed during initial stage of the 3-prong protocol

- *Family history of alcoholism, depression, and suicide.*
- *Extreme parental mis-attunement and emotional neglect, e.g. John's isolated, unsafe conditions at home frightened and overwhelmed him. When he tried to communicate his fear to his parents, they minimized him and told him "how easy he had it compared to them".*

Table 5.4 John's negative and positive cognitions and cluster types

Negative cognitions (NC)	Positive cognitions (PC)	Cluster types
"I am permanently damaged"	"I am fine as I am"	Responsibility
"There's something really wrong with me"	"I am fine as I am"	Responsibility
"I'm not safe"	"I can keep myself safe now"	Safety
"I can't trust"	"I can learn to trust"	Safety
"I am powerless"	"I have choices now"	Choices
"I can't stand it"	"I can handle it"	Choices

- *This ongoing invalidation was later revealed as the earliest contributor for the present-day over-reactivity to wife's communications with him.*
- *Extended periods of isolation and loneliness.*
- *Sexual assault from age 11 to 13 by his 18-year-old male cousin.*

John reported that his preoccupation with pornography and substance abuse emerged in his early teens, shortly after the molestation began. This is the most commonly reported temporal relationship between trauma and substance abuse (Steward and Conrod 2003).

Early relational mis-attunement, poor attachment, parental neglect, and extended periods of isolation would be expected to decrease John's developing ability to manage affect in childhood and into adulthood (Perry 1999; Schore 2002; Siegel 1999; Van der Kolk et al. 1996). The Adaptive Information Processing (AIP) model would see John's symptoms as being an expression of his genetic, environmental, and experiential factors that fostered the later development of his mood disorders and substance abuse (Felitti et al. 1998; Shapiro 1995, 2001).

The negative, irrational beliefs or Negative Cognitions (NCs) that often emerge from a history such as John's are a focus of treatment in EMDR therapy. Both the SUD level and the VOC rating are re-assessed and re-measured after the reprocessing and installation phases 4–6 of EMDR therapy. A decrease in the SUD rating to "0" or ecological validity associated with the memory, along with an increased, felt-sense rating of the VOC to a 7, indicates a positive treatment effect as a result of reprocessing traumatic material in EMDR therapy.

John's negative belief clusters related to the sexual assault are listed below. Each belief was targeted through the complete 3-prong approach of past contributors, present triggers, and desired future states and behaviors (Table 5.4).

Present triggers: To be processed during the second phase of the 3-prong protocol

1. *Feeling "criticized"*
2. *Feeling "misunderstood" and "not able to be heard"*
3. *Feeling "unimportant" to his wife*

Phase 2 of EMDR Therapy: Preparation

Safety, stabilization, and resource development

Readiness for EMDR therapy reprocessing (Phases 4–6) includes:

- The ability to access and use safe coping skills (Najavits 2002; Shapiro 1995, 2001) to soothe high levels of distress
- The ability to have a dual awareness of the past traumatic material while still maintaining present-moment orientation
- The willingness to engage available resources such as a 12-step program, sober living, family, and/or other personal support systems—this is crucial when clients are still using substances
- Sobriety of at least 30 days or until symptoms of withdrawal are minimized, whenever possible—this recommendation has exceptions, see the section "Early Trauma and Other Adverse Life Experiences Treatment in Addictions: Guidelines and Exceptions" later in this chapter

Safety and stabilization with any population comes first in treatment, but because of the potentially evocative nature of EMDR therapy, and the risk for relapse with co-occurring disorders, the timing of the reprocessing (phases 4–6) is carefully assessed. When EMDR therapy is used to treat single incident traumas, such as a motor vehicle accident, dog-bite, or a one-time assault, reprocessing with EMDR therapy can be an exceedingly brief, effective intervention consisting of 1–3 (90-min) sessions (Marcus et al. 1997; Rothbaum 1997; Shapiro 2001). There are also clients who have strong personal strengths and resources who may not need a lengthy preparation phase. Sobriety and self-soothing are often enough to move forward into trauma processing when clients have less complex histories.

For clients with complex trauma histories

For those who have confounding variables of long-term, complex childhood trauma, and exhibit a more severe and chronic course of symptoms, extensive preparation is *strongly recommended* to promote the safest trauma reprocessing experience. Here, reprocessing with EMDR therapy may have both a longer preparation phase and longer reprocessing phases.

Additional resource development is needed when clients are missing resources that may interfere with their ability to tolerate reprocessing. Resource Development and Installation (RDI; Korn and Leeds 2002), for example, which accesses and incorporates a variety of positive affective and somatic states, can accomplish this. Other grounding and self-soothing exercises may include visualizations in which people are able to imagine themselves behaving in a more positive, adaptive way. This manner of preparation for trauma treatment is a variation of the 3rd-prong, or Future Template, of EMDR therapy.

More structured interventions may be integrated with EMDR therapy in environments where group work or more intensive individualized preparatory experience is needed prior to individual trauma processing, for example: Seeking Safety

(Najavits 2002), Motivational Interviewing (M.I.; Miller and Rollnick 1991), Desensitization of Triggers and Urge Reprocessing (DeTUR; Popky 1998), and Dialectical Behavior Therapy (DBT; Linehan 1993).

John's Preparation

Personal strengths and resources

- *Creative and artistic*
- *Intelligent*
- *Sensitive and warm*
- *Long-term friendships from high school*
- *Supportive wife*

Resources needed

- *Ability to self-soothe (Safe Place)*
- *Willingness to commit to sobriety*

When John initially sought treatment, he was not sober and had suicidal thoughts. Substance abuse can confound assessments and trigger or prolong symptoms; therefore, a psychiatrist conducted a medical evaluation and concluded, in collaboration with the treating therapist, that John required medically managed stabilization prior to initiating any trauma processing with EMDR therapy. John agreed to take medication and enter into a course of sobriety to allow the clinical picture to clear. He was able to remain clean for 30 days and the co-occurring Bipolar, PTSD, and Substance Use Disorders were confirmed.

John was now able to demonstrate, along with other self-soothing techniques, his use of the Safe/Calm Place exercise and an ability to shift from a state of high distress to a state of calm. This, along with his sobriety and medical stabilization, allowed the client and clinician to move forward and reprocess his first EMDR therapy target.

STAGE TWO (Phases 3–6 in EMDR Therapy)

Phases 3–6 in EMDR Therapy (assessment, desensitization, installation, body scan) use the 3 prongs of past, present, and future

- Assess, desensitize, and reprocess all *past* adverse life experiences and *present* symptoms and triggers until they no longer cause cognitive, affective, or somatic distress
- Teach necessary skills and imaginally rehearse future reactions and behaviors with BLS in order to develop *future* templates for more adaptive choices

Phase 3 of EMDR Therapy: Assessment

John collaborated in his treatment planning, and with the clinical agreement of his therapist, chose the first of the sexual assaults against him as his first target for memory reprocessing.

Setting up and activating the target

- Identify the most disturbing image associated with the event:
  The first time he was held captive in a closet and sexually assaulted by his older cousin
- Identify the irrational negative belief (NC) related to the event:
  "There's something really wrong with me"
- Identify the desired positive, more accurate belief (PC):
  "I'm fine the way I am"
- Assess the Validity of Cognition (VOC) with the image held in mind, on a scale of 1–7, where 1 feels totally gut-level false and 7 feels completely gut-level true *now*:
  John reported a VOC of 2
- Assess the Subjective Units of Distress (SUD) on a scale of 0–10, where 0 is no disturbance and 10 is the highest disturbance imaginable:
  John reported a SUD of 9
- Identify where in the body the distress is noticed:
  John reported tightness in chest, nausea, stomach cramping, and "head spinning"

Phase 4 of EMDR Therapy: Desensitization

The desensitization and reprocessing phases use an initial set of 18-24 eye-movement passes while asking the client to mindfully "just notice" what is emerging during and between sets. The length of subsequent sets of eye-movements is based upon the clinician's assessments of the client's affective and cognitive responses. A deep breath is taken when BLS is stopped, and the client then reports what is being experienced. The clinician then helps guide the client to the focus of attention for the next set. After approximately 20 sets, John stated with clear conviction that he was only 11 years old, that his cousin was "almost an adult" at 18, and that he could not imagine an 11-year-old child "causing or being responsible for their own molest." He also noted that the "absence of his parents' supervision" during much of his childhood left him at greater risk for exploitation. Clearing those networks revealed John's additional NCs such as "I'm unimportant" and "I can't trust" and the insight that he inappropriately managed "feeling misunderstood or unduly criticized" by becoming explosive and abusive toward his wife.

The Treatment of Present Triggers and Urges to Use

John's present triggers and urges to use alcohol, marijuana, pornography, and verbally abuse his wife were reprocessed. It should be emphasized that in order to prevent relapse, it is also necessary to reprocess any other early memories and their triggers that might contribute to setting the groundwork for pathology (Table 5.5).

When exploring John's triggers, they were revealed to be directly associated with the experiences and emotions he had first felt as a child in response to his parents' behavior. His parents' insensitive responses to him frequently left him feeling misunderstood, unheard, unimportant, and extremely frustrated.

In EMDR therapy's Standard Protocol, triggers are identified and reprocessed as an individual EMDR target. For example, the "feeling of being misunderstood" was set up as follows:

Target image   Arguing with his wife

NC   I'm not important
PC   I am important and deserve to be heard
VOC   3
Emotions   Extreme frustration, anger, sadness, fear
SUD   8
Location   Tightness in chest and stomach

The target was reprocessed to SUD of 0 and VOC of 7 with clear body scan.

As a result, John saw that his parents were "good people" who often communicated with criticism due to their own anxiety, not his shortcomings. They also left him alone for long periods of time because both worked long hours to support the child they loved, not because he was unimportant. These clarifications spontaneously emerged during reprocessing and were keys to John's establishing positive, loving connections within and for himself and for his wife.

Additional outgrowths of reprocessing included desensitization of his triggers. They no longer activated his urge to use substances or pornography and his nervous system was cleared of the old feelings associated with the belief that he didn't matter. As expected, he also no longer incorrectly perceived his wife's intentions as critical, demeaning, or mistrustful. John was then able to respond more appropriately and non-defensively to her communications and her needs and their marriage improved.

Table 5.5 Triggers and addictions of choice

Triggers	Addiction of choice
Perception of being criticized	Marijuana (calming)
Feeling misunderstood	Marijuana, alcohol (calming, and to relieve tension)
Social events	Marijuana and alcohol (felt more social)
Loneliness and isolation	Pornography (felt more connected)

Phase 5 of EMDR Therapy: Installation

Once a SUD of 0 (or with some ecological exceptions, a 1) is reported, installation of the PC is continued until a VOC of 7 is reached. John's original NC was, "It's my fault." John's PC evolved into, "I was just a child; it wasn't my fault" and was reported to be felt at a VOC of 7.

Phase 6 of EMDR Therapy: Body Scan

During the body scan the client brings up the original target, their positive belief, and scans their body for any remaining distress or sensation. If anything even slight is reported, reprocessing continues until no remaining discomfort or body sensations can be identified. John reported he was clear and had no remaining bodily distress.

Future Template: At this point, if possible, a future imaginal rehearsal can be conducted. In John's case, he was asked to think about a future time that he might run into his cousin and notice whether he sensed any distress connected with that possibility. John was able to imagine the scene without much problem, until the therapist tested his Future Template by suggesting that he visualize his cousin chatting with another young male family member. This triggered some distress and feelings of protectiveness toward the younger male family member. John stated that, as an adult, he would do whatever might be necessary to keep a child safe from his cousin. The visualization was continued until John could imagine himself thinking, feeling, and behaving as he wished: calmly and assertively with no physical, emotional, or cognitive disturbance.

Phase 7 of EMDR Therapy: Closure

Close down complete or incomplete sessions by using the Safe/Calm Place and positive resources developed and strengthened by the client in the preparation phase of EMDR therapy. John's session, having arrived at a SUD of 0 and VOC of 7 with a clear body scan, was closed down safely. The desensitization and reprocessing of his triggers and Future Templates would come at later sessions. John left the session confident in the truth of his words, "I was just a child; it wasn't my fault."

Phase 8 of EMDR Therapy: Re-evaluation

Treatment targets are re-evaluated at the following session to see whether any change has occurred. The client is asked to "bring up the memory" that was worked on and "notice what comes up for you today." If the client reports any distressing imagery, thoughts, feelings, or body sensations, they are reprocessed until complete (SUD of 0, VOC of 7) using the same procedures noted during assessment and desensitization. When no further disturbance is reported, Phase 3 is revisited and the next target in the treatment plan is selected.

At John's follow-up visit, the target was reassessed and remained at a SUD of 0, a VOC of 7, with a clear body scan. He also reported he experienced a sense of "lightness" between sessions when he would think of the molestation, as if the weight of a boulder had been lifted from his chest.

STAGE THREE All Phases of EMDR Therapy's 8-phases and 3-prongs

Reconnection, Integration, and Relapse Prevention

Reconnection and reintegration takes place in all phases of EMDR therapy. When traumatic memories are successfully reprocessed and one's personal strengths and resources are fully accessible, this then allows for the freedom to be a more honest, open, and authentic "self."

Stage 3 involves and may result in:

- A felt-sense of integration with oneself, along with an enhanced ability to connect or reconnect with others which is believed to be a natural result of reprocessing and integrating distressing material
- Preparation of the neural networks for future adaptive action—without the use of substances or other self-destructive behaviors

Future Template: 3rd-prong of the 3-prong Protocol

Use of the Future Template (imaginal rehearsal) gives clients an opportunity to systematically *imagine* the future, as if running a movie, focusing on potentially relapse-triggering situations, people, places, rituals, and/or internal states. These targets are reprocessed with bilateral stimulation until they can be imagined without distress and the positive, self-referencing statement (e.g., "I am deserving") feels true at a "felt-sense" level.

The therapist asks: "With respect to these issues, how would you like to see yourself thinking, feeling, and behaving in the future?"

- *Calm and rational communications with wife*
- *Able to hear and receive feedback without interpreting it all as critical*
- *Clean and sober from substances and pornography*
- *Able to be alone or connect with others and be comfortable either way*

John's Future Template Target: Remaining calm when in disagreement with his wife.

John was asked to imagine a movie scene of he and his wife disagreeing about the social plans she made without first consulting him. This triggered his belief, "I don't matter" along with anger and tension in his chest. The image, emotion, and body sensation were reprocessed until he reported they were neutral and no longer disturbing. Asked if there was any level of urge to use substances at the thought of arguing with his wife, John said, "No." It is expected that successful use of the Future Template will lower the risk of relapse because it reduces or eliminates identified motivators to self-medicate.

Early Trauma and Other Adverse Life Experiences Treatment in Addictions: Guidelines and Exceptions

Treating clinicians must be experienced as both chemical addiction and behavioral compulsion specialists in addition to EMDR therapy, or be under close supervision of someone with those qualifications. The common guideline in addiction treatment has been to wait for a period of stabilization and sobriety, generally 30 days, before working through disturbing memories. However, although there clearly are risks in treating trauma prior to sobriety or early in recovery, there are also cases where reprocessing a traumatic memory can reduce the risk that unresolved trauma will interfere with attempts to sustain sobriety (Zweben and Yeary 2006).

Case Example: EMDR Therapy Before the Client Has Attained Sobriety

Jeannie (not her real name) had a rocky childhood with adoptive parents who had decided, "They really didn't want a child after all." She was physically cared for but was emotionally neglected and verbally berated. An alcoholic, sex, and cocaine addict since her teens, she was now 41, married, with a teenage son.

At 15 years of age, Jeannie's parents, who often fought violently with one another, went through a bitter divorce. She blamed herself for their marital failure since she was often the subject of their fights. Jeannie lived with her mother who made it clear that she was not to open the door to her father if she was not present. Her father, who suffered from severe emphysema, came by one day hauling his oxygen tank behind him. He became angry and escalated into a rage when Jeannie refused to open the door. The angrier he got the more impaired his breathing became. Terrified of her mother, Jeannie did not let him in. Later that week, her father was hospitalized and died shortly thereafter. She blamed herself for his death and her mother blamed her as well. Jeannie soon began to use substances to cope with her perception of these childhood events, and her addictions quickly spiraled out of control. She found herself unable to manage without the use of substances.

Jeannie had numerous previous attempts at counseling and sobriety, but when sober, the flashbacks and anxieties stemming from her childhood overwhelmed her. After several months of phased preparation: teaching safe coping skills, strengthening inner resources, and developing emotional management skills, she was still unable to establish sobriety for more than a few days and could not maintain a serious recovery program. While sobriety is preferable before beginning EMDR therapy reprocessing phases, in Jeannie's case the therapist and client collaboratively decided to proceed and target her belief that she was responsible for her father dying, in the hope that lessening the distress of that memory would promote her efforts at sobriety.

The reprocessing was successful within two sessions and freed Jeannie from her 26-year belief that she caused her father's death. She also came to know that the way her parents treated her in childhood was not because something was wrong with her, but was a consequence of her parents' own issues which were not her fault. With these deeply felt perceptual changes, Jeannie was finally able to enter into and sustain recovery. She said that resolving that experience had given her hope that the remainder of her traumatic past could be reprocessed as well. It took over a year to target her remaining issues with one relapse early in recovery. Jeannie is now in her tenth year of uninterrupted sobriety.

An Integrated Trauma Treatment Program (ITTP) Using EMDR Therapy and Seeking Safety in an American Drug Court Program

An Integrated Trauma Treatment Program (ITTP; Brown et al. 2015) combining two evidence-based, empirically validated treatments: EMDR therapy (Shapiro 2001) and Seeking Safey (Najavits 2002), was implemented as an enhancement to the Thurston County Drug court program in Olympia, Washington, which previously had no trauma-focused component. The ITTP included 3 phases (early, middle, and later recovery) over a period of 12–18 months and offered treatment in lieu of incarceration to nonviolent individuals arrested for drug-related offenses. Data was collected from 220 participants from 2004–2009. Since unresolved trauma is believed to underlie addiction, the objective of the ITTP was to determine if adding a trauma-specific treatment component to the program as usual (PAU) would improve program outcomes such as graduation and recidivism. Drug court program completion and graduation are the strongest predictors of lower post-program recidivism rates (National Institute of Justice 2006).

Seeking Safety (SS) is a manualized, CBT-based treatment program for PTSD and substance abuse that focuses on the present rather than delving into past trauma. SS can be conducted as a group intervention or individually by trained, non-licensed support staff. SS has demonstrated signficant treatment effects (Hien et al. 2010; Najavits and Hien 2013). See www.seekingsafety.org for a comprehensive list of SS studies. SS is listed as a Best Practice through the Substance Abuse and Mental Health Services Administration (SAMHSA 2005) and is composed of 25 topics that provide education, safety skills-building, and stabilization techniques. Same-gender groups were a mandatory addition to the PAU for those endorsing a trauma history. Fifteen pre-selected topics were used in the ITTP as a more formal part of Phase 2 in EMDR therapy (Preparation, Safety, and Stabilization) to prepare participants for individual trauma treatment with EMDR therapy, including exploration and reprocessing of past trauma. Completion of all SS groups was required prior to receiving voluntary EMDR therapy. Participants' sobriety was assessed via random urine drug screens throughout the entirety of the drug court program.

Out of the 220 participants assessed with either the Clinican Administered Posttraumatic Stress Scale (CAPS; Blake et al. 1995) or the Detailed Assessment of Posttraumatic Stress (DAPS; Briere 2001), 68 % endorsed a criterion A trauma sometime in their life. Program graduation outcomes revealed that participants in the PAU who did not endorse any trauma history graduated at a rate of 60 %. Those who endorsed trauma and completed the Seeking Safety portion of the ITTP but declined EMDR therapy, graduated at a rate of 57 %. Those who went on to complete EMDR therapy, graduated at a rate of 91 %. Post-program recidivism rates were 10 % for PAU graduates, 12 % for those receiving EMDR therapy and 33 % for those completing SS groups but declining individual EMDR therapy.

Case Example of Drug Court Participant

One Drug court participant, Tom, (not his real name) had been arrested 14 times for felony drug possession. He was in his third, and final, Drug court program opportunity when EMDR therapy was introduced. His history revealed two alcoholic parents, and other adverse childhood experiences, including his father's early death from cancer. Tom's substance abuse began in adolescence and included alcohol, marijuana, and his primary drug of choice: methamphetamine. At the age of 31, Tom and his brother were cross-country tractor-trailer truck driving partners. They engaged in a bitter argument while driving drunk. In a fit of rage, Tom's brother unbuckled his seat belt and stepped out of the truck as it was going 65 miles (105 km) per hour. He died in Tom's arms at the side of the road.

Tom blamed himself for his brother's death. His addictions increased and led to the loss of his family, business, and freedom. Tom never had treatment for his traumatic past, nor did he know that unprocessed adverse experiences fueled his addictions. Successfully targeting and reprocessing the death of his brother with EMDR therapy was the beginning of a long-lasting recovery for Tom, now 12 years sober. One of the first successful participants of the ITTP, Tom has been an avid spokesperson and role model for the program and often speaks publically to inspire other Drug court participants.

The following case example illustrates the importance of considering small-t traumas, or adverse life experiences, as well as the Big-T traumas when treating this population.

Case Example: Co-occurring Panic and Substance Use Disorder Rooted in a Small-T Trauma

Karen (not her real name) was 47 years old when she was referred for EMDR therapy. She was nine months sober from poly-substance abuse, but was still sexually compulsive and continued to have panic attacks, that despite several trials of psychotropic medication, caused her to use again. She thought choosing her own drugs was more effective than medication, even though using only deepened her sense of guilt, shame, and isolation.

She had more than 10 years of unsuccessful treatment for her panic attacks before her earliest memories of them were targeted and reprocessed with EMDR therapy. She focused on the "fear in her body" as the target and within a few moments connected with a memory from age four of being dropped off at a park with instructions to care for her 2-year-old sister. It seemed to Karen that her parents left her there the entire day. By the time they returned, Karen was in a panic, vomiting, sobbing, and unable to catch her breath. Her father screamed at her to "knock it off and quit acting like a baby." Her panic shifted to shame and humiliation when his rage changed to laughter about how "wimpy" she was.

The developing brain of a child requires a certain level of attunement and safety in order to develop its emotional regulation capacities (Schore 2002; Siegel 1999) without which a child is more vulnerable to later substance use (Linehan 1993). Thus, 4-year-old Karen tried to regulate her emotions in the absence of supportive parenting. In less than a year, at age 5, Karen took her first sip of beer at an unsupervised party of her parents and from that point, continued to drink as opportunities at home presented themselves. At age 12, she began smoking marijuana. She entered treatment for alcohol and marijuana abuse at age 46.

More serious traumatic and adverse experiences occurred throughout her childhood, including multiple molestations by her brother's friends such as sexually inappropriate touching. However, Karen states she experienced the park incident as the first and most overwhelming experience that set the tone for the "rest of my life." That memory felt just like the panic attacks she continued to experience in adulthood and attempted to medicate with drugs, alcohol, and compulsive sex; by all clinical standards the adverse childhood experience at the park was a small-t trauma.

The intensity and frequency of Karen's panic attacks diminished after reprocessing of this pivotal memory easing her urges to use marijuana and alcohol to medicate them. This case underscores the importance of reprocessing memories responsible for not only the faulty cognitive beliefs one holds about one's self, but also the body sensations that are reported, such as in panic attacks, that may or may not have a specific negative cognition associated with them. This example illuminates the importance of not only reprocessing Big-T traumas, but also all of the relevant adverse life experiences we consider to be small-t traumas.

Conclusion and Summary: Why Use EMDR Therapy to Treat Co-occurring Disorders?

"Although the world is full of suffering, it is also full of overcoming it." Helen Keller

As research and clinical experience suggest, the incidence of co-occurring disorders within the criminal justice system (Substance Abuse and Mental Health Services Administration (SAMHSA) 2005) and substance abuse treatment centers across the nation indicates the need for specialized treatment programs designed specifically for this challenging population. The personal, family, social, health, and economic consequences as a result of failing to treat these individuals have been staggering and seems remediable.

Co-occurring disorders are a unique treatment challenge and EMDR therapy is a unique response to that challenge. EMDR therapy's 8-phases and 3-prongs, along with the informing AIP model, predicts that early trauma and other adverse life experiences are primary contributors to the emergence of clinical symptoms and disorders, and are often the leading causes for the use of substances designed to regulate distress. The 3-prong approach of EMDR therapy is ideally suited to the treatment of co-occurring disorders and targets: (1) the *past* experiential contributors to present-day symptoms, (2) *present*-day triggers that activate distress, and (3) *future* templates of desired states and behavior.

The third prong (Future Template) in EMDR therapy gives clients an opportunity to imagine encountering many possible relapse-triggering situations (people, places, and things) as well as internally triggering negative emotions in the future. These future targets are then reprocessed with BLS until the future can be visualized without distress and the client's positive self-referencing statements feel true at that "felt-sense" level. It is believed that the treatment effects observed with EMDR therapy offer co-occurring disordered clients an extra measure of protection against future relapse with drugs, alcohol, or other self-destructive behaviors originally intended to help the client "feel better." The temporary solution of addiction eventually displaces a person's true self with a sense of powerlessness and self-loathing that impacts the not only the individual, but their family and the next generation in the vicious cycle introduced at the beginning of this chapter. Therefore, we call to attention the hypothesis that society's number one problem is not substance abuse and other harmful behaviors, but rather, unresolved trauma, neglect, and other adverse life experience that with effective treatment can transform a person and allow for a life free of past suffering and worth living substance free.

References

American Psychiatric Association. (2004). *Practice guideline for the treatment of patients with acute stress disorder and posttraumatic stress disorder.* American Psychiatric Publishing: Arlington, VA.

American Psychiatric Association. (2013). *Diagnostic and statistical manual of mental disorders* (5th Ed.) Arlington, VA: American Psychiatric Publishing

Beck, A. T., Ward, C., & Mendelson, M. (1961). Beck depression inventory (BDI). *Archives of General Psychiatry, 4*, 561–571.

Beer R. (2005). *Symposium: EMDR and eating disorders—EMDR for adolescents with anorexia nervosa: Evolution of conceptualization and illustration of clinical applications.* EMDR European Association Conference, Brussels, Belgium, June 2005.

Bergmann, U. (2000). Further thoughts on the neurobiology of EMDR: The role of the cerebellum in accelerated information processing. *Traumatology, 6*(3), 175–200.

Bergmann, U. (2008). The neurobiology of EMDR: Exploring the thalamus and neural integration. *Journal of EMDR Practice and Research, 2*(4), 300–314.

Bernstein, E. M., & Putnam, F. W. (1986). Development, reliability and validity of a dissociation scale. *Journal of Nervous and Mental Disease, 174*, 727–735.

Bisson, J., & Andrew, M. (2007). Psychological treatment of post-traumatic stress disorder (PTSD). *Cochrane Database of Systematic Reviews,* Art. No.: CD003388. doi:10.1002/14651858.CD003388.pub3

Blake, D. D., Weathers, F. W., Nagy, L. M., Kaloupek, D. G., Gusman, F. D., Charney, D. S., et al. (1995). The development of a Clinician-Administered PTSD Scale. *Journal of Traumatic Stress, 8*(1), 75–90.

Bloomgarden, A., & Calogero, R. M. (2008). A randomized experimental test of the efficacy of EMDR treatment on negative body image in eating disorder inpatients. *Eating Disorders, 16*(5), 418–427.

Brady, K. T., Killeen, T., Saladin, M. E., Dansky, G., & Becker, S. (1994). Comorbid substance abuse and posttraumatic stress disorder: Characteristics of women in treatment. *The American Journal on Addictions, 3*, 160–164.

Briere, J. (2001). *Detailed Assessment of Posttraumatic Stress (DAPS).* Odessa, Florida: Psychological Assessment Resources.

Brown, S. H., Gilman, S. G., Goodman, E. G., Adler-Tapia, R. & Freng. (2015). Integrated trauma treatment in drug court: Combining EMDR therapy and Seeking Safety. *Journal of EMDR Practice and Research, 9*(3), 123–136.

Brown, K. W., McGoldrick, T., & Buchanan, R. (1997). Body dysmorphic disorder: Seven cases treated with eye movement desensitization and reprocessing. *Behavioural and Cognitive Psychotherapy, 25*(2), 203–207.

Brown, S., & Shapiro, F. (2006). EMDR in the treatment of borderline personality disorder. *Clinical Case Studies, 5*(5), 403–420.

Brown, P. J., Stout, R., & Mueller, T. (1996). Post-traumatic stress disorder and substance abuse relapse among women: A pilot study. *Psychology of Addictive Behaviors, 10*, 124–128.

Christman, S. D., Garvey, K. J., Propper, R. E., & Phaneuf, K. A. (2003). Bilateral eye movements enhance the retrieval of episodic memories. *Neuropsychology, 17*, 221–229.

de Jongh, A. (2003). Anxiety disorders—Treatment of phobias with EMDR. In *Proceedings of the EMDR European association conference*. Rome, Italy.

de Jongh, A., & ten Broeke, E. (2007). Treatment of specific phobias with EMDR: Conceptualization and strategies for the selection of appropriate memories. *Journal of EMDR Practice and Research. 1*(1), 46–56.

de Roos, C., & de Jongh, A. (2008). EMDR treatment of children and adolescents with a choking Phobia. *Journal of EMDR Practice and Research, 2*(3), 201–211.

Department of Veterans Affairs & Department of Defense. (2004). *VA/DoD clinical practice guideline for the management of post-traumatic stress*. Washington, DC.

Felitti, V. J. (2004). The origins of addiction: Evidence from the adverse childhood experiences study. English version of the article published in Germany as: Felitti VJ. *Ursprunge des Suchtverhaltens—Evidenzen au seiner Studies u belastenden Kindheitserfahrungen Praxis der Kinderpsychologie under Kinderpsychiatrie, 52*, 547–559.

Felitti, V. J., Anda, R. F., Nordenberg, D., Williamson, D. F., Spitz, A. M., Edwards, V., et al. (1998). Relationship of childhood abuse and household dysfunction to many of the leading causes of death in adults: The adverse childhood experiences (ACE) study. *American Journal of Preventive Medicine, 14*(4), 245–258.

Fernandez, I., & Faretta, E. (2007). Eye movement desensitization and reprocessing in the treatment of panic disorder with agoraphobia. *Clinical Case Studies, 6*(1), 44–63.

Feske, U., & Goldstein, A. (1997). Eye movement desensitization and reprocessing treatment for panic disorder: A controlled outcome and partial dismantling study. *Journal of Consulting and Clinical Psychology, 65*(6), 1026–1035.

Foa, E. B., Hembree, E. A., & Rothbaum, B. O. (2007). *Prolonged exposure therapy for PTSD: Emotional processing of traumatic experiences therapist guide (treatments that work)*. Oxford: Oxford University Press.

Forgash, C., & Copeley, M. (Eds.). (2008). *Healing the heart of trauma and dissociation with EMDR and ego state therapy*. New York: Springer Publishing.

Grant, J., Brewer, J., & Potenza, M. (2006). The neurobiology of substance and behavioral addictions. *CNS Spectrum, 11*(12), 924–930.

Hase, M., Schallmayer, S., & Sack, M. (2008). EMDR reprocessing of the addiction memory: Pretreatment, posttreatment, and 1-month follow-up. *Journal of EMDR Practice and Research, 2*, 170–179.

Henry, S. (1996). Pathological gambling: Etiologic considerations and treatment efficacy of eye movement desensitization/reprocessing. *Journal of Gambling Studies, 12*(4), 395–405.

Herman, J. (1992). *Trauma and recovery: The aftermath of violence—From domestic abuse to political terror*. New York: Basic Books.

Hien, D. A., Jiang, H., Campbell, A. N. C., Hu, M.-C., Miele, G. M., Nunes, E. V., et al. (2010). Do treatment improvements in PTSD severity affect substance use outcomes? A secondary analysis from a randomized clinical trial in NIDA's Clinical Trials Network. *American Journal of Psychiatry, 167*(1), 95–101.

Hucker, S. J. (2004). Disorders of impulse control. In O'Donohue & Levensky (Eds.), *Forensic psychology*. New York: Academic Press.

Hudson, W. W., & Ricketts, W. A. (1993). *Index of self esteem*. Tallahassee, FL: Walmyr Publishing.

Ironson, G. I., Freund, B., Strauss, J. L., & Williams, J. (2002). Comparison of two treatments for traumatic stress: A community-based study of EMDR and prolonged exposure. *Journal of Clinical Psychology, 58*, 113–128.

Jaberghaderi, N., Greenwald, R., Rubin, A., Dolatabadim, S., & Zand, S. O. (2004). A comparison of CBT and EMDR for sexually abused Iranian girls. *Clinical Psychology and Psychotherapy, 11*, 358–368.

Janet, P. (1907). *The major symptoms of hysteria*. London: Macmillan.

Kessler, R. C., Sonnega, A., Bromet, E., Hughes, M., & Nelson, C. B. (1995). Posttraumatic stress disorder in the National Comorbidity Survey. *Archives of General Psychiatry, 52*, 1048–1060.

Khantzian, E. J. (1985). The self-medication hypothesis of addictive disorders: Focus on heroin and cocaine dependence. *American Journal of Psychiatry, 142*, 1259–1264.

Korn, D., & Leeds, A. (2002). Preliminary evidence of efficacy for EMDR resource development and installation in the stabilization phase of treatment of complex posttraumatic stress disorder. *Journal of Clinical Psychology, 58*(12), 1465–1487.

Lee, C. W., & Cuijpers, P. (2013). A meta-analysis of the contribution of eye movements in processing emotional memories. *Journal of Behavior Therapy and Experimental Psychiatry, 44*, 231–239.

Lee, C., Gavriel, H., Drummond, P., Richards, J., & Greenwald, R. (2002). Treatment of post-traumatic stress disorder: A comparison of stress inoculation training with prolonged exposure and eye movement desensitization and reprocessing. *Journal of Clinical Psychology, 58*, 1071–1089.

Linehan, M. (1993). *Cognitive-behavioral treatment of borderline personality disorder.* New York: Guilford Press.

Marcus, S., Marquis, P., & Sakai, C. (1997). Controlled study of treatment of PTSD using EMDR in an HMO setting. *Psychotherapy, 34*, 307–315.

Marich, J. (2009). EMDR in the addiction continuing care process: Case study of a cross-addicted female's treatment and recovery. *Journal of EMDR Practice and Research, 3*, 98–106.

Marich, J. (2010). EMDR in addiction continuing care: A phenomenological study of women in recovery. *Psychology of Addictive Behaviors, 24*(3), 498–507.

McLaughlin, D., McGowan, I., Paterson, M., & Miller, P. (2008). Cessation of deliberate self harm following eye movement desensitization and reprocessing: A case report. *Case Journal, 1*, 177. http://www.casesjournal.com/content/1/1/177. Accessed 28 Feb 2009.

Miller, W. R., & Rollnick, S. (1991). *Motivational interviewing: Preparing people to change addictive behavior.* New York: The Guildford Press.

Mol, S., Arntz, A., Metsemakers, J., Dinant, G., Vilters-Van Montfort, P., & Knottnerus, A. (2005). Symptoms of posttraumatic stress disorder after non-traumatic events: Evidence from an open population study. *British Journal of Psychiatry, 186*, 494–499.

Najavits, L. (2002). *Seeking safety: A treatment manual for PTSD and substance abuse.* New York: Guilford Press.

Najavits, L. M. & Hien, D. (2013). Helping vulnerable populations: A comprehensive review of the treatment outcome literature on substance use disorder and PTSD. *Journal of Clinical Psychology: In Session, 69*(5), 433–479.

Najavits, L. M., Weiss, R. D., & Shaw, S. R. (1999). A clinical profile of women with PTSD and substance dependence. *Psychology of Addictive Behaviors, 13*, 98–104.

National Child Traumatic Stress Network (NCSTN). (2008). *Making the connection: Trauma and substance abuse; understanding the links between adolescent trauma and substance abuse.*

National Institute for Clinical Excellence. (2005). *Post traumatic stress disorder (PTSD): The management of adults and children in primary and secondary care.* London: NICE Guidelines.

National Institute of Justice. (2006). *Drug courts: The second decade.* U.S. Dept of Justice, Office of Justice Programs.

Ouimette, P., & Brown, P. (Eds.). (2003). *Trauma and substance abuse: Causes, consequences and treatment of comorbid disorders.* Washington: American Psychological Association.

Pallanti, S. (2006). From impulse-control disorders toward behavioral addictions. *CNS Spectrum, 11*(12), 921–922.

Perry, B. (1999). Memories of fear: How the brain stores and retrieves physiologic states, feelings, behaviors and thoughts from traumatic events. In J. Goodwin & R. Attias (Eds.), *Splintered reflections: Images of the body in trauma.* New York: Basic Books.

Popky, A. J. (2005). Desensitization of triggers and urge reprocessing; 1998 (DeTUR). In R. Shapiro (Ed.), *EMDR solutions, Chapter 7.* W.W. Norton.

Power, K. G., McGoldrick, T., Brown, K., et al. (2002). A controlled comparison of eye movement desensitization and reprocessing versus exposure plus cognitive restructuring, versus waiting list in the treatment of post-traumatic stress disorder. *Journal of Clinical Psychology and Psychotherapy, 9*, 299–318.

Prochaska, J., & DiClemente, C. (1983). Stages and processes of self-change of smoking: Toward an integrative model of change. *Journal of Consulting and Clinical Psychology, 51*, 390–395.

Ricci, R. J. (2006). Trauma resolution using Eye Movement Desensitization and Reprocessing with an incestuous sex offender. *Clinical Case Studies, 5*(3), 248–265.

Ricci, R. J., Clayton, C. A., & Shapiro, F. (2006). Some effects of EMDR on previously abused child molesters: Theoretical reviews and preliminary findings. *The Journal of Forensic Psychiatry and Psychology, 17*(4), 538–562.

Rothbaum, B. (1997). A controlled study of eye movement desensitization and reprocessing in the treatment of post-traumatic stress disordered sexual assault victims. *Bulletin of the Menninger Clinic, 61*, 317–334.

Russell, M. C. (2008). Treating traumatic amputation-related phantom limb pain: A case study utilizing eye movement desensitization and reprocessing within the Armed Services. *Clinical Case Studies, 7*(2), 136–153.

Schneider, J., Hofmann, A., Rost, C., & Shapiro, F. (2007). EMDR and phantom limb pain: Theoretical implications, case study, and treatment guidelines. *Journal of EMDR Practice and Research, 1*(1), 31–45.

Schore, A. (2002). Dysregulation of the right brain: A fundamental mechanism of traumatic attachment and the psychopathogensis of posttraumatic stress disorder. *Australian and New Zealand Journal of Psychiatry, 36*, 9–30.

Schurmans, K. (2007). A clinical vignette: EMDR treatment of choking phobia. *Journal of EMDR Practice and Research, 1*(2), 118–121.

Shapiro, F. (1995). *Eye movement desensitization and reprocessing: Basic principles, protocols, and procedures*. New York: Guilford Press.

Shapiro, F. (2001). *Eye movement desensitization and reprocessing: Basic principles, protocols and procedures*, (2nd edn). New York: Guilford Press.

Shapiro, F. (2005). *Eye movement desensitization and reprocessing (EMDR) training manual*. Watsonville, CA: EMDR Institute.

Shapiro, F. (2007a). EMDR, adaptive information processing, and case conceptualization. In F. Shapiro, F. Kaslow, & L. Maxfield (Eds.), *Handbook of EMDR and family therapy processes*. New York: Wiley.

Shapiro, F. (2007b). EMDR, adaptive information processing, and case conceptualization. *Journal of EMDR Practice and Research, 1*, 68–87.

Shapiro, F. (2014). The role of eye movement desensitization & reprocessing (EMDR) therapy in medicine: Addressing the psychological and physical symptoms stemming from adverse life experiences. *The Permanente Journal, 18*, 71–77.

Shapiro, F., Vogelmann-Sine, S., & Sine, L. F. (1994). Eye movement desensitization and reprocessing: Treating trauma and substance abuse. *Journal of Psychoactive Drugs, 26*(4), 379–391.

Siegel, D. (1999). *The developing mind: Toward a neurobiology of interpersonal experience*. New York & London: The Guilford Press.

Solomon, R., & Shapiro, F. (2008). EMDR and the adaptive information processing model: Potential mechanisms of change. *Journal of EMDR Practice and Research, 2*, 315–325.

Steward, S. H., & Conrod, P. J. (2003). Psychosocial models of functional associations between posttraumatic stress disorder and substance use disorder. In P. Ouimette & P. Brown (Eds.), *Trauma and substance Abuse: Causes, consequences, and treatment of comorbid disorders*. Washington, DC: APA.

Stickgold, R. (2002). EMDR: A putative neurobiological mechanism of action. *Journal of Clinical Psychology, 58*, 61–75.

Stowasser, J. (2007). EMDR and family therapy in the treatment of domestic violence. In F. Kaslow, F. Shapiro, & L. Maxfield (Eds.), *The integration of EMDR and family therapy processes*. New York: Wiley.

Substance Abuse and Mental Health Services Administration (SAMHSA). (2005). *Substance Abuse treatment for persons with co-occurring disorders. Treatment improvement protocol*

(TIP) series 42. Center for Substance Abuse Treatment. U.S. D HHS Publication No. (SMA) 05-3922.

Sun, T. F., & Chiu, N. M. (2006). Synergism between mindfulness meditation and eye movement desensitization and reprocessing in psychotherapy of social phobia. *Chang Gung Medical Journal, 29*(4), 1–4.

Tinker, R. H., & Wilson, S. A. (2005). The phantom limb pain protocol. In R. Shapiro (Ed.), *EMDR solutions: Pathways to healing* (pp. 147–159). New York: W W Norton & Co.

Van der Kolk, B., Pelcovitz, D., Roth, S., Mandel, F., McFarlane, A., & Herman, J. (1996). Dissociation, affect dysregulation and somatization: The complex nature of adaptation to trauma. *American Journal of Psychiatry, 153*(7), Festschrigt Supplement, 83–93.

Van Etten, M. L., & Taylor, S. (1998). Comparative efficacy of treatments for posttraumatic stress disorder: A meta-analysis. *Clinical Psychology & Psychotherapy, 5*, 126–144.

Vogelmann-Sinn, S., Sine, L. F., Smyth, N. J., & Popky, A. J. (1998). *EMDR chemical dependency treatment manual.* New Hope, PA: EMDR Humanitarian Assistance Programs.

Volkow, N. (2007). *Addiction and the brain's pleasure pathway: Beyond willpower.* The addiction project; 2007. http://www.addictioninfo.org/articles/1376/1/Addiction-and-the-Brains-Pleasure-Pathway-Beyond-Willpower/Page1.html

Whisman, M. (1997). An integrative treatment of panic disorder and OCD. In *Proceedings of the EMDR international association annual conference.* San Francisco, CA.

Whisman, M., & Keller, M. (1999). Integrating EMDR in the treatment of obsessive-compulsive disorder. In *Proceedings of the EMDR international association annual conference.* Las Vegas, NV.

Wilensky, M. (2006). Eye movement desensitization and reprocessing (EMDR) as a treatment for phantom limb pain. *Journal of Brief Therapy, 5*(1), 31–44.

Wolpe, J. (1969). *The practice of behavior therapy.* New York: Pergamon Press.

World Health Organization. (2004). *Neuroscience of psychoactive substance use and dependence.* Geneva: WHO Library.

World Health Organization. (2013). *Guidelines for the management of conditions that are specifically related to stress.* Geneva: WHO.

Zweben, J., & Yeary, J. (2006). EMDR in the treatment of addiction. Co-published simultaneously. *Journal of Chemical Dependency Treatment: Psychological Trauma and Addiction Treatment, 8*(2), 115–127 (editor: Bruce Carruth). Philadelphia: The Haworth Press.

Chapter 6
Mindfulness and Substance Abuse

Elisa Harumi Kozasa, Isabel Cristina Weiss de Souza,
Víviam Vargas de Barros and Ana Regina Noto

Introduction

Metacognition, or *cognition about cognition*, one of our highest brain functions, involves attention, conflict solving, error correction, inhibitory control, and emotional regulation being therefore fundamental in learning processes. These aspects of cognition are presumably mediated by frontal brain areas (Shimamura 2000). By contributing to the development of awareness of one's own thoughts and actions, mindfulness practices (full awareness or attention) are related to the development of the ability of metacognition. According to Baer (2003), mindfulness practices are those in which the subject becomes intentionally attentive to the internal and external experiences that are happening in the present moment, without judgment. There have been several researches in this area that suggest such practices lead subjects to a state of aware observation of their own perceptions, rather than being dragged by the turmoil of their emotions and thoughts.

Consequently, mindfulness practices represent an instrument of subjective investigation and monitoring of experiences that serves as an interesting resource

E.H. Kozasa
Neurociências, Hospital Israelita Albert Einstein, Av. Albert Einstein,
627/701- Bloco A- 2o Subsolo (Sala de Pesquisadores), São Paulo
SP 05601-901, Brazil
e-mail: ehkozasa@gmail.com

I.C.W. de Souza · V.V. de Barros · A.R. Noto (✉)
Departamento de Psicobiologia, Universidade Federal de São Paulo, Rua Botucatu,
862 - 1° Andar, Edifício de Ciências Biomédicas, São Paulo, SP 04023-062, Brazil
e-mail: anareginanoto@gmail.com; ana.noto@unifesp.br

I.C.W. de Souza
e-mail: isabel.weiss8@gmail.com

V.V. de Barros
e-mail: viviamvb@yahoo.com.br

© Springer International Publishing Switzerland 2016
A.L.M. Andrade and D. De Micheli (eds.), *Innovations in the Treatment
of Substance Addiction*, DOI 10.1007/978-3-319-43172-7_6

for self-care and self-knowledge. Various studies that will be dealt with in this chapter have explored its potential in the promotion of health as well as in the treatment of physical and mental illnesses.

There is, however, certain difficulty to understand the meaning of mindfulness, since its original concept in Buddhism does not correspond to that used in psychology and Western medicine. Moreover, the term has been used as a construct, a mental state, and a number of practices devised to help individuals reach that state (Chiesa and Malinowski 2011).

The word *mindfulness* originates from the word *sati*, from the Pali language of the ancient Buddhist texts. A literal translation of *sati* would be *remembering*. *Remembering*, in this case, refers to *remembering the object of one's attention*, which can be one's own breathing, or mental and emotional processes, or even the landscape observed during a walk. Developing this ability to remember the object of one's attention and, when one perceives himself/herself distracted, returning to it, prevents the mind from entering a process of rumination or anxiety and promotes mental stillness. This might lead to a state of mental presence which, in turn, leads the practitioner to see internal and external phenomena as they really are (Analayo 2006). Meditation practices are recommended for the development of this state of mental presence. This component of memory or recollection is not often mentioned in the *modern* definitions of mindfulness.

Jon Kabat-Zinn proposed one of them and developed the first mindfulness-based program, the *Mindfulness-Based Stress Reduction* (MBSR): "paying attention in a specific, purposeful way, to the present moment, and without judgement" (Kabat-Zinn 1994, p. 4). When he proposed MBSR, he did it as an attempt to integrate the Buddhist philosophy and the practice of the Mahayana and Theravada traditions with the psychology and medical practice of the West in a secular format, that is, not religious. It is worth remembering that Kabat-Zinn has never been a scholar in Buddhist texts, which might have contributed to a certain diversity regarding the concept of mindfulness in the West, when compared to the original meaning from the texts in Pali.

Bishop et al. (2004), by operationalizing the definition of Kabat-Zinn, suggest that mindfulness should be considered a particular form of focus attention, characterized by a component that involves self-regulation of attention to the present moment, while a second component would concern the adoption of an orientation marked by curiosity, opening, and acceptance. The first component would be related to a mental state or ability that emerges when the individual purposefully focuses his/her attention on the experiences of the present moment, and the second component takes into account the personality characteristics underlying the tendencies to be mindful.

There is no consensus as to how to measure mindfulness. The Mindful Attention Awareness Scale (MAAS), devised by Brown and Ryan (2003), measures mindfulness as a trait and has a single main component, which is attention/awareness focused on the present moment. In another example, Baer et al. (2006) combining different scales to measure mindfulness, propose the *Five Facets Mindfulness*

Questionnaire (FFMQ), in which they identify non-reactivity, observation, action with awareness, description, and non-judgment as its components (Baer et al. 2008).

There is, however, no consensus as regards the concept of mindfulness. The component *sustained attention to the present moment* is the one most authors agree on. As regards other components, such as non-reactivity and non-judgment, there is no consensus. For example, non-reactivity to a situation, or even non-judgment to it, might be considered characteristics related to an undesirable level of awareness and mental clarity, which would reflect a lower level of mindfulness. Non-reactivity, when considered as avoidance of automatic responses, might be an important ability to be developed, as well as not judging or labeling people or situations instantly. Those aspects, on the other hand, are not qualities per se without the maturity required for one to have discernment.

General Physiological Effects and Clinical Applications of Mindfulness Practices

If we consider the component *sustained attention to the present moment*, several meditative practices involve mindfulness. Wallace (1970) published a pioneer study in a journal of high impact factor. The meditative state evaluated in that study was induced by the practice of transcendental meditation, in which the focus of attention is a mantra. As a result of the practice, participants developed a differentiated state of awareness that would be responsible for several metabolic alterations, such as the reduction of oxygen consumption, increase in galvanic skin resistance, increase in the intensity of alpha waves, and occasional increase in the activity of theta waves (Wallace 1970).

As years went by, researchers realized that meditation techniques seemed to contribute to the treatment of cardiovascular problems in patients with coronary disorders (Zamarra et al. 1996) and hypertension (Wallace et al. 1983), for example. There are also reports on regulatory processes of hormone and neurotransmitter levels that might be associated with such practices (Stefano et al. 2006). Improvements in immune responses have been associated with the practice of mindfulness as well (Davidson et al. 2003).

From the perspective of mental health, meditation techniques that help foster the mindfulness state are used so that individuals can develop distancing from thoughts and emotions, recognizing them simply as mental events. Through the training of mindfulness practice, people develop skills to reduce their identification with thoughts and emotions during stressful events, rather than engaging in anxious concerns or other negative thought patterns that might be the beginning of a cycle of reactivity to stress and contribute to increase it (Teasdale et al. 1995, 2000).

Practitioners go through different phases that include the development of the ability to keep their attention sustained, observe their thoughts and emotions without identifying with them, and observe both the adequate thoughts and the non-adaptive ones the moment they emerge and disappear, as well as their triggers and consequences (Rapgay and Bystrisky 2009).

As a result, there is a decrease in negative affects and an increase in positive affects, as well as improvement in subjective well being (Schroevers and Brandsma 2010). As regards depression, mindfulness-based interventions have presented great efficacy concerning relapse prevention (Segal et al. 2010). Those interventions are also effective in the treatment of bipolar disorder (Weber et al. 2010), chronic pain (Morone et al. 2008), and insomnia (Gross et al. 2011).

Neurobiology of Mindfulness Practices

Functional neuroimaging techniques opened up new possibilities for the investigation of meditative states, as in the study of Newberg and Iversen (2003). In spite of the scanty publications in the literature when their study was published, those authors proposed a hypothesis on their possible neural mechanism. According to them, there is the activation of the pre-frontal cortex, along with that of the cingulate gyrus, due to the need for the individuals to willingly focus their attention during the process.

Brefczynski-Lewis et al. (2007), in a study with functional magnetic resonance, compared experienced meditators (Tibetan monks) with novices. They observed that those who had practiced it for a long time presented higher activity in several regions associated with attention, such as the frontoparietal, cerebellar, temporal, parahippocampal, and posterior occipital cortex during the practice of meditation with focused attention. The novices, on the other hand, presented higher activation in the medial frontal gyrus, anterior cingulate, and insula in its right medial to posterior region, areas that are negatively correlated with the performance in tasks of sustained attention.

In another study comparing the two types of meditators, the authors observed a higher increase in the electric activity in the left pre-frontal cortex, a higher proportion of gamma waves, and synchrony of the brain hemispheres of very experienced meditators than of novices (Lutz et al. 2004).

Lazar et al. (2005) observed that the cortical thickness in the pre-frontal areas and the right anterior insula (regions associated with attention, introception, and sensory processing) of individuals who had been practicing meditation for at least 10 years, about 40 min a day (insight meditation, which involves focused attention to internal perceptions) is higher than that in non-practitioners. Such differences were more pronounced in elderly individuals, and the thickness correlated with the time they had been practicing meditation.

Kozasa et al. (2012) compared the performance of individuals who practiced meditation regularly (three times a week for at least three years) with individuals who did not. Those researchers used the *Stroop Word-Color Task*, a test of attention and impulse control that was applied during a magnetic resonance imaging exam. Even though all the participants had a high educational level, it was possible to observe that those who did not meditate showed higher activity than the meditators in the frontal medial, temporal medial, pre-central and post-central gyri, and the lentiform nucleus during the incongruent condition. This task is the most complex one, in which the word *blue*, for instance, is printed in red, and the individual is supposed to choose the color. In the same experiment, no other regions were more activated in meditators than in non-meditators, which suggest that meditators might be more efficient in tasks that require sustained attention and impulse control. Regarding those abilities, mindfulness practices might contribute in the treatment of drug abuse.

Mindfulness and Craving

Drug dependence is constantly characterized as a chronic condition that entails several relapses (Leshner 1999). Relapse is a great challenge in the treatment of behavioral disorders in general. According to the original model of relapse prevention (RP), proposed by Marlatt and Donovan (2009, p. 16), it is a "return to the target behavior in the patterns presented prior to treatment." It differs from lapse, which is "a brief return to the target behavior."

Several strategies for relapse prevention based on the cognitive-behavioral model have been largely used in randomized clinical trials (Hajek et al. 2009). That model focuses on the individual's response to a risk situation, which can be related to an intrapersonal factor (affections, coping with problems, self-efficacy, expectation of results) of factors related to the external environment (social influences, access to substance, exposure to triggers) (Marlatt and Donovan 2009).

The idea is that if the individuals lack the resources that comprise a coping response to a risk situation (low self-efficacy) (Bandura 1977), they become vulnerable to relapse. Using the drug or not, in that situation, will depend on the expectations they have regarding the expected effects of use (Marlatt and Donovan 2009).

When they give into a risk situation without using coping alternatives, they are considered to have become vulnerable to the "abstinence violation effect" (AVE), which generally entails feelings of guilt, shame, and weakening of their faith that they would be able to remain (affective components of AVE). However, this model considers that if the subjects attribute their lapse to internal factors over which they have no control, the risk of relapse increases. If they consider that lapse is related to external factors, on the other hand, the odds of a lapse decrease (cognitive attributions for AVE decrease) (Marlatt and Gordon 1985).

In this perspective, lapse can be understood as a learning experience that might help individuals better understand their vulnerable points, evaluating which resources they have available, and which ones they still have to develop and train to be able to deal with risk situations (Marlatt and Gordon 1985).

In order to facilitate understanding the concept of lapse, craving, and their implications, we are going to use the example of tobacco. The outcome measure considered appropriate for studies that involve the evaluation of treatments for tobacco dependence would be the complete absence of lapses within a period of 6 months after the treatment (Hajek et al. 2009). Therefore, becoming occasional smokers is not a valid option, since there is no evidence that the decrease in tobacco use, or even a strategy based on damage reduction, is safe to health (Marlatt and Donovan 2009). Moreover, studies show that 85 % of the lapses lead to relapse (Kenford et al. 1994).

Still regarding tobacco use, several treatment models might help promote its abstinence. The best known and tested ones are based on pharmacological treatments (such as nicotine replacement and the use of antidepressants) as well as behavioral and motivational approaches that aim at developing coping skills for risk situations. In spite of the relative success of those approaches, the rate of treatment dropout and relapses is still high. Additionally, the number of studies that test alternative approaches for the treatment is scanty (Instituto Nacional de Câncer 2004; Hajek et al. 2009; Zgierska et al. 2009). The success of those approaches is still modest, with abstinence rates in treatments based on the cognitive model ranging from 20 to 30 % in the last three decades (Fiore et al. 2008).

Some of the problems that lead to the low abstinence rate are relapse and craving. The concept of craving involves several affective, biological, and cognitive motivational factors. According to Witkiewitz et al. (2013), relapse can be understood as a subjective experience of urge to use a drug, often experienced as intrusive thoughts, an impulse to use, strong desire, with physical sensations, and other manifestations, with positive expectations as to the effect the drug might produce.

In the perspective of mindfulness, craving is an attempt of holding, keeping, or hindering the cognitive, affective, and physical experience. The practice of mindfulness includes observing craving without fighting against it, since it is considered a transient phenomenon, such as many others in our lives (Witkiewitz et al. 2013).

Several studies on craving and tobacco addiction are available and might greatly help understand this relation between both, not always a successful one. Craving is also an issue in other drugs abuse. Nevertheless, in this part of this chapter, we will focus on the impact of mindfulness-based practices among smokers only.

According to the literature, the best known risk factors for tobacco relapse are smoking triggers, strong emotions, stressful situations, addictive thoughts (for instance: *A cigarette would calm me down now!*), craving, and withdrawal symptoms (Davis et al. 2013).

It is widely recognized that the tobacco dependence trajectory is complex and that all the factors mentioned above are directly involved in relapse. As we mentioned before, there are several tested treatments to lead to smoking cessation. However, review articles point to a severe lack of studies, randomized clinical trials that are robust, and evaluate strategies that enable smokers to deal with smoking cues (Hajek et al. 2009).

A therapy based on the exposure to those stimuli (such as smell, sight, relevant situations) aims at minimizing the link between the triggers and the conditioned response to use the drug, allowing drug dependents to put in practice their coping skills when facing triggers. This type of therapy, known as exposure therapy, yields relative success in the prevention of relapse to other drugs. Yet, the same is not true as regards smoking cessation (Niaura et al. 1999). Only the use of nicotine gum seems to promote some relief in the face of exposure to stimuli that trigger craving (cue-induced craving), but the substitution of cigarette for gum helps keep the link with the addictive behavior, rather than extinguish it (Brewer et al. 2013).

The reinforcing properties of nicotine might be positive (i.e., enhancement of concentration and attention, appetite reduction to keep low weight) or negative (i.e., relief of aversive states as abstinence, reduction of anxiety and sadness). Those reinforcing conditions end up creating memories. Consequently, stimuli that trigger those affective states become associated with the act of smoking, which in turn induces to cigarette craving (Brewer et al. 2013; Elwafi et al. 2013).

We might say that craving is the end of this chain of conditioning, being considered as a broader concept and at the same time the least understood in the studies on drug dependence. It may even be considered the central idea for one to understand the process of drug dependence and the greatest obstacle for individuals with drug addiction to remain abstinent (Robinson and Berridge 1993). This is the reason why we chose to emphasize this issue in this chapter.

Treatments that focus on craving control can certainly offer a major contribution to reduce relapse, since craving and negative affects are predictors of such event. Behavioral-based treatments available so far address the factors associated with craving without treating craving itself (Elwafi et al. 2013).

Recent evidence shows that mindfulness-based treatments can act on the interface between the stimulus and the response (Brewer et al. 2013), since it helps practitioners regulate attention, increase body awareness, regulate affects, and change perspective of themselves. Body awareness detects signs of emotional responses to stimuli. The process of emotional regulation, sustained by the maintenance of full attention, helps prevent the occurrence of habitual and hyperlearned responses. With training and time, this might eventually result in the extinction of those responses and in the prevention of relapses of maladaptive behaviors, as in drug use (Bowen et al. 2014; Penberthy et al. 2013).

In short, craving takes place as a result of affective reactions triggered by a perceived stimulus. When the senses register environmental stimuli, an affective reaction arises and is immediately perceived as pleasant or unpleasant. This experience is validated by the memory of previous experiences. Craving arises immediately, felt as intense, urgent, and uncontrollable. Therefore, the perception of an object is influenced by previous experiences and the formation of related memories strengthens the habit, which will provide a "registry" of what might function in the future, for example, when the individual is facing unpleasant situations ("I'll feel better if I smoke!"). Craving itself, as well as the sensations related to abstinence, is in the field of the unpleasant ones, and hence feed the process back (Brewer et al. 2013).

Craving is a key element for the understanding of some of the main evidence of how mindfulness might contribute to the treatment of dependence and other compulsive behaviors. According to Brewer et al. (2013), craving is perceived as an unpleasant sensation that pushes the individual to act (in order to relieve the ill being). Within this dynamics, the contribution of mindfulness consists of teaching the individual to explore the physical sensations associated with craving. With that observation, the individual learns two lessons: (1) that craving involves physical sensations and (2) that those sensations are transient. This apparently simple learning allows the individuals to coexist with those unpleasant physical sensations, without necessarily acting on them immediately (impulsively). The participants learn to pause ("give it some time") and not react immediately when facing craving. This pause is fundamental, since it helps disrupt the automatic associative process typical of dependence.

One of the main indicators that mindfulness practice might help individuals to dissociate dependence from craving is based on a study with smokers under treatment. Brewer et al. (2013) reported that when smokers started mindfulness practices, they showed a strong positive association between the daily mean number of cigarettes smoked and craving. Four weeks later, this correlation gradually decreased until it reached statistical nonsignificance. By the end of the treatment, those who had stopped smoking presented craving scores similar to those of the individuals who continued smoking. The difference between the two groups, however, was observed in the subsequent weeks. Those who had quit smoking presented craving decrease, while those who had continued smoking presented increase. That study not only shows the potential impact of mindfulness on craving, but the way through which the relation between craving and dependence is established as well (Brewer et al. 2013).

More recently, the role of craving and negative affects on relapse to drug use has also been studied in the context of neurobiology. A review study endorses the view that mindfulness might affect brain systems related to craving, thus contributing to the decrease in reactivity to the stimuli associated with it. Considering the decrease in the activation of the areas in the pre-frontal region involved in top-down processing, one might suggest that mindfulness allows the individual to operate in the bottom-up processing in the event of craving, based essentially on sensory information, as opposed to previous contextualization (top down). This in turn might favor the exploration of the craving experience in a different way, reducing the reactivity to stressing stimuli (Witkiewitz et al. 2013).

The same review (Witkiewitz et al. 2013) mentions studies involving specifically the protocol of Mindfulness-based Relapse Prevention (Bowen et al. 2011), where the authors found suggestive results that corroborate those mentioned above (Brewer et al. 2009; Lustyk 2012), and confirming the decrease in the reactivity to stimuli associated with craving (Westbrook et al. 2013).

The effects of mindfulness-based treatments in the medium- and long-term show that participants in clinical trials broaden their skills to recognize and tolerate the discomfort associated with craving and negative affects, defusing the automatic response to use the drug. This improvement takes place as the patients get in touch with the discomfort but engage in a non-judging perspective of their physical, affective, and cognitive experience, and in the acceptance of their craving state rather than automatically or simply avoiding the experience. Through repeated experiences of exposure and non-reaction, the patients develop a new repertoire of responses to those stimuli that they previously felt indefensible (Bowen et al. 2014; Witkiewitz et al. 2013).

The techniques based on mindfulness meditation integrate the practices of cognitive-behavioral therapy and mindfulness. They are consistent with them in several aspects, namely they help patients develop self-handling and facilitate their process of sustaining exposure to unpleasant sensations, thoughts, and emotions, which results in desensitization to conditioned responses, as in the case of drug use (Baer 2003).

Interventions that foster acceptance and broaden awareness help patients develop a non-judging attitude about their experiences, thus increasing their repertoire of action when facing the phenomenon of craving. We will now present studies that involve mindfulness practices in the prevention of relapse to drug use.

Scientific Evidence of Mindfulness-Based Interventions for Substance Use and Abuse

In the 1970s, encouraged by positive results of meditation for mental health, Marlatt and Marques (1977) and Marlatt (2002) began to explore this possibility among alcohol users. The results they observed were promising and provided the foundation for subsequent randomized and more robust studies. The first studies were performed using relaxation techniques (transcendental meditation) and, later on, evolved to studies with mindfulness meditation (Marlatt et al. 1984; Marlatt 2002).

Almost two decades later, Breslin et al. (2002), in a review of the scientific literature on the theory and cognitive treatment of substance dependence, reinforced that idea by concluding that there is strong scientific basis to understand the potential benefits of mindfulness meditation in the treatment of dependences, especially as a complementary strategy for relapse reduction. As reported by the authors, even though the use of meditation for the treatment of such problems is not a novel idea, several studies presented theoretical and methodological limitations. More recent studies evolved, as those by Bowen et al. (2014), mainly anchored in cognitive-behavioral therapy (Breslin et al. 2002).

Several limitations remain to be overcome. As regards tobacco dependence, for instance, most of the researches comprised small samples; often had no control group, and used a very short follow-up time, no longer than 4 months. Many are based on the MBSR, not specifically for relapse prevention—MBRP (Vidrine et al. 2009).

In spite of the limitations, the number of scientific studies that involve the use of mindfulness-based interventions has grown exponentially in the last decade (Black 2014). An interesting point is that this growth came along with improvement in the quality of the studies with respect to longer follow-ups, larger samples and studies that compare them with interventions considered gold standard, such as cognitive therapy and relapse prevention. Those comparisons allow researchers to identify and describe the specific contribution of mindfulness more clearly, beyond what had already been achieved by other interventions. This evolution in research has also facilitated the comprehension of the possible mechanisms of interventions involved in the recovery of substance users, as well as in the prevention of relapse. In order to make it possible for the reader to understand this evolution in the researches, we should go on to a brief history on the applicability of mindfulness-based interventions for the treatment of substance use.

As mentioned previously, Alan Marlatt was the pioneer in the studies on meditation and the use of drugs. His great motivation was his own personal contact with the Buddhist philosophy and his curiosity about how this philosophy might help in the definition of the mechanisms of addictive behaviors in general, more specifically substance use. Therefore, it would be essential to understand how the mind works and how thoughts and expectations might both facilitate and reduce the occurrence of addictive behaviors (Marlatt 2002).

For that purpose, before creating the protocol of *Mindfulness-Based Relapse Prevention*, Marlatt (2002) started a contextualization of drug use (or addictive behaviors), from the perspective of the Buddhist philosophy. It states that those behaviors are a *false refuge*, since they are motivated by a strong wish or craving that aims at alleviating suffering (in the short term), even though the continuous engagement in those behaviors increases the pain and suffering. In this sense, people learn and rely on this strategy that supply them with a *refuge* and tend to resort to it more frequently so as to anticipate some relief to a potential suffering. Cognitive therapy defines this behavior as craving. By making use of those strategies, people would become less skilled in the presence of discomfort, reinforcing the belief that they have to do something to free themselves from this suffering, hence keeping this vicious circle.

Following this line of thought, the attitude of acceptance and the metacognitive skill to observe how the mind works, that is, how thoughts are linked to emotions and, consequently, to behaviors, and to recognize the impermanence of things, developed by meditation practices, might provide instruments for individuals to recognize triggers and how their minds react to them. This strategy would help them break the vicious circle and favor their release from the suffering that, in the case of drug use, could refer to negative mood states, craving or uncomfortable sensations generated by the drug abstinence. For this reason, the objective of mindfulness practice would not be to change the individuals' thought, as in the cognitive-behavioral therapy (CBT), but rather to allow them to develop a different attitude or relation regarding thoughts and emotions as they spring to mind. From this perspective, the concept is that, instead of *sick* and *handicapped*, individuals are seen as having the ability to choose and being responsible for their own actions. The focus of this practice is to foster more skilled mental states and behaviors that in turn generate well being (Marlatt 2002).

After this integration of the Buddhist concepts and mindfulness practices to the psychological model of addiction, Witkiewitz et al. (2005) published a study in which they described the components of relapse prevention, the mechanisms of change according to CBT and made a brief introduction of MBRP, with preliminary empiric results, highlighting the efficacy of this new approach for addictive behaviors.

Those results regard a training in Vipassana meditation among an incarcerated male population who had a history of heavy use of alcohol and other drugs. Even though the results were preliminary and presented a series of limitations due to the great loss of participants during the study, the results were the starting point for the creation of MBRP. In that study, they observed that self-monitoring in itself did not guarantee the development of self-regulation skills, and consequently of the components which are the basis of the mindfulness concept, as the focus on the present, the acceptance, and the non-judgment (Witkiewitz et al. 2005).

With the promising results of that first study in the penitentiary, Marlatt and his team enlarged the study. They continued comparing the Vipassana course with other usual treatments, such as the 12 steps and psychoeducation. However, that time they included female participants and increased the follow-up time to 6 months after participants had finished the Vipassana course. The results showed that after being released from prison, the participants presented more significant reductions in their use of alcohol, marijuana, and cocaine/crack than their control counterparts. Moreover, those participants reported fewer alcohol-related problems and psychiatric symptoms and had significant increase in positive psychosocial measures, such as optimism and locus of control in the use of drugs (Bowen et al. 2006).

As to the efficacy and effectiveness of the MBRP protocol specifically, two special studies deserve attention and illustrate the evolution of the studies in that area. The first was a pilot study, and the first randomized clinical trial that tested the viability and the efficacy of MBRP, in comparison with conventional treatment. The study comprised 168 participants, mostly males (64 %), users of various types of drugs: alcohol (46 %); cocaine/crack (26 %); methamphetamine (14 %); heroin/opioids (7 %); marijuana (5 %); and others (2 %), who had undergone at least 1 month of treatment for drug use, either inpatient or intensive outpatient treatment. Important data about the sample are that they had average school level, up to high school (71 %), and most of them were unemployed. They received some government benefit or less than $500.00 a month, had unstable housing conditions, or no housing (Bowen et al. 2009).

All the measures were taken before the beginning of interventions, immediately after them, and 2 and 4 months after they ended. The experimental group received the MBRP protocol, and the control group received the usual maintenance treatment, mainly the 12 steps or psychoeducation, at the service where they had completed the treatment. The viability of the study was assessed by the performance of formal practices (4.74 days a week, approximately 30 min a day); activities meant to be performed between the sessions, participation in the sessions (65 %, Mean = 5.1 sessions, SD = 2.4), and satisfaction of the participants. The initial efficacy could be detected by the significantly lower rates of substance use in the experimental group in comparison with the control, a trend that remained until the 4-month follow-up. Additionally, the participants who received MBRP showed greater decrease in the intensity of craving, and increase in the ability to accept and act with awareness than the participants in the control group (Bowen et al. 2009).

In a subsequent study, the authors showed that craving mediated the relation between depressive symptoms and the use of substances in the group that received the usual treatment, but not in the group that received MBRP. Therefore, it is possible to assert that MBRP had attenuated the relation between post-intervention depressive symptoms and craving by the time of the 2-month follow-up. This moderating effect was an important predictor of substance use 4 months after the intervention. In other words, through the practice of mindfulness, the participants were able to change their responses to depressive symptoms, which in turn ceased to work as a potential trigger of craving, breaking the vicious circle among negative emotional states, craving and substance use (Witkiewitz and Bowen 2010).

The most recent and robust study that evaluated the efficacy of MBRP in relapse prevention and substance use was recently published in the *Journal of American Medical Association* (JAMA—Psychiatry). It aimed at comparing three groups: MBRP, the standard protocol of relapse prevention (RP) or treatment as usual (12 steps and psychoeducation), comprising 286 participants (Bowen et al. 2014). This study, similar to previous ones, comprised a predominantly male population, multiple drug users (82 %), and low socioeconomic status. The major difference is that it included follow-ups of 2, 4, 6, and 12 months after the intervention and clarified very important points in the differentiation among interventions and possible mechanisms of change related to substance use (Bowen et al. 2014).

Their results showed that after 6 months of the end of intervention, both the group that received MBRP, and the RP group had a significantly lower mean number of days on which they had used the substances and made heavy use of alcohol than the group that received the usual treatment. The group that received RP had 21 % lower chances of relapse than the MBRP after 6 months. After 12 months, however, the group that received MBRP kept their relapse rates, number of days on which they used the drugs and episodes of heavy drinking at a level similar to that they showed after 6 months. Those values were therefore significantly lower than those in the groups of RP and treatment as usual, who increased significantly as of the sixth month. The MBRP group presented 31 % fewer days of drug use, and significantly lower odds of participants that did not engage in any episode of heavy drinking after the 12 months (Bowen et al. 2014).

However, what might have happened between the sixth and the twelfth months to cause this difference between the protocols? The authors argue that those differences might be accounted for by the skills the participants in the MBRP develop to recognize and experience discomfort associated with craving and negative affects. Moreover, the MBRP intervention integrates empirically tested approaches, such as CBT and mindfulness, to increase the awareness of individual and environmental events that might trigger relapse and alter the responses to craving and negative affects through the processes based on exposure, a reaction that is possible through the practices of mindfulness. The continuous practice over time strengthens one's ability to monitor and understand the factors that contribute to the individual well being, which gives support to longer term results (Bowen et al. 2014).

Even though so far we have endeavored to better explore MBRP, there is a wide range of studies that used other mindfulness-based interventions that show positive results in the treatment of substance use.

We will now explore the main findings of two systematic reviews that aimed at evaluating the application and effectiveness of these interventions for substance use.

The first was carried out in 2009 and included 25 articles that contain randomized clinical trials, non-randomized controlled studies, case studies, and other qualitative studies. There was no standardization of the mindfulness-based interventions used in those studies. Consequently, the authors included both studies that really are based on the practices of mindfulness, such as *Mindfulness-Based Stress Reduction* (MBSR) and Vipassana, and other interventions that used components of mindfulness, but are based on therapy, other concepts, as the *Acceptance and Commitment Therapy* (ACT) and *Dialectical Behavior Therapy* (DBT). The studies show that even though there was evidence on the safety and efficacy of those interventions for the treatment of substance use, there was still lack of more robust evidence, since methodological problems were detected in most of the studies. Those problems were identified precisely because they are a field in which studies are still in a preliminary phase, and the systematization of their methodologies is still in its early stages. The main limitations found then were very small samples (most were pilot studies) and very heterogeneous populations, which made it difficult for researchers to safely establish what type of users might benefit from mindfulness-based interventions. In addition, it was not possible to establish which mindfulness mechanisms would be involved in the behavior change, neither to evaluating the effect size of the interventions (Zgierska et al. 2009).

The second review was published more recently, and once 5 years had gone by since the previous one, the studies grew progressively, and the authors managed to focus only on clinical trials and those that had actually used mindfulness-based interventions for the treatment of substance use (Chiesa and Serretti 2014).

That review included 24 studies, and its main results are that mindfulness-based interventions promote a reduction in the use of several substances (alcohol, marijuana, cocaine, opioids amphetamines, and tobacco), in a significantly better way than in the control groups (waiting list, psychoeducation, and other interventions). It also showed that structural changes in the brain and the activation of brain areas are associated with the reduction of ruminative thoughts which, in turn, reduces the odds of relapse. Another important finding was that the participants who received mindfulness increased their ability to reduce reactivity to stimuli related to craving (Chiesa and Serretti 2014).

Although the quality of the evidence greatly improved between the two reviews, Chiesa and Serretti (2014) still point to severe limitations that must be addressed in future studies. Some of them are larger samples, a more detailed description of the study and intervention methodology, strategies to keep adherence of participants to the protocol, longer follow-ups, and better structured measures of both mindfulness and the use of substances.

There is evidence that mindfulness may be effective in the treatment of compulsive behaviors other than drug use. Spinella et al. (2013) evaluated, in a community sample, the relation between the components of mindfulness and several compulsive behaviors, such as alcohol abuse, pathological gambling, compulsive shopping, and sexual behavior. They observed inverse correlations between the "non-judging attitude" and alcohol abuse, compulsive sex and pathological gambling. Compulsive shopping presented an inverse relation with *acting with awareness*. Their results suggest that mindfulness might be useful in the treatment of substance abuse as well as other compulsive behaviors (Spinella et al. 2013).

Finally, mindfulness practices seem to be a very promising tool in the treatment of drug dependency and substance abuse, offering resources for individuals with addictive behavior to take a leading role in their own prevention process and impulse management.

References

Analayo, V. (2006). Mindfulness in the Pali Nikayas. In D. K. Nauriyal, D. K. Drummond, & Y. B. Lal (Eds.), *Buddhist thought and applied psychological research: Transcending the boundaries* (pp. 229–249). London: Routledge.

Baer, R. A. (2003). Mindfulness training as a clinical intervention: A conceptual and empirical review. *Clinical Psychology: Science and Practice, 10*(2), 125–143.

Baer, R. A., Smith, G. T., Hopkins, J., Krietemeyer, J., & Toney, L. (2006). Using self-report assessment methods to explore facets of mindfulness. *Assessment, 13*(1), 27–45.

Baer, R. A., Smith, G. T., Lykins, E., Button, D., Krietemeyer, J., Sauer, S., et al. (2008). Construct validity of the five facets mindfulness questionnaire in meditating and nonmeditating samples. *Assessment, 15*(3), 329–342.

Bandura, A. (1977). Self-efficacy: Toward a unifying theory of behavioral change. *Psychological Review, 84*(2), 191–215.

Bishop, S. R., Lau, M., Shapiro, S., Carlson, L., Anderson, N. D., Carmody, J., et al. (2004). Mindfulness: A proposed operational definition. *Clinical Psychology, 11*(3), 230–241.

Black, D. S. (2014). Mindfulness-based interventions: An antidote to suffering in the context of substance use, misuse, and addiction. *Substance Use and Misuse, 49*(5), 487.

Bowen, S., Chawla, N., Collins, S. E., Witkiewitz, K., Hsu, S., Grow, J., et al. (2009). Mindfulness-based relapse prevention for substance use disorders: A pilot efficacy trial. *Substance Abuse, 30*(4), 295–305.

Bowen, S., Chawla, N., & Marlatt, G. A. (2011). *Mindfulness-based relapse prevention for addictive behaviors: A clinician's guide.* New York: The Guilford Press.

Bowen, S., Witkiewitz, K., Clifasefi, S. L., Grow, J., Chawla, N., Hsu, S. H., et al. (2014). Relative efficacy of mindfulness-based relapse prevention, standard relapse prevention, and treatment as usual for substance use disorders: A randomized clinical trial. *JAMA Psychiatry, 71*(5), 547–556.

Bowen, S., Witkiewitz, K., Dillworth, T. M., Chawla, N., Simpson, T. L., Ostafin, B. D., et al. (2006). Mindfulness meditation and substance use in an incarcerated population. *Psychology of Addictive Behaviors, 20*(3), 343–347.

Brefczynski-Lewis, J. A., Lutz, A., Schaefer, H. S., Levinson, D. B., & Davidson, R. (2007). Neural correlates of attentional expertise in long-term meditation practitioners. *Proceedings of the National Academy of Sciences of the United States of America, 104*(27), 11483–11488.

Breslin, F. C., Zack, M., & McMain, S. (2002). An information-processing analysis of mindfulness: Implications for relapse prevention in the treatment of substance abuse. *Clinical Psychology: Science and Practice, 9*(3), 275–299.

Brewer, J. A., Elwafi, H. M., & Davis, J. H. (2013). Craving to quit: Psychological models and neurobiological mechanisms of mindfulness training as treatment for addictions. *Psychology of Addictive Behaviors, 27*(2), 366–379.

Brewer, J. A., Sinha, R., Chen, J. A., Michalsen, R. N., Babuscio, T. A., Nich, C., et al. (2009). Mindfulness training and stress reactivity in substance abuse: Results from a randomized, controlled stage I pilot study. *Substance Abuse., 30*(4), 306–317.

Brown, K. W., & Ryan, R. M. (2003). The benefits of being present: The role of mindfulness in psychological well-being. *Journal of Personality and Social Psychology, 84*(4), 822–848.

Chiesa, A., & Malinowski, P. (2011). Mindfulness-based approaches: Are they all the same? *Journal of Clinical Psychology, 67*(4), 404–424.

Chiesa, A., & Serretti, A. (2014). Are mindfulness-based interventions effective for substance use disorders? A systematic review of the evidence. *Substance Use and Misuse, 49*(5), 492–512.

Davidson, R. J., Kabat-Zinn, J., Schumacher, J., Rosenkranz, M., Muller, D., Santorelli, S. F., et al. (2003). Alterations in brain and immune function produced by mindfulness meditation. *Psychosom Medicine, 65*(4), 564–570.

Davis, J. M., Mills, D. M., Stankevitz, K. A., Manley, A. R., Majeskie, M. R., & Smith, S. S. (2013). Pilot randomized trial on mindfulness training for smokers in young adult binge drinkers. *BMC Complementary and Alternative Medicine, 13*, 215.

Elwafi, H. M., Witkiewitz, K., Mallik, S., Thornhill, T. A, 4th, & Brewer, J. A. (2013). Mindfulness training for smoking cessation: Moderation of the relationship between craving and cigarette use. *Drug and Alcohol Dependence, 130*(1–3), 222–229.

Fiore, M., Jaén, C. R., Baker, T. B., Bailey, W. C., Bennett, G., Benowitz, N. L., et al. (2008). A clinical practice guideline for treating tobacco use and dependence: 2008. *American Journal of Preventive Medicine, 35*(2), 158–176.

Gross, C. R., Kreitzer, M. J., Reilly-Spong, M., Wall, M., Winbush, N. Y., Patterson, R., et al. (2011). Mindfulness-based stress reduction versus pharmacotherapy for chronic primary insomnia: A randomized controlled clinical trial. *Explore (NY), 7*(2), 76–87.

Hajek, P., Stead, L. F., West, R., Jarvis, M., & Lancaster, T. (2009). Relapse prevention interventions for smoking cessation. *The Cochrane Database of Systematic Reviews, 25*(1), CD003999.

Instituto Nacional de Câncer. (2004). *Deixando de fumar sem mistérios*. Rio de Janeiro: Ministério da Saúde.

Kabat-Zinn, J. (1994). *Wherever you go, there you are: Mindfulness meditation in everyday life.* New York: Hyperion.

Kenford, S. L., Fiore, M. C., Jorenby, D. E., Smith, S. S., Wetter, D., & Baker, T. B. (1994). Predicting smoking cessation: Who will quit with and without the nicotine path. *Journal of the American Medical Association, 271*(8), 589–594.

Kozasa, E. H., Sato, J. R., Lacerda, S. S., Barreiros, M. A., Radvany, J., Russell, T. A., et al. (2012). Meditation training increases brain efficiency in an attention task. *Neuroimage, 59*(1), 745–749.

Lazar, S. W., Kerr, C. E., Wasserman, R. H., Gray, J. R., Greve, D. N., Treadway, M. T., et al. (2005). Meditation experience is associated with increased cortical thickness. *NeuroReport, 16*(17), 1893–1897.

Leshner, A. I. (1999). Science is revolutionizing our view of addiction—and what to do about it. *American Journal of Psychiatry, 156*(1), 1–3.

Lustyk, M. K. B. (2012). *Hemodynamic response to a laboratory challenge in substance abusers treated with mindfulness-based relapse prevention.* Paper presented at the International Research Congress on Integrative Medicine and Health, Portland, OR.

Lutz, A., Greischar, L. L., Rawlings, N. B., Ricard, M., & Davidson, R. J. (2004). Long-term meditators self-induce high-amplitude gamma synchrony during mental practice. *Proceedings of the National Academy of Sciences of the United States of America. 101*(46), 16369–16373.

Marlatt, G. A. (2002). Buddhist philosophy and the treatment of addictive behavior. *Cognitive and Behavioral Practice, 9*(1), 44–50.

Marlatt, G. A., & Donovan, D. M. (2009). *Prevenção de Recaída: estratégias de manutenção no tratamento de comportamentos aditivos*. Porto Alegre: Artmed.

Marlatt, G. A., & Gordon, J. R. (Eds.). (1985). *Relapse prevention: Maintenance strategies in the treatment of addictive behaviors*. New York: Guilford Press.

Marlatt, G. A., & Marques, J. K. (1977). Meditation, self-control, and alcohol use. In R. B. Stuart (Ed.), *Behavioral self-management: Strategies, techniques, and outcomes* (pp. 117–153). New York: Brunner/Mazel.

Marlatt, G. A., Pagano, R. R., Rose, R. M., & Marques, J. K. (1984). Effects of meditation and relaxation training upon alcohol use in male social drinkers. In D. H. Shapiro & R. N. Walsh (Eds.), *Meditation: Classic and contemporary perspectives* (pp. 105–120). New York: Aldine Press.

Morone, N. E., Lynch, C. S., Greco, C. M., Tindle, H. A., & Weiner, D. K. (2008). "I felt like a new person." The effects of mindfulness meditation on older adults with chronic pain: Qualitative narrative analysis of diary entries. *The Journal of Pain, 9*(9), 841–848.

Newberg, A. B., & Iversen, J. (2003). The neural basis of the complex mental task of meditation: Neurotransmitter and neurochemical considerations. *Medical Hypotheses, 61*(2), 282–291.

Niaura, R., Abrams, D. B., Shadel, W. G., Rohsenow, D. J., Monti, P. M., & Sirota, A. D. (1999). Cue exposure treatment for smoking relapse prevention: A controlled clinical trial. *Addiction, 94*(5), 685–695.

Penberthy, J. K., Konig, A., Gioia, C. J., Rodríguez, V. M., Starr, J. A., Meese, W. et al. (2013). Mindfulness-based relapse prevention: History, mechanisms of action, and effects. *Mindfulness*. Acesso em 00 de mês por extenso de 2014, em. http://link.springer.com/article/10.1007%2Fs12671-013-0239-1.

Rapgay, L., & Bystrisky, A. (2009). Classical mindfulness: An introduction to its theory and practice for clinical application. *Annals of the New York Academy of Sciences, 1172*(1), 148–162.

Robinson, T. E., & Berridge, K. C. (1993). The neural basis of drug craving: An incentive-sensation theory of addiction. *Brain Research Reviews, 18*(3), 247–291.

Schroevers, M. J., & Brandsma, R. (2010). Is learning mindfulness associated with improved affect after mindfulness-based cognitive therapy? *British Journal of Psychology, 101*(Pt 1), 95–107.

Segal, Z. V., Bieling, P., Young, T., MacQueen, G., Cooke, R., Martin, L., et al. (2010). Antidepressant monotherapy vs sequential pharmacotherapy and mindfulness-based cognitive therapy, or placebo, for relapse prophylaxis in recurrent depression. *Archives of General Psychiatry, 67*(12), 1256–1264.

Shimamura, A. P. (2000). Toward a cognitive neuroscience of metacognition. *Consciousness and Cognition, 9*(2 Pt 1), 313–323.

Spinella, M., Martino, S., & Ferri, C. (2013). Mindfulness and Addictive behaviors. *Journal of Behavioral Health, 2*(1), 1–7.

Stefano, G. D., Fricchione, G. L., & Esch, T. (2006). Relaxation: Molecular and physiological significance. *Medical Science Monitor, 12*(9), HY21–HY31.

Teasdale, J. D., Segal, Z. V., Williams, J. M. G., Ridgeway, V. A., Soulsby, J. M., & Lau, M. A. (2000). Prevention of relapse/recurrence in major depression by mindfulness-based cognitive therapy. *Journal of Consulting and Clinical Psychology, 68*(4), 615–623.

Teasdale, J. D., Segal, Z., Williams, J., & Mark, G. (1995). How does cognitive therapy prevent depressive relapse and why should attentional control (mindfulness) training help? *Behaviour Research and Therapy, 33*(1), 25–39.

Vidrine, J. I., Businelle, M. S., Cinciripini, P., Li, Y., Marcus, M. T., Waters, A. J., et al. (2009). Associations of mindfulness with nicotine dependence, withdrawal, and agency. *Substance Abuse: Official publication of the Association for Medical Education and Research in Substance Abuse, 30*(4), 318–327.

Wallace, R. K. (1970). Physiological effects of transcendental meditation. *Science, 167*(3926), 1751–1754.

Wallace, R. K., Silver, J., Mills, P. J., Dillbeck, M. C., & Wagoner, D. E. (1983). Systolic blood pressure and long-term practice of the transcendental meditation and TM-Sidhi program: Effects of TM on systolic blood pressure. *Psychosomatic Medicine, 45*(1), 41–46.

Weber, B., Jermann, F., Gex-Fabry, M., Nallet, A., Bondolfi, G., & Aubry, J. M. (2010). Mindfulness-based cognitive therapy for bipolar disorder: A feasibility trial. *European Psychiatry, 25*(6), 334–337.

Westbrook, C., Creswell, J. D., Tabibnia, G., Julson, E., Kober, H., & Tindle, H. A. (2013). Mindful attention reduces neural and self-reported cue-induced craving in smokers. *Social Cognitive and Affective Neuroscience, 8*(1), 73–84.

Witkiewitz, K., & Bowen, S. (2010). Depression, craving, and substance use following a randomized trial of mindfulness-based relapse prevention. *Journal of Consulting and Clinical Psychology, 78*(3), 362–374.

Witkiewitz, K., Bowen, S., Douglas, H., & Hsu, S. H. (2013a). Mindfulness-based relapse prevention for substance craving. *Addict Addictive behaviors, 38*(2), 1563–1571.

Witkiewitz, K., Bowen, S., & Lustyk, M. K. B. (2013b). Retraining the addicted brain: A review of the hypothesized neurobiological mechanisms of mindfulness-based relapse prevention. *Psychology of Addictive Behaviors, 27*(2), 351–365.

Witkiewitz, K., Marlatt, G. A., & Walker, D. (2005). Mindfulness-based relapse prevention for alcohol and substance use disorders. *Journal of Cognitive Psychotherapy: An International Quarterly, 19*, 211–228.

Zamarra, J. W., Schneider, R. H., Besseghini, I., Robinson, D. K., & Salerno, J. W. (1996). Usefulness of the transcendental meditation program in the treatment of patients with coronary artery disease. *The American Journal of Cardiology, 77*(10), 867–870.

Zgierska, A., Rabago, D., Chawla, N., Kushner, K., Koehler, R., & Marlatt, A. (2009). Mindfulness meditation for substance use disorders: A systematic review. *Substance Abuse, 30*(4), 266–294.

Chapter 7
Micro- and Macronutrients on Dependence

Juçara Xavier Zaparoli

Over the past decades, several studies have shown the role, effects, and importance of different nutrients, such as vitamins and other compounds in the proper functioning of our body. Some of these substances, such as omega-3 fatty acids, besides the fundamental role in the proper functioning of our organism, have been studied as tools for reduction of withdrawal symptoms and/or addiction treatment. Throughout this chapter, we will see some examples of nutrients with potential for this purpose.

Omega-3 Fatty Acids

The fatty acids have shown various functions such as storage and power generation, production of specific phospholipid and sphingolipid of the cell membrane (specific types of lipids found in cell membrane), and covalent modification of several regulatory proteins (Spector 1999).

Fatty acids can be saturated, monounsaturated, and polyunsaturated. Fatty acids can be nominated, besides the official name for organic chemistry compounds, using the omega format. On these cases, the numerals (e.g., n3, n6, and n9) indicate the position of double-bond carbon–carbon, counting from the methyl end of the chain.

Some of the most important polyunsaturated fatty acids (PUFAs) for our body are the linoleic acid (LA) and alpha-linolenic acid (ALA). These PUFAs are the precursors of two different series of fatty acids: omega-3 series, derived from ALA, and omega-6 derived from LA (Spector 1999; Haag 2003). The most abundant fatty acids

J.X. Zaparoli (✉)
Departamento de Psicobiologia, Universidade Federal de São Paulo, Rua Botucatu, 862 - 1° Andar, Edifício de Ciências Biomédicas, São Paulo, SP 04023-062, Brazil
e-mail: jxzaparoli@gmail.com

© Springer International Publishing Switzerland 2016
A.L.M. Andrade and D. De Micheli (eds.), *Innovations in the Treatment of Substance Addiction*, DOI 10.1007/978-3-319-43172-7_7

belonging to the omega-3 series are eicosapentaenoic acid (EPA) and docosahexaenoic acid (DHA). In addition, some of the representatives of the omega-6 series are as follows: arachidonic acid (AA), gamma-linoleic acid, and docosadienoic acid (Spector 1999; Haag 2003; Bourre 2005; Dyall and Michael-Titus 2008).

Polyunsaturated fatty acids are produced by a series of biochemical steps that occur in specific cell structures called organelles. Specifically, two of them actively participate in this process: the endoplasmic reticulum and peroxisomes. To illustrate this biochemical process, in a very simplistic way, we will take as an example the production of the omega-3 fatty acid series. The precursor, ALA, after passing through a series of steps, will be converted to EPA, and this after following a package of similar steps (enzymatic conversions) will be converted to DHA. So, after the end of the process, we will have the production of DHA, where EPA is an intermediate product. It is important to keep in mind that this process consists of several steps and includes the participation of different enzymes and may be influenced by other processes (Spector 1999). As the discussion of this issue is beyond the scope of this chapter, it is suggested further reading elsewhere (supporting literature at the end of the chapter).

Omega-3 and omega-6 fatty acids are physiologically and metabolically distinct; however, the same enzymes can metabolize their precursors, ALA and LA, leading to a competition between them. An example of this process is the competition between EPA and AA for the synthesis of certain compounds. The compounds produced by the fatty acids may be pro- or anti-inflammatory. In a situation with higher intake of omega-3 fatty acids, we will have, in summary, an increase in production of anti-inflammatory compounds and a decrease in pro-inflammatory compounds (these compounds favor inflammation). On the contrary, in a situation where there is an increased intake of omega-6 fatty acids (and a decrease in omega-3 fatty acids), an increased production of pro-inflammatory compounds will happened (and a decrease in anti-inflammatory compounds) (Simopoulos 2011). Since this subject escapes from the interest of this chapter, it is suggested to search other sources for more information.

Fatty acids receive the essential term because mammalian cells are unable to produce them completely, so they must be obtained through the diet (Spector 1999; Freeman 2000; Bourre 2005), and in the same way that some of the amino acids (proteins "building blocks") are classified as essential. The omega-3 fatty acid series can be found in same plants and sea animals (Spector 1999; Freeman 2000; Bourre 2005; Mazza et al. 2007), and the main source of omega-3 fatty acids is fish oil (Hallahan et al. 2007; Rusca et al. 2009; Kapoor and Patil 2011). A large percentage of omega-6 fatty acids can be found in vegetable oils, nuts, and cereals. Some examples of vegetable oils containing these fatty acids are linseed oil, soybean oil, and sunflower seed oil, among others.

Unlike the saturated and trans-fatty acids, which have shown some negative health effects, omega-3 fatty acids have been associated with numerous benefits, for example, in the treatment of hypertension, Crohn's disease, rheumatoid arthritis, age-related macular degeneration, and asthma. There also have reports of efficacy in reducing the primary cardiac risk of coronary heart disease and decrease in triglycerides (Freeman 2000; Mazza et al. 2007).

It is important to emphasis that more beneficial effects are been enlightened, as in the described cases above; however, in the Western diets, the omega-3 fatty acid consumption is reduced. In the UK and Western Europe, intake of omega-3 and omega-6 reaches 1:15 (omega-3: omega-6) proportion, whereas some studies indicates that these proportion can reach 1:20 ratio in some countries (Simopoulos 2011). The diet with high sugar intake and deficiency in nutritious foods such as omega-3 fatty acids, vegetables, and vitamins is known as Western diet (Simopoulos 2011; Prior and Galduróz 2012). Some studies show that standard dietary ratio should be 3–3.5:1 (omega-3: omega-6) (Richardson 2004; Bourre 2005; Garland et al. 2007; and Simopoulos 2011). Some studies show that the balance between omega-3 fatty acids/omega-6 is of utmost importance for health; a possible consequence for this unbalanced could be a likely increase in the production of pro-inflammatory compounds, for example (Simopoulos 2011).

Analyzing the lipid percentage of all the human body organs, the central nervous system (CNS), excluding the adipose tissue, is the organ that has the largest amount of lipids (Haag 2003; Bourre 2005). Approximately 50–60 % of the dry weight of an adult brain is from lipids, whereas almost 30 % of the polyunsaturated fatty acids found in its constitution are from the omega-3 series. This high concentration demonstrates the important role of these PUFAs to this tissue and for its proper functioning (Haag 2003; Bourre 2005).

Some clinical studies suggests that a reduction in the percentage of omega-3 fatty acids can be associated with various diseases, such as attention deficit disorder, depression, Alzheimer's disease, and multiple sclerosis (Spector 1999; Dyall and Michael-Titus 2008), and that dietary supplementation can improve the clinical condition of the patients with those diseases (Hallahan et al. 2007; Lakhan and Vieira 2008; Ross 2009).

Polyunsaturated fatty acids are compounds that participate in the constitution of membrane cells from almost all cells. Neurons require an adequate amount of omega-3 and omega-6 fatty acid series in their membranes for proper functioning (Spector 1999; Chalon et al. 2001; Haag 2003; Dyall and Michael-Titus 2008). Besides participating in the constitution of the neuronal membranes, omega-3 and omega-6 fatty acids affect the neuronal function either by direct relationship with its compounds (other constituents of the cell membrane), or through modulation of the biophysical properties of the membranes, as well as by producing biochemical messengers (Chalon et al. 2001; Dyall and Michael-Titus 2008).

The EPA and DHA fatty acids (compounds of omega-3 fatty acid family) have neuroprotective effects, that is, resulting in processes that culminate in the protection of neurons. These actions are related to different mechanisms, some of which are as follows: (1) direct action on the cell membrane (e.g., influence proteins such as ion channels and receptors present on the membrane), (2) alteration of inflammatory response, and (3) control over gene expression. The alteration of the inflammatory response is due to the competition between the arachidonic acid and EPA, in which higher concentration of EPA favors the synthesis of anti-inflammatory mediators. In addition, an example of control over gene expression is the synthesis of anti-inflammatory resolvins derived from EPA and DHA, which inhibit pro-apoptotic proteins and increase the activity of antiapoptotic proteins (Spector 1999; Haag 2003; Dyall and Michael-Titus 2008; Simopoulos 2011).

As PUFAs of omega-3 series (and omega-6 series) are compounds obtained solely from nutrition, variations in the diet can result in small changes in the concentration of these compounds in various body tissues, such as the central nervous system (CNS). Small changes on the concentration of these compounds could be responsible for causing an imbalance and malfunction of this tissue (Haag 2003). Studies using animal models have shown that chronic dietary deficiency of ALA (omega-3 precursor) in rodents affects the composition of the neuronal membranes (Zimmer et al. 1998, 2000a, b; Chalon et al. 2001; Chalon 2006; and Lakhan and Vieira 2008).

Possible Role for Omega-3 Fatty Acids on Dependence

For a better understanding of the possible omega-3's role on dependence follows a brief reminder about the processes and related structures.

The reward system, related with pleasure, welfare (and reward), is usually stimulated by neurotransmitters after a natural stimuli, such as food intake, water, and sex. Psychoactive substances (such as nicotine, alcohol, and cocaine) are also capable of stimulating this system, but, more intensely, resulting in a more intense pleasure (Ventulani 2001). The interaction of these psychoactive substances with specific brain structures [such as the ventral tegmental area (VTA)] triggers the direct release of neurotransmitters (chemical compounds responsible for the communication between neurons), such as dopamine (DA) in a region known as the center of the reward (Stahl 2010). The DA released in reward center (such as nucleus accumbens and the amygdala) is responsible for pleasure, satisfaction, and euphoria states. This process when often stimulated can result in adaptations on these brain structures, and this can lead to dependence (Ventulani 2001; Rosemberg 2003).

As previously mentioned, studies performed with animal models show that omega-3 deficiency results in structural changes in the nervous tissue (Zimmer et al. 1998, 2000a; Chalon et al. 2001; Chalon 2006). In studies conducted in the years 1998 and 2000, a group of researchers demonstrated that rodents deprived of omega-3 precursor (alpha-linolenic acid, ALA) present abnormal functioning of the dopaminergic system (related to the reward system described in the previous paragraph). This is due to the reduction of the number of vesicles that stores and protects this neurotransmitter (DA) (Zimmer et al. 1998, 2000a). Using a similar experimental approach, another study showed that these changes also occur in the serotonergic system (mediated by serotonin). This system also plays a role in sense of well-being. Importantly, the losses described above were reversed after the omega-3 precursor was restored in the experimental animal diet (Chalon 2006).

Deficiency of essential fatty acids (omega-3 or omega-6 subtype) have been associated with impulsivity states and compulsive behaviors (Buydens-Branchey et al. 2003a, b), affecting the healthiness of the neural systems (Chalon et al. 2001; Das and Fams 2003).

As the deficiency of omega-3 influences the functioning of different neurotransmitters (such as dopamine and serotonin) in several systems, including those related to the reward center, it is possible that the orally administered omega-3 fatty acids increase their bioavailability. Consequently, its concentration in the whole body and in CNS could increase, thus favoring the balance between the involved structures (in the reward center) and reducing the compulsion and addiction.

The commonly employed dosage in clinical studies to evaluate the effects of omega-3 (using marine supplements) is 3 g/daily, divided into three intakes for an approximate 90 days (3 months) (Hallahan et al. 2007; Rusca et al. 2009; Kapoor and Patil 2011). So far, there is no consensus on the optimal therapeutic dosage, and we can find difference between the doses and duration of treatment (Lakhan and Vieira 2008; Nitta et al. 2007; Fogaça et al. 2011). Another important parameter to consider is the amount of EPA and DHA acids present in the capsules. To illustrate this point, let us take the example of two studies: The study conducted by researcher Rabinovitz used capsules containing 542 mg of EPA and 408 mg DHA, and in a study conducted by the group led by Barbadoro, the capsules contained 60 mg of EPA and 252 mg DHA. Beyond this point, it is necessary to consider the amount of ingested capsules per day. Thus, considering the mentioned factors, when analyzing a study (and the treatment or intervention that it proposes), one of the points to be considered is the daily dose (Barbadoro et al. 2013; Rabinovitz 2014).

Considering fish oil as a major source of omega-3, the possible side effects of their use in treatment are dose-dependent increase in bleeding time (due to change in the concentration of the compounds involved in platelet aggregation), fishy aftertaste in the mouth and gastrointestinal disorders, the latter two being the most common (Rusca et al. 2009; Kapoor and Patil 2011); however no reports of abnormal bleeding even in super dosages associated with anticoagulant therapy (Kapoor and Patil 2011).

One issue to be considered during the decision of the dosage is the influence that some substances, such as alcohol and the free radicals present in cigarette smoke, can cause the metabolism of polyunsaturated fatty acids.

Several studies show that due to the elevate number of unsaturated bonds present in omega-3 molecule, this compound is highly susceptible to oxidation by free radicals and increased oxidative stress caused by cigarette smoke. Omega-3 oxidation process can also occur due to increased inflammatory response of the body to the aggression of smoke and compounds of cigarette (Morrow et al. 1995; Zappacosta et al. 1999; Pawlosky et al. 2007; Pasupathi et al. 2009; Abdolsamadi et al. 2011). In a study that aimed to investigate the effects of cigarette compounds on omega-3 fatty acids, the researchers found that smokers had lower concentrations of DHA and other polyunsaturated fatty acids such as linoleic acid and arachidonic acid, compared with non-smokers (Simon et al. 1996).

The same effect can be found in studies investigating the effects of alcohol on the metabolism of omega-3. In a review published in 2008, the authors discuss the harmful effects of alcohol, which are as follows: changing the environment of the neuronal membrane, changing its permeability through the lipid portion (Goldsteim cited Borsonelo and Galduróz 2008), and also changing the absorption and metabolism of essential fatty acids due to the inhibition of enzymes that perform the process (desaturation and elongation) for the production of EPA and DHA (Borsonelo and Galduróz 2008).

Below is a brief description of studies that evaluated the effects of the use of omega-3 fatty acids in different applications.

According to Ross (2009), supplementation with omega-3 PUFAs proved to be effective in treating anxiety disorders and led to improvements in depression ratings, suicide, and daily stress (Hallahan et al. 2007). In a review about omega-3, published in 2012, it argued that studies have shown that a low intake of omega-3 fatty acids is related to a higher prevalence of mood disorders and instability (Prior and Galduróz 2012). This same review mentions a study in which patients with depression have an altered metabolism of omega-3 fatty acids, and the conventional treatment with antidepressants was not able to reverse the clinical status (Prior and Galduróz 2012).

In a study whose objective was to examine the associations between aggressive and impulsive behaviors in patients with major depressive disorder without treatment, it was identified that low concentrations of the EPA fatty acid were associated with aggression and impulsivity only in patients suffering from this disorder associated with substance-use disorder, although this, in most cases, was in remission (Beier et al. 2014).

A study that evaluated the effects of PUFAs and other antioxidant nutrients under stress in a smoking population identified improvements in psychosocial stress. Treatment consisted in the use of capsules containing vitamins, minerals, and PUFAs (5.6 g) for approximately 30 days. The study suggests that the psychosocial stress relief obtained at the end of treatment could be related to the effects of DHA present in the used capsules. Importantly, this study identified improvements in psychosocial stress, but did not make use of a special series of fatty acids in particular, but a combination of PUFAs (Nitta et al. 2007).

In a different approach to the above studies, Buydens-Branchey et al. (2003a, b) investigated the association between omega-3 and omega-6 levels of cocaine addicts with relapse after a period of hospitalization and detoxification. The researchers found that individuals who had relapsed in the first 3 months after detoxification had lower concentrations of omega-3 series and omega-6 series (Buydens-Branchey et al. 2003a).

This same group of researchers conducted another study with a population of substance abusers. Subjects were treated with fatty acids of the omega-3 series (approximate amount of 2.250 mg EPA, 500 mg DHA, and 250 mg of other PUFAs per day) for 3 months, and at the end of the intervention, those receiving active treatment showed a progressive decline in anxiety levels (Buydens-Branchey and Branchey 2006).

In another study conducted by the same group, it was investigated the relationship between the aggression levels and the concentration of omega-3 and omega-6 of cocaine-dependent inpatients. Patients were treated with capsules containing an approximate amount of 2.250 mg of EPA, 500 mg DHA, and 250 mg of other PUFAs per day for 3 months. At the beginning of the trial before the treatment, it was identified that among the most aggressive inpatients, the concentrations of omega-3 fatty acids, particularly DHA, were lower when compared with non-aggressive inpatient. Moreover, after treatment, inpatients treated with capsules containing a combination of PUFA showed a reduction in levels of aggression (Buydens-Branchey and Branchey 2008).

The results of these studies suggest evidences of the relationship between omega-3 and omega-6 fatty acids and behaviors related to addiction, relapses, and aggressiveness (Buydens-Branchey et al. 2003a; Buydens-Branchey and Branchey 2008).

A study led by Rabinovitz (2014), treated a group of smokers, who had no intention of quitting, during a month with capsules containing a combination of omega-3 fatty acids (2.710 mg EPA/day and 2.040 mg DHA/day) and vitamin E. This study identified a decrease in craving after the exposure of participants to smoking clues, and a reduction in the number of cigarettes smoked per day (Rabinovitz 2014).

In a study conducted with inpatients of a treatment program for alcohol dependence, participants (abstinent during the intervention) were treated during 3 weeks with omega-3 fatty acids (60 mg of EPA/day and 252 mg of DHA/day), and it was found that after the intervention, a reduction of stress and anxiety levels occurred when compared with the initial values (Barbadoro et al. 2013).

Another example of positive effects of the use of PUFAs in the treatment of alcohol dependence is the work by Fogaça et al. (2011), in which they performed the treatment by supplementing with a combination of PUFAs (derived from a vegetable oil—400 mg of EPA + DHA, and fish oil—160 mg EPA and 240 mg DHA). At the end of the intervention, it was identified an improvement in the symptoms associated with dependency compared to pretreatment values (Fogaça et al. 2011).

Importance of Other Nutrients

Studies show that individuals who have dependent, due to different reasons, have deficient nutrient intake (Prior et al. 2014; Alberg 2002). Many of these micronutrients are components of utmost importance to the proper functioning of our body. An example is the importance of compounds such as zinc, magnesium, and the vitamins A and D, in the stabilization of glutamatergic, serotonergic, and dopaminergic pathways, all related to the reward system (Prior et al. 2014).

Another important example is the role of B vitamins, in particular B1. The B1 thiamine) deficiency, although rare, is associated with a severe neurological condition. Neurological syndrome of alcohol dependents is typically manifested by progressive loss of white matter of the central and peripheral nervous system and is probably correlated with thiamine deficiency (B1). This condition may be related to the fact that the B vitamins are water soluble, which hinders the body reserve, because many of them takes part during the metabolism of carbohydrates and are preferably depleted during high rates of alcohol metabolism (Manzardo et al. 2013).

Aiming to evaluate the effect of benfotiamine (a synthetic liposoluble analogue of thiamine), a study tested the supplementation on alcohol dependents (who did not seeking for treatment) during 24 weeks. The capsules contained 600 mg benfotiamine and were ingested once a day. After the completion of treatment, the researchers identified a gender difference, in which women who received benfotiamine showed a decrease in alcohol consumption when compared with women who did not take this compound (placebo group), while treated men did not showed the same effect. The researchers reported that benfotiamine was well tolerated (no serious adverse events were reported) and that this compound could be used as an adjunct therapy in treating thiamine deficiency in alcohol dependence (Manzardo et al. 2013).

In a study published in 2014, researchers have shown a possible correlation between micronutrient deficiencies and severity of alcohol withdrawal syndrome. Researchers found that individuals with alcohol withdrawal syndrome had low concentrations of several micronutrients, including magnesium and vitamin D. It is suggested that supplementation of these nutrients to those patients can benefit the evolution of symptoms (Prior et al. 2014).

The nutritional strategies described in this chapter can be used on different approaches within addiction treatment context, for example, (1) under relief acute symptoms of withdrawal (abstinence syndrome) and/or (2) in an attempt to reduce the compulsive behavior of psychoactive substances use in long term, and/or (3) prevention of the deleterious effects caused by exposure of those substances (e.g., alcohol and tobacco).

References

Alberg, A. (2002). The influence of cigarette smoking on circulating concentrations of antioxidant micronutrients. *Toxicology, 180*(2), 121–137.

Abdolsamadi, H. R., Goodarzi, M. T., Mortazavi, H., Robati, M., & Ahmadi-Motemaye, F. (2011). Comparison of salivary antioxidants in healthy smoking and non-smoking men. *Chang Gung Medical Journal, 34*(6), 607–611.

Barbadoro, P., Annino, I., Ponzio, E., Romanelli, R. M. L., D'Errico, M. M., Prospero, E., et al. (2013). Fish oil supplementation reduces cortisol basal levels and perceived stress: A randomized, placebo-controlled trial in abstinent alcoholics. *Molecular Nutrition & Food Research, 57*, 1110–1114.

Beier, A. M., Lauritzen, L., Galfalvy, H. C., Cooper, T. B., Oquendo, M. A., Grunebaum, M. F., et al. (2014). Low plasma eicosapentaenoic acid levels are associated with elevated trait aggression and impulsivity in major depressive disorder with a history of comorbid substance use disorder. *Journal of Psychiatric Research, 57*, 133–140.

Borsonelo, E. C., & Galduróz, J. C. F. (2008). The role of polyunsaturated fatty acids (PUFAs) in development, aging and substance abuse disorders: Review and propositions. *Prostaglandins Leukotrienes and Essential Fatty Acids, 78*, 237–245.

Bourre, J. M. (2005). Dietary omega-3 fatty acids and psychiatry: Mood, behaviour, stress, depression, dementia and aging. *The Journal of Nutrition, Health and Aging, 9*(1), 31–38.

Buydens-Branchey, L., Branchey, M., McMakin, D. L., & Hibbeln, J. R. (2003a). Polyunsaturated fatty acid status and relapse vulnerability in cocaine addicts. *Psychiatry Research, 120*(1), 29–35.

Buydens-Branchey, L., Branchey, M., McMakin, D. L., & Hibbeln, J. R. (2003b). Polyunsaturated fatty acid status and aggression in cocaine addicts. *Drug and Alcohol Dependence, 71*(3), 319–323.

Buydens-Branchey, L., & Branchey, M. (2006). n-3 Polyunsaturated fatty acids decrease anxiety feelings in a population of substance abusers. *Journal of Clinical Psychopharmacology, 26*(6), 661–665.

Buydens-Branchey, L., & Branchey, M. (2008). Long chain n-3 polyunsaturated fatty acids decrease feelings of anger in substance abusers. *Psychiatry Research, 157*(1–3), 95–104.

Chalon, S., Vancassel, S., Zimmer, L., Guilloteau, D., & Durand, G. (2001). Polyunsaturated fatty acids and cerebral function: Focus on monoaminergic neurotransmission. *Lipids, 36*(9), 937–944.

Chalon, S. (2006). Omega-3 fatty acids and monoamine neurotransmission. *Prostaglandins Leukotrienes and Essential Fatty Acids, 75*(4–5), 259–269.

Das, U. N., & Fams, M. D. (2003). Long-chain polyunsaturated fatty acids in the growth and development of the brain and memory. *Nutrition, 19*(1), 62–65.

Dyall, S. C., & Michael-Titus, A. T. (2008). Neurological benefits of omega-3 fatty acids. *Neuromolecular Medicine, 10*(4), 219–235.

Freeman, M. P. (2000). Omega-3 fatty acids in psychiatry: A review. *Annals of Clinical Psychiatry, 12*(3), 159–165.

Fogaça, M. N., Santos-Galduróz, R. F., Eserian, J. K., & Galduróz, J. C. F. (2011). The effects of polyunsaturated fatty acids in alcohol dependence treatement—A double blind, placebo-controlled pilot study. *BMC Clinical and Pharmacology, 11*, 10.

Garland, M. R., Hallahan, B., McNamara, M., Carney, P. A., Grimes, H., Hibbeln, A., et al. (2007). Lipids and essential fatty acids in patients presenting with self-harm. *British Journal of Psychiatry, 190*, 112–117.

Haag, M. (2003). Essential fatty acids and the brain. *Canadian Journal of Psychiatry, 48*(3), 195–203.

Hallahan, B., Hibbeln, J. R., Davis, J. M., & Garland, M. R. (2007). Omega-3 fatty acid supplementation in patients with recurrent self-harm. *British Journal of Psychiatry, 190*, 118–122.

Kapoor, R., & Patil, U. K. (2011). Importance and production of omega-3 fatty acids from natural sources. *International Food Research Journal, 18*, 493–499.

Lakhan, S. E., & Vieira, K. F. (2008). Nutritional therapies for mental disorders. *Nutrition Journal, 21*(7), 2.

Manzardo, A. M., He, J., Poje, A., Penick, C. E., Campbell, J., & Butler, M. G. (2013). Double-blind, randomized placebo-controlled clinical trial of benfotiamine for severe alcohol dependence. *Drug Alcohol Depend, 133*(2), 562–570.

Mazza, M., Pomponi, M., Janiri, L., Bria, P., & Mazza, S. (2007). Omega-3 fatty acids and antioxidants in neurological and psychiatric diseases: An overview. *Progress in Neuropsychopharmacology and Biological Psychiatry, 31*(1), 12–26.

Morrow, J. D., Frei, B., Longmire, A. W., Gaziano, J. M., Lynch, S. M., Shyr, Y., et al. (1995). Increase in circulating products of lipid peroxidation (F2-isoprostanes) in smokers. Smoking as a cause of oxidative damage. *New England Journal of Medicine, 332*(18), 1198–1203.

Nitta, H., Kinoyama, M., Watanabe, A., Shirao, K., Kihara, H., & Arai, M. (2007). Effects of nutritional supplementation with antioxidant vitamins and minerals and fish oil on antioxidant status and psychosocial stress in smokers: An open trial. *Clinical and Experimental Medicine,* 7(4), 179–183.

Pasupathi, P., Saravanan, G., & Farook, J. (2009). Oxidative stress bio markers and antioxidant status in cigarette smokers compared to nonsmokers. *Journal of Pharmaceutical Sciences and Research, 1*(2), 55–62.

Pawlosky, R. J., Hibbeln, J. R., & Salem, N, Jr. (2007). Compartmental analyses of plasma n-3 essential fatty acids among male and female smokers and nonsmokers. *Journal of Lipid Research, 48*(4), 935–943.

Prior, P. L., & Galduróz, J. C. F. (2012). (N-3) Fatty acids: Molecular role and clinical uses in psychiatric disorders. American Society for Nutrition. *Advances in Nutrition, 3,* 257–265.

Prior, P. L., Vaz, M. J., Ramos, A. C., & Galduróz, J. C. F. (2014). Influence of microelement concentration on the intensity of alcohol withdrawal syndrome. *Alcohol and Alcoholism, 50*(2), 152–156.

Rabinovitz, S. (2014). Effects of omega-3 fatty acids on tobacco craving in cigarette smokers: A double-blind, randomized, placebo-controlled pilot study. *Journal of Psychopharmacology, 28* (8), 804–809.

Richardson, A. J. (2004). Long-chain polyunsaturated fatty acids in childhood developmental and psychiatric disorders. *Lipids, 39*(12), 1215–1222.

Ross, B. M. (2009). Omega-3 polyunsaturated fatty acids and anxiety disorders. *Prostaglandins Leukotrienes and Essential Fatty Acids, 81*(5–6), 309–312.

Rosemberg, J. (2003). *Nicotina droga universal.* São Paulo: INCA—Instituto Nacional do Câncer.

Rusca, A., Di Stefano, A. F., Diog, M. V., Scarsi, C., & Perucca, E. (2009). Relative bioavailability and pharmacokinetics of two oral formulations of docosahexaenoic acid/eicosapentaenoic acid after multiple-dose administration in healthy volunteers. *European Journal of Clinical Pharmacology, 65*(5), 503–510.

Simon, J. A., Fong, J., Bernert, J. T, Jr., & Browner, W. S. (1996). Relation of smoking and alcohol consumption to serum fatty acids. *American Journal of Epidemiology, 144*(4), 325–334.

Simopoulos, A. P. (2011). Evolutionary aspects of diet: The omega-6/omega-3 ratio and the brain. *Molecular Neurobiology, 44,* 203–215.

Spector, A. A. (1999). Essentiality of fatty acids. *Lipids, 34 Suppl,* S1–S3.

Stahl, S. M. (2010). Transtornos de Recompensa, Abuso de Drogas e seus tratamentos. In Stephen M. Stahl (autor 3ª edição). *Psicofarmacologia. Bases neurocientíficas e Aplicações práticas* (pp. 639–644). Rio de Janeiro: Guanabara Koogan.

Ventulani, J. (2001). Drug addiction. Part II. Neurobiology of addiction. *Polish Journal of Pharmacology, 53*(4), 303–317.

Zappacosta, B., Persichilli, S., De Sole, P., Mordente, A., & Giardina, B. (1999). Effect of smoking one cigarette on antioxidant metabolites in the saliva of healthy smokers. *Archives of Oral Biology, 44*(6), 485–488.

Zimmer, L., Hembert, S., Durand, G., et al. (1998). Chronic n-3 polyunsaturated fatty acid diet-deficiency acts on dopamine metabolism in the rat frontal cortex: A microdialysis study. *Neuroscience Letters, 240*(3), 177–181.

Zimmer, L., Delion-Vancassel, S., Durant, G., et al. (2000a). Modification of dopamine neurotransmission in the nucleus accumbens of rats deficient in n-3 polyunsaturated fatty acids. *Journal of Lipid Research, 41*(1), 32–40.

Zimmer, L., Delpal, S., Guilloteau, D., Aïoun, A., Durand, G., & Chalon, S. (2000b). Chronic n-3 polyunsaturated fatty acid deficiency alters dopamine vesicle density in the rat frontal cortex. *Neuroscience Letters, 284*(1–2), 25–28.

Chapter 8
How Do Interventions and Brief Psychotherapies Work? Evaluating the Change Processes in Drug User's Interventions

Laisa Marcorela Andreoli Sartes, Erica Cruvinel and Maira Leon Ferreira

Introduction

The brief intervention was firstly proposed in 1972, in Canada, by Sanchez-Craig and collaborators as a reference to a psychotherapy approach supposed to motivate alcohol users to change their drinking behavior in the short term. The four-session intervention is based on the cognitive and behavioral theories, and it presented better results among alcohol dependents under treatment than among those who have received no treatment. A series of studies conducted in the last decades assessed the effects of different interventions using this nomenclature. However, it is necessary to separate the brief intervention (BI) from the brief psychotherapy. The brief intervention is focused on prevention; i.e., it helps abusive or under-risk users to reduce or stop consuming due to its motivational profile. The brief therapies, in their turn, focus on substance-dependent treatments. Marques and Furtado (2004) describe these modalities as an attention continuum, which changes depending on the individual's substance consumption severity. We will address in the current text two modalities that, along with other modalities, are usually called "brief interventions."

We can find a significant set of research about the effects of brief interventions on drug consumption reduction. Most of these researches assess interventions' effectiveness and efficiency, but little is known about how these interventions

L.M.A. Sartes (✉) · E. Cruvinel · M.L. Ferreira
Psychology Department, Universidade Federal de Juiz de Fora,
Rua José Lourenço Kelmer, s/n - Campus Universitário, Juiz de Fora,
MG 36036-900, Brazil
e-mail: laisa.sartes@ufjf.edu.br

E. Cruvinel
e-mail: ecruvinel@yahoo.com.br

M.L. Ferreira
e-mail: mleonferreira2014@gmail.com

© Springer International Publishing Switzerland 2016
A.L.M. Andrade and D. De Micheli (eds.), *Innovations in the Treatment of Substance Addiction*, DOI 10.1007/978-3-319-43172-7_8

actually work. A new trend focused on assessing the intervention processes has been in place for the last 15 years, and it is focused on identifying the specific elements adapted to each individual able to influence results. The first part of the present chapter regards a brief review about the knowledge on brief interventions focused on prevention through the identification of specific components mentioned in previous studies. The second and larger part of the present chapter is a review of the advances in the intervention studies focused on understanding how these interventions actually work.

Brief Intervention Components

The first definitions given to the term brief intervention (BI) head toward the understanding of a practice that aims to identify real or potential problems associated with alcohol or other drugs use, as well as to identify strategies to motivate individuals to change their relation with such consumption (Babor and Higgins-Biddle 2003). Many studies cite the FRAMES method as the technique used to guide their interventions. This acronym refers to the brief intervention principles (feedback, responsibility, advice, menu of options, empathy, and self-efficacy), which will be further described in the current chapter. However, since the very first studies, the heterogeneity of these definitions has been highlighted through the plurality of the time dedicated to the approach, to the content, to the way the intervention is developed, to the profile of professionals involved with the implementation of techniques, and to the target group (Heather 1995). This plurality of definitions may be explained, for instance, by the different terms and acronyms found in international publications, such as brief intervention for alcohol; brief intervention; identification and brief advice; extended brief intervention; brief advice; screening and brief intervention; screening, brief intervention, and referral to specialized services; brief motivational interviews; and brief cognitive–behavioral therapy, among others. All these approaches are performed in a limited period of time, and they are focused on behavior change, but they must fulfill the expected aims of a brief intervention. However, there are specific aspects that differentiate the highlighted nomenclatures.

The difficulty in formally conceptualizing the term brief intervention has been deeply discussed and guided to advances in the herein described thematic in recent years. The author of the text "Brief Intervention content matters," which was published in 2013 (McCambridge 2013), questions the remaining knowledge gap in the content of this intervention, due to the different results presented in recent studies. The text mentions a randomized clinical study conducted in the UK. The study compared the effect of alcohol consumption reduction among patients from two experimental groups who have just received an informative flyer about alcohol. The first group received the same flyer plus 5 min of brief advice, whereas the second intervention group got 20 min of additional advice. The results of this research do not show the best results in groups that have received intensive advice.

Can we then conclude that the brief intervention does not work? This type of result has motivated researchers, as well as the author of the previously cited text, to try to understand in details what we are defining here as brief intervention and, mainly, to question the components involved with the interventions as a way to understand these results and to clearly measure the impact of the most effective aspects.

A systematic review published in a Brazilian journal (Pereira et al. 2013) highlighted 30 researches that used brief intervention strategies to treat the abusive use of alcohol or other drugs, published between 1997 and 2010 in different countries. We assessed the full texts of the six studies conducted within the Brazilian context mentioned in the current review as an attempt of getting to know the definition of brief intervention. Table 8.1 highlights the four studies that

Table 8.1 Brief intervention components in Brazilian studies

Study 1: De Micheli et al. (2004)	
Target group	108 adolescents; 10–19 years old, outpatient
BI components	Frames (feedback, responsibility, advice, menu of options, empathy, and self-efficacy)
Duration	Single session, 20 min
Professionals conducting BI	4 doctors previously trained on the application of the screening instruments and on BI
Study 2: Andretta and Oliveira (2008)	
Target group	50 adolescents, specialized institutions to follow the protective measures to adolescents
BI components	Motivational interview
Duration	Non-specified time, 5 motivation interview sessions (first session defined as feedback)
Professionals conducting BI	It is mentioned that it was performed by a therapist, but his/her specialization was not mentioned
Study 3: Oliveira et al. (2008)	
Target group	152 patients, dependence treatment center
BI components	Motivational interview
Duration	Non-specified time, 5 motivational interview sessions (it mentions that the feedback was given during the session)
Professional conducting BI	It does not mention the profile of the professionals, but it highlights the training on the motivational interview and a supervisor with great expertise on the approach
Study 4: Castro and Laranjeira (2009)	
Target group	71 patients, outpatients
BI components	Non-specified
Duration	Non-specified
Professionals conducting BI	Non-specified

Data extracted from the review study by Pereira et al. (2013)

assessed the intervention impacts. The other two researches will not be mentioned since they were a transversal study and an experience report.

The aim of the four studies was to assess the effect of intervention, and they highlighted participants' positive results in alcohol or drug consumption behavior change, even if different target groups and consumption patterns were adopted. However, although the results corroborate the intervention's impact, just one of these studies cites the FRAMES method as the technique adopted in the intervention. Two studies used the motivational interviews, and the last article did not mention the used approach. Besides, the herein described researches were distinguished by the necessary treatment to apply the approach; the study by De Micheli et al. (2004) mentions that the professionals received a brief training, whereas the study by Oliveira et al. (2008) points out the continuous supervision conducted by specialists on motivational interviews. It is worth mentioning that the two studies using motivational interview adopted five sessions. Differently from the study by De Micheli et al. (2004), who used a single session (of approximately 20 min) as brief intervention model, the intervention model and duration of these sessions were not highlighted in the article. The three studies cited the feedback as a way to inform the patient—in a single session or throughout the other motivational interview meetings—about the use pattern and the associated issues.

It is known that the four studies just show part of the Brazilian publications and that they do not depict the data in the international literature. However, even with the limitation on the range of the present discussion, it is noticed that there is no clearness or standardization of what a brief intervention would actually be. The studies have used the FRAMES method, the motivational interview, the single session, as well as the multiple sessions to refer to brief interventions. Maybe, the results of these interventions are related to specific aspects that are not detailed in the studies.

The systematic review published by O'Donnell et al. (2014) corroborates this idea; it points out the efficacy of brief intervention on the reduction of problems related to alcohol use in the international scenario through the analysis of 56 randomized clinical studies that involve a large number of patients in the primary care service. However, the authors point out that there is need to set BI ideal duration, frequency, and content, so that the effects remain in the long term. The studies seem to indicate that the structured feedback and the written information have positive effect in changing some behaviors.

The importance given to brief interventions as instruments used to help patients changing their behavior regarding drug consumption is already known. However, understanding their components is crucial for guiding the practices of the professionals involved in it, mainly due to time limitation and to the overload of activities in many potential services at the time to put these approaches in practice, such as primary health care.

Brief Intervention as Prevention

Nowadays, studies about BI efficacy have been broadly spread within different contexts. However, it is known that the largest number of studies about this intervention has been done in primary health care. The BI proposal in these places is focused on performing drug consumption screening followed by the BI in risk use and treatment refer cases when the suggestive substance dependence use is detected. The initial researches about BI were focused on assessing this intervention's efficacy by comparing them to other longer approaches (Formigoni 1992). They also aimed to analyze which key elements found in the BIs were directly related to behavior change (Bien et al. 1993). As time went by, the performed studies started to focus on the barriers and on the obstructions to their dissemination, besides the BI testing in other contexts and populations. If we take into account the advancements in the BI research field, it is possible to see a critic to the adopted methodologies. It is considered that BI is not totally based on evidences, due to the lack of pattern in the studies, to the lack of control groups, and to the fact that many studies are not based on randomized clinical assays.

According to Babor et al. (2006), many randomized clinical studies about brief interventions were conducted in the last decades in different healthcare environments. The accumulated evidence basis about the efficacy and effectiveness of BI has been documented in many systematic reviews since 1993 (Agerwala and McCance-Katz 2012; Ballesteros et al. 2004; Bien et al. 1993; Kahan et al. 1995; Kaner et al. 2007; Nilsen et al. 2008; Moyer et al. 2002; Pereira et al. 2013; Whitlock et al. 2004; Wilk et al. 1997).

One of the first systematic review articles about the evidence of BIs was suggested by Bien et al. (1993). Their study comprises 32 studies involving a sample encompassing 6000 patients from 14 countries. It was evidenced that the BI does not differ from the longer approaches when it comes to its effectiveness. The authors have indicated that the BI can be performed in primary care contexts and in assistance programs given to employees. At this time, the authors also identified common key elements able to encourage behavior changing. The principles often seen in interventions called brief interventions gathered the same components previously suggested by Miller and Sanchez (1993), namely FRAMES, as it is described in Table 8.2. The "feedback" is related to a feedback session given to the individual about the consumption pattern related to drug use. It refers to the screening, to the evaluation, and to the feedback about the score ranked through screening instruments. According to Miller and Rollnick (2001), the feedback is an essential element to the motivation to change, since it provides patients with the clear knowledge about their current situation. The "responsibility" emphasizes the individuals' autonomy and responsibility to the decisions to change or not their dug use behavior. It also implies commitment to the change. The "advice" refers to the advice provided by professionals as a way to guide the individuals in the search for problem solving. The advices work as a set of information about drug use for health, personal problems, and legal problems, among others. The "menu of

Table 8.2 Specifying FRAMES components in BI evaluations

	Feedb.	Respon.	Advises	Menu	Empat.	Self-ef.	Results
[a]Anderson and Scott (1992)	Yes	Yes	Yes	Yes	Yes	Yes	BI > no advice
[a]Babor and Grant (1992)	Yes	Yes	Yes	Manual	Yes	Yes	BI > no advice
[a]Bien (1992)	Yes	Yes	Yes	No	Yes	Yes	BI > no advice
[a]Brown and Miller (1993)	Yes	Yes	Yes	No	Yes	Yes	BI > no advice
[a]Carpenter et al. (1985)	Yes	No	Yes	No	No	No	BI = extensive advice
[a]Chapman and Hygens (1988)	Yes	Yes	Yes	Yes	No	Yes	BI = IPT = OPT treatment
[a]Chick et al. (1985)	Yes	Yes	Yes	No	Yes	Yes	BI > no advice
[a]Chick et al. (1988)	No	No	Yes	No	No	No	BI = extensive motiv. advice
Daniels et al. (1992)	Yes	No	Yes	Manual	No	No	Advices + manual = no advice
Drummond et al. (1990)	Yes	No	Yes	No	No	No	BI = OPT treatment
Edwards et al. (1977)	Yes	Yes	Yes	No	Yes	Yes	BI = OPT/IP treatment
Elvy et al. (1988)	Yes	No	Yes	No	No	No	BI > no advice
[a]Harris and Miller (1990)	No	Yes	Yes	Manual	Yes	Yes	BI = extensive > no advice
[a]Heather et al. (1986)	Yes	Yes	Manual	Manual	No	No	Manual > non-manual
[a]Heather et al. (1987)	Yes	Yes	Yes	Manual	No	No	BI = no advice
[a]Heather et al. (1990)	Yes	Yes	Yes	Manual	No	No	Manual > non-manual
[a]Kristenson et al. (1983)	Yes	Yes	Yes	No	Yes	Yes	BI > no advice
Kichipudi et al. (1990)	Yes	No	Yes	Yes	No	No	BI = no advice
Maheswaran et al. (1992)	Yes	No	Yes	No	No	No	BI > no advice
[a]Miller and Taylor (1980)	No	Yes	Yes	Manual	Yes	Yes	BI = behavioral advice
[a]Miller et al. (1980)	No	Yes	Yes	Manual	Yes	Yes	BI = behavioral advice
[a]Miller et al. (1981)	No	Yes	Yes	Manual	Yes	Yes	BI = behavioral advice
[a]Miller et al. (1988)	Yes	Yes	Yes	Yes	Yes	Yes	BI > no advice
[a]Miller et al. (1991)	Yes	Yes	Yes	Yes	Yes	Yes	BI > no advice

(continued)

Table 8.2 (continued)

	Feedb.	Respon.	Advises	Menu	Empat.	Self-ef.	Results
[a]Persson and Magnusson (1989)	Yes	Yes	Yes	No	Yes	Yes	BI > no advice
[a]Robertson et al. (1986)	Yes	Yes	Yes	Yes	Yes	Yes	BI < behavioral advice
[a]Romelsjö et al. (1989)	Yes	Yes	Yes	No	Yes	Yes	BI = OPT treatment
[a]Sannibale (1988)	Yes	Yes	Yes	No	Yes	Yes	BI = OPT treatment
[a]Scott and Anderson (1990)	Yes	Yes	Yes	Yes	Yes	Yes	BI = no advice
Skutle and Berg (1987)	Yes	Yes	Yes	Yes + Man	Yes	Yes	BI = behavioral advice
[a]Wallace et al. (1988)	Yes	Yes	Yes	Manual	Yes	Yes	BI > no advice
[a]Zweben et al. (1988)	Yes	Yes	Yes	Yes	No	Yes	BI = combined therapy
% Yes	81 %	81 %	100 %	59 %	63 %	69 %	

The table was translated and adapted from the study by Bien et al. (1993), by the authors

Notes The listed components are typical of the brief intervention in each study

[a]Additional information may be gathered with the authors

options" is given to patients along with many strategies in order to change or stop their drug use behavior. According to Miller and Rollnick (2001), it is necessary to offer a set of strategies to patients in order to create conditions for them to select those that best fulfill their needs. The "empathy" means showing to patients the understanding of their difficulties about drug use, without being confrontational. It is important not to "force" patients to change their behavior; the professional must be comprehensive and welcoming. The "self-efficacy" refers to the encouragement that must be given to the patient; the professional must help the patient to trust in his/her own resources and to be optimistic toward behavior changing. The professional must promote the self-perception of personal efficacy and of the achievement of established targets.

The number of studies about BI efficacy and effectiveness in the following years has multiplied in the literature; some bring the identification of moderators, such as gender, which could influence the results. Kahan et al. (1995) assessed articles about BI in the health context, which were published between 1966 and 1972. The authors observed that BI was effective in reducing alcohol consumption among men in a gender comparison, but the results about women were inconsistent. Wilk et al. (1997) also performed a meta-analysis involving outpatients and evidenced BI effectiveness within the referred context.

Given such results, in 2004, BI emerged as recommendation by The United States Preventive Services Task Force, due to the nonexistence of evidences that the benefits of this intervention would overcome its damages. However, the current study considered that the participants reduced from 13 to 34 % the mean number of doses per week when they were compared to the control groups. Nilsen et al. (2008), in a systematic review about BI in the last three decades, established that these researches pointed toward significant reduction of risky and damaging alcohol consumption. The authors reported that despite the existing solid basis evidencing BI's effectiveness, the barriers to disseminate this strategy have been challenging.

Agerwala and McCance-Katz (2012) reinforced that, nowadays, SBIRT (screening, brief intervention, and referral to treatment) is not a practice totally based on evidences. These authors' main critics refer to the methodological limitations of the studies. Although some studies found reduction in alcohol use through the follow-up assessment performed 6 months after the BI, some of these studies lack control group. They have recommended the performance of randomized clinical assays to corroborate the BI efficacy hypothesis.

Throughout the years, the studies about BI went beyond the health context; they covered other environments (Pereira et al. 2013). The study conducted by Thom et al. (2014) provided a general view over BI application beyond health care. These authors reported that although the evidence of BI in other contexts is less clear, when it is applied to pharmacies (remove the word "drugstore") **drugstores**, to criminal justice, and to the college environment, it might reduce the damaging alcohol use. On the other hand, the authors pointed out that there are few evidences about the BI impact on the dental context, on working places, and on the young and homeless populations. Thus, they highlighted the barriers to BI application in other contexts, mainly in regard to the absence of long-term investments.

Despite the fact that the researches about BI are predominantly positive when it comes to alcohol use reduction, some studies did not present significant differences between the standard advice and the BI application. The study by Pengpid et al. (2013) about the hospital context concluded that there was no significant difference in consumption reduction between the control group and the group that received BI, thus stating that the screening instruments and the distribution of an educational handout may, by themselves, cause consumption reduction. The study by McCambridge and Day (2008) about the college context also showed similar results. The study by Lock et al. (2006) about primary health care also concluded that BI did not overcome the standard advice effects. A prominent conclusion in these studies takes into account the possible fundamental effects of feedback—the first specific component of FRAMES—on BI effectiveness, fact that could explain the lack of differences in the results between groups (Donovan et al. 2012).

The Brief Motivational Interview

The motivational interview (MI) was developed by Miller and Rollnick, and it aims to help the individual in behavior change processes through ambivalence reduction. The MI, which is also known as motivational enhancement therapy (MET) or as brief motivational interview (BMI), is often the beginning of a treatment, since this intervention opens a path to the change that supports the way to future treatments (Miller and Rollnick 2001).

Miller and Rollnick (2001) described five principles to guide the MI technique, namely expressing empathy, which means having a reflexive and cozy hearing; developing the discrepancy between the desired targets and the behaviors to be changed; avoiding confrontation in order to not increase resistance to treatment; monitoring the resistance in order to use it in one's own benefit, thus facilitating ambivalence solution; and encouraging the self-efficacy so that the individual becomes aware of his/her conditions and strategies to deal with difficult situations and to succeed. The MI is based on the trans-theoretical model suggested by Prochaska and DiClemente (1992), who describe a model of readiness to change through motivational stages followed by the individuals. The motivational stages are pre-contemplation, contemplation, determination or preparation, action, maintenance, and relapse.

In a systematic review elaborated by Sales and Figlie (2009), MI appeared to be effective in reducing alcohol consumption and in increasing motivation to behavior change. The MI is also related to the increased search for and adhesion to alcohol dependence treatments. It is a low-cost intervention, which is easily applicable to any health environment or community. Studies showed that the brief MI is supported by 6- to 12-month periods, but the specific factors contributing to these data sustain are not known. According to Carey et al. (2006), when MI is offered along with other techniques, it is more effective than when it is offered alone.

Advances in Studies About Brief Interventions and Brief Psychotherapies

Despite the dubious results found in recent decades about the efficacy and effectiveness of brief interventions, much has been discussed about the elements that indicate these differences. The hypothesis that specific ingredients may forcefully interfere in the results began to be taken into consideration, not only in studies about BI focused on prevention, but also in brief interventions focused on treating alcohol and other drug dependents or abusive users, as in the case of the brief motivational interview and the brief cognitive–behavioral therapies.

Bricker (2015) points out that professionals working with drug users use a number of evidence-based interventions and instruments that may guide their practice. Although it is good news, the interventions show small-to-moderate effect size in most efficacy studies. Assessing the effect size means that in addition to the statistical significance—which tells us whether the results of two interventions, for example, are statistically different—it is necessary to check whether the positive effects of the intervention are large enough for it to be considered useful. What concerns the researchers in the field is the fact that the effects of specific and innovative interventions that have been tested in clinical trials do not differ much, in terms of effect size, from the treatments usually used in outpatient clinics and in hospitals. According to the author, the comprehensive assessment of the ingredients that really encompass the services would be a real contribution to future studies. Another common concern regards the effects of the therapist/professional's features, such as his/her discernment to make comments at the right time, his/her time of clinical experience, and how much it affects the results.

In recent years, a new trend has emerged in order to evaluate the brief interventions offered to substance users. According to Longabaugh and Magill (2012), until the twentieth century, the studies about the behavioral treatments for addition were mainly focused on developing and evaluating the efficacy and effectiveness of different interventions. However, the authors argue that in the twenty-first century, the studies' priority is to understand the treatment processes, i.e., the changing mechanisms and the active ingredients. The goal is to understand how the treatment works and for whom, and not just whether it works.

Kazdin and Nock (2003) conducted a review on the methods used to assess the therapy offered to children and adolescents and found that studies about treatment mechanisms were probably the best short- and long-term investments to improve clinical practice and patient care. Many questions may be answered through studies about therapy, such as "why," "how," and "for whom" the treatment works and what components and combinations may contribute to the result. The authors argue that understanding why the treatment works could maximize its effects and ensure that essential features are generalized in order to obtain a practical intervention. The mechanisms are defined as processes and events that lead to therapeutic changes. It means that a causal relationship is established between the intervention and the treatment outcomes, which itself is not enough because it does not explain why the relationship happened. For example, evaluating a treatment approach is not enough to identify the specific components (such as behavioral skills, readiness to change, cognitive restructuring, and promotion of hope) that promoted the change. Understanding the treatment processes may minimize the differences among the several interventions proposed in the literature, as well as promote, optimize, and maximize the patients' improvement. Finally, the authors highlight that knowing how an intervention works may help identifying treatment moderators, i.e., the variables whose results depend, for example, on the age of drug use onset and on the dependence severity, among others.

Much of this change of interest due to the limited results found when different treatment modalities were compared, such as the results reported in the Match Project (Donovan and Mattson 1994). The Match Project was a large randomized clinical trial conducted in the 1990s, in several American centers. It tested the hypothesis that different types of problematic alcohol users would respond differently to three types of treatment for consumption reduction, namely the motivational interview, the cognitive–behavioral therapy, and the twelve steps. The effects of the concept called "treatment matching"—the direction to different treatment approaches according to the individual needs and features of each patient—on the primary results related to alcohol consumption reduction ended up getting little empirical support (Project MATCH Research Group 1998). For example, according to one of the numerous hypotheses, the motivational interview would bring better results for those who had less readiness to change. However, it did not occur because patients with the same level of readiness to change (some high, others low) showed similar results in any modality. According to Longabaugh and Magill (2012), the treatment moderating effect hypothesis did not allow identifying the mechanisms through which the moderation occurred. In this case, the moderation would be a feature of the patient. Longabaugh and Wirtz (2001) conducted a comprehensive review of the project and concluded that the theoretical approach was at odds with what had been empirically observed. The authors cited the active ingredients, which have been targeted by studies in the field since then. Based on the hypothesis that active ingredients are fundamental mechanisms that generate effect on results, one explanation for this similar result among the three Match Project approaches lies on the fact that they often do not differ from one another in their emphasis on some ingredients. Thus, the hypothesis that a subtype of patient would respond differently was not substantiated, since an active ingredient was present in all the approaches, such as in the case of readiness to change (Longabaugh and Wirtz 2001). Therefore, Longabaugh and Magill (2012) understand that it is necessary to develop more sophisticated models in order to test the theory. Magill and Longabaugh (2013) point out a new movement in the evaluation of treatments for substance users—the need to include a new criterion in the list of evidence-based interventions for this population. An intervention based on the brief cognitive–behavioral therapy is considered as evidence-based when well-conducted randomized controlled trials are considered the gold standard to show its effectiveness. However, it would be necessary, but not sufficient, since the identification of the so-called active ingredients would be of great relevance. The hypothesized active ingredients refer to the key elements of the treatment. They are processes and interventions within the treatment. In addition, they predict incremental results and are different from the individuals' mechanisms, i.e., the individuals' internal changing processes. According to the authors, the impact of the active ingredients on the treatment outcome would be an important criterion to clarify an evidence-based practice. Several elements are part of the treatment, namely the patient's features, the life context, the therapeutic alliance, the promotion of hope in the individual, the professional empathy, and many other unknown ingredients that could affect the results; the professional must be aware of them. The proposal consists of empirically validating these active ingredients, i.e., to consider them active as predictors of the individuals' mechanisms and of the treatment outcomes. Changes should be observed at each stage of the clinical trial, even if they occurred in all study conditions or groups. For example, during the pre-treatment or pre-randomization, the attitude change may simply occur because the individuals sign a consent term to participate in the study and in the evaluations that will take place later. Therefore, an assessment would be helpful at this point. Another example relates to the treatment dose, namely the differences between the experimental and control groups regarding the number of sessions they get, a factor that is often neglected in the studies. These ingredients may affect all groups; however, they may also affect the effect size in the studies about the effectiveness of interventions. In the final analysis, it is important to take into consideration and to control covariables, such as the number of sessions the individual attended to or the individual features of the therapist. Therefore, the idea would be to dismantle the main sources of variation in the measurement of the treatment effect size—in other words, in the evaluation of its efficacy or effectiveness.

In 2004, Longabaugh, Donovan, Karno, McGrady, Morgenstern, and Tonigan organized a symposium in Canada to discuss evidences of active ingredients in behavioral therapies and summed up what was discussed in a manuscript published the following year (Longabaugh et al. 2005). The authors argued that although there were already good evidences about treatments for alcohol and other drugs users, little was discussed about how they worked. Overall, the researchers assumed that when a treatment was effective, they already knew how and why it worked. In 2001, the limited evidence about the intervention working processes led the National Institute on Alcohol Abuse and Alcoholism to encourage studies on the alcoholism treatment working mechanisms, by justifying that it was difficult to use evidence-based treatments in clinical practice without knowing how they worked. With regard to the cognitive–behavioral therapy (CBT), Donovan recalled some key elements of the approach, such as the increased self-efficacy and coping skills used as strategies to reduce drug use. He pointed out that there are reports in the literature of what is called proximal results, i.e., specific changes in attitudes, beliefs, and behaviors that according to the theory, patients should undergo or achieve as a consequence of their commitment to the therapy. The evolution in the proximal result variables allows assuming that there will be best "final results," such as alcohol consumption reduction, and they may stand out as active ingredients. Among some primary CBT active ingredients, the author cites the increased self-efficacy to remain abstinent in high-risk situations, the reduction of positive expectations of substance use, and the increased expectations related to the benefits of stop consuming the substance.

A study conducted by Finney et al. (1998) showed that the proximal results (self-efficacy, coping strategies) were the same among hospitalized patients subjected to the 12-step intervention in comparison with those subjected to the CBT. It shows that although one of the CBT priorities encompasses the development of self-efficacy and coping strategies, it is not necessarily the only therapy developing them. The authors argue that the fragile support of the specific CBT elements to the results may due to methodological failures. For example, the classical evaluation generally done in three or four steps (baseline, final line, and follow-up evaluations) may not be a good strategy. Performing several measurements in the course of a treatment, for example, may be a better strategy to identify mediators in a more subtle way. The authors suggested, for future studies, identifying possible CBT-specific mechanisms such as self-efficacy, readiness to change, overall commitment to the treatment, as well as therapeutic alliance. On the other hand, the article also discusses the good results of the twelve-step facilitation therapy, which are mostly compared to the CBT. Some specific elements identified in this approach were the link with the anonymous alcoholics, the commitment to abstinence, the spirituality, the character transformation, and the social learning factors. Social learning factors are also used by CBT. In short, most of the studies conducted so far identified the existence of active ingredients, but little was known about the way they worked. The authors point out the need for conceptual models that demonstrate the ways mediators can be identified.

Since then, the same proposal has been used in several studies in order to evaluate the processes and to identify the mediators of brief motivational interviews. A study compared the MI effectiveness versus the personalized feedback (alone) to young adult drinkers in an American emergency room. One group was subjected to one MI session, and the other just received personalized feedback. Both groups also received reinforcement by phone one and three months after the intervention. Results showed that the MI was able to reduce alcohol consumption, which was checked at the follow-up assessments performed 6 and 12 months after the intervention, using aggregate data (Monti et al. 2007). According to Gwaltney et al. (2011), although the strategy of using aggregate data to compare the groups (e.g., mean number of doses consumed in the last 6 months) is an interesting way to evaluate the MI efficacy results, it provides few details about the treatment dynamics over time. For example, the MI attempts to increase the motivation to stop or reduce alcohol consumption, which may occur immediately after the intervention or after 1 or 2 months, or even after the reinforcement by telephone. It is not possible to know, by just using an aggregate data 6 months later, or by comparing the mean number of doses consumed after the intervention, for example. Refined measurements may possibly find fluctuations over time better than the summary or aggregate measures (Neal et al. 2006). Thus, the research group suggested, in this same experiment, using the alcohol consumption data from a diary interview, in which the consumption of doses was recorded by the participants on a daily basis during the six evaluation months and also during 30 days before hospitalization. The main goal was to understand at what point the MI effects and those of the personalized feedback differed from each other. In a first attempt, differences were not observed between the groups when the data concerning all the post-intervention period days were analyzed. However, differences emerged when the intervals were individually analyzed. During the first 3 months after the intervention, there was no association between the type of treatment and alcohol consumption. However, in the 6-month assessment, i.e., after the reinforcement by phone at 3 months, the personalized feedback was associated with increased likelihood of drinking (Gwaltney et al. 2011). Therefore, the differences between groups only emerged after the reinforcement session conducted after 3 months and before 6 months, so that the possibility of heavy drinking in 1 day was significantly greater in the group that just received the personalized feedback. It means that both interventions were able to reduce the consumption within 3 months of assessment; however, the MI effect was stronger in the long term and the reinforcement session was more effective in this group. Results such as these show that investing in the MI and in the 3-month reinforcement session is valid when one wants to encourage alcohol consumption reduction in young drinkers at the hospital emergency room, although the personalized feedback is a simpler and probably lower-cost intervention.

Barnett et al. (2011), aiming to differentiate the MI effects from those of the personalized feedback in the emergency room of the aforementioned study, sought to identify possible intervention effectiveness moderators such as the patient's gender, the importance of the event that led him/her to the emergency room (if it was related to alcohol use), the alcohol use severity, and the degree of readiness to change the drinking behavior. In addition, the authors attempted to evaluate the behavior change mediators in the MI. The mediator was understood as a variable that temporarily intervenes between the intervention and the outcome assessment and that totally or partly explains their relationship. The main reason that justified this study was the lack of clarity as well as of consistent data supporting the brief intervention therapeutic effects on behavior change (Burke et al. 2003).

Most studies on the subject separately evaluate the elements, and they rarely include the effects of different possible elements (Apodaca and Longabaugh 2009). This study evaluated the effects of readiness to change, of the perceived risks and benefits, of self-efficacy, and of the search for additional treatment. All variables, except for alcohol consumption, were measured using just one question. The results showed that the patients admitted to the emergency room, due to alcohol use or not, may better benefit from interventions that take into consideration the alcohol consumption severity and the readiness to change. Thus, if the patient has drunk before entering the emergency room and/or score in the AUDIT as risk use pattern, a single question about the readiness to change could be added in order to provide the most appropriate intervention. Barnett et al. (2011) justify that the moderators and mediators evaluated in their study have contradictory effects toward the results of studies described in the literature.

As for the perceived risks and benefits, it is known that the development of discrepancy, which is one of the MI principles, aims to clarify to the individual the disconnection between the consequences of alcohol consumption and his/her goals and values. It suggests that the perception of risks and benefits may influence the behavior change.

As for self-efficacy, which in theory is one of the central MI elements, it is worth highlighting that increasing the drug user's self-efficacy perception may provide good results in changing his/her consumption behavior. However, studies have found conflicting results when they compared the groups subjected to MI and the control group (Galbraith 1989; Rohsenow et al. 2004). According to Rohsenow et al. (2004), the MI did not significantly change the self-efficacy of cocaine addicts in comparison with the control group. Galbraith (1989) compared the MI and an advice-interview for problematic alcohol users and found significant self-efficacy increase, which was measured by applying the Situational Confidence Questionnaire to those who were subjected to MI. According to the authors, it suggests that self-efficacy might not have been properly measured in some studies. The question regarding the search for additional treatment as a result of MI also appears in the literature with conflicting results (Barnett et al. 2007; Bernstein et al. 2005). According to the study by Barnett et al. (2007), the search for treatment in order to reduce alcohol consumption among college students was higher among those who were subjected to one brief MI session than among those who were subjected to computerized intervention. However, according to Bernstein et al. (2005), one MI session had no effect on the search for additional treatment among cocaine and heroin users. Identifying how the MI works could allow improving the knowledge and increasing health services' effectiveness. The authors recommend that further studies should be performed, especially among populations with different ages. However, these results highlight the fact that from the cost-effective perspective, the intervention itself, even if it is held in a single meeting, appears to be more cost-effective than an extremely brief intervention such as feedback alone.

Some studies focus on the effects mediators have on interventions performed with specific groups, such as college students and children and adolescents. Barnett et al. (2007) assessed the effects that mediators, in a brief motivational interview, had on the alcohol consumption by college students who had already had problems related to alcohol use. At the third-month follow-up, it was found that using behavioral strategies helped reducing alcohol consumption among the students subjected to MI in comparison with that of the control group. In other words, the amount of alcohol consumption was mediated by the use of behavioral strategies among those subjected to MI. On the other hand, other assessed variables such as motivation to change and the drinking perception by peers did not work as mediators in alcohol consumption. However, before the herein presented study, Fromme and Corbin (2004) found no study assessing the readiness to change drinking as a possible mediator of brief motivational interventions among young drinkers and college students. Thus, the authors tested the effectiveness of a program based on a motivational intervention and on behavioral techniques of CBT as a strategy to prevent alcohol consumption among college students. In addition, the group hypothesized that a high readiness to change would be predictive of good results in the program based on the results of the aforementioned Match Project. As it was previously mentioned, one of the Match Project hypotheses was that those who had low readiness to change would show better results in one of the three evaluated interventions, namely the MI. However, according to the study results, all the individuals who showed high readiness to change had positive results in the three intervention modalities (DiClemente et al. 2001). Thus, Fromme and Corbin (2004) also hypothesized that participating in the intervention could increase their motivation to change later. The first hypothesis was corroborated, since the high level of readiness to change influenced the reduction in heavy alcohol consumption. However, the study provided little evidence that the intervention improved motivation in those who showed low readiness to change.

The last mechanism we would like to address in the current chapter is the therapeutic alliance. The quality of the therapeutic relationship is identified as a significant predictor of good outcomes in psychotherapies and counseling techniques (Horvath and Symonds 1991). One of the major concerns among researchers in recent decades is trying to better understand how the therapeutic relationship factors work together with other specific and common factors. The factors have been described in the literature for a long time as improvement expectations, treatment ritual, and therapeutic relationship (Gilbert and Leahy 2007). Among the treatments for drug users within the Match Project, for example, it was found that a strong therapeutic alliance could better predict outcomes and adherence to treatment (Connors et al. 1997). A literature review that included peer-reviewed articles published between 1985 and 2005 (Meier et al. 2005) also found that early alliances seem to be a consistent predictor of commitment and adherence to treatment among drug users. The early-established alliance seems to favor more rapid improvement during treatment. However, it is not clear that the alliance directly influences the post-treatment results. The authors also found that until that year, there were few studies assessing the alliance determinants. The available studies showed that demographic features and drug use severity were not determinant aspects for the alliance. It was concluded that the alliance has to do with the results, but the alliance formation determinants are not yet clear in the literature. A study using the Match Project data published in 2015 (Maisto et al. 2015) showed that self-efficacy (measured after the treatment) was a mediator in the alcohol consumption reduction, thus reinforcing the effects of the good therapeutic alliance evaluated by the patient and by the therapist. The study reinforced the importance of the therapeutic alliance and self-efficacy to the treatment outcomes. However, the authors suggest that future research should examine the changes in the therapeutic alliance during treatment and how these changes relate to the self-efficacy and treatment results over time. These results seem to indicate that although the relationship influence in the results is clear, the scientific literature still does not answer how the alliance process happens and how it affects the results.

Final Considerations

MacKinnon et al. (2007) explain that the mediating variables have become the subject of interest of several studies in the psychological and social field. Two types of studies have been conducted to evaluate the mediators. The first study investigates how a particular effect happens. According to the authors, these studies take place after the completion of previous researches that found some relationship between two variables, such as X is related to Y. Next, another variable is added in order to improve the understanding about the relationship. A good example is the one in which several studies associate childhood physical abuse with violence in adulthood. One explanation for this pattern is that children exposed to physical violence acquire deviant patterns of social information processing that lead to violent behavior later in life. Authors such as Dodge et al. (1990) found evidence for this theory mediation process, because the social processing measurements explained the relation between the child physical abuse and the subsequent emergence of aggressive behavior. A second group of researchers uses the theory of mediators in experiments—those typically used to evaluate interventions and psychological treatments. In these cases, an intervention is developed to change one mediating variable that, in turn, will change the final result.

Despite the numerous studies performed to evaluate efficacy, to this day, very little is known about how brief evidence-based interventions for problems with alcohol and other drugs achieve their effects. The new movement toward the understanding of the specific elements that interfere in the results of brief interventions presented in the current chapter seems to be a promising way. Identifying the features associated with the better response to brief interventions could explain a number of inconsistencies found in studies, improve the intervention and the screening effectiveness, as well as increase the dissemination of brief intervention approaches. However, it is noteworthy that the process investigation is more advanced in treatment-focused interventions than in the BI used for primary or secondary prevention, although it is also interesting to researchers in this field. On the one hand, this review gives the impression that there is a good way for studies about intervention mechanisms to develop an appropriate conceptual model. On the other hand, it shows that understanding the treatment mechanisms may provide rich information to foster an evidence-based clinical practice.

References

Agerwala, S. M., & McCance-Katz, E. F. (2012). Integrating screening, brief intervention, and referral to treatment (SBIRT) into clinical practice settings: A brief review. *Journal of Psychoactive Drugs, 44*(4), 307–317.

Anderson, P., & Scott, E. (1992). The effect of general practitioners' advice to heavy drinking men. *British journal of addiction, 87*(6), 891–900.

Andretta, I., & Oliveira, M. S. (2008). Efeitos da entrevista motivacional em adolescentes infratores. *Estudos de Psicologia, 25*(1), 45–53.

Apodaca, T. R., & Longabaugh, R. (2009). Mechanisms of change in motivational interviewing: A review and preliminary evaluation of the evidence. *Addiction, 104*(5), 705–715.

Babor, T. F., & Grant, F. (Eds.). (1992). *Project on identification and management of alcohol-related problems: Report on phase II: A randomized clinical trial of brief interventions in primary health care.* Geneva, Switzerland, World Health Organization, Programme on Substance Abuse.

Babor, T. F., & Higgins-Biddle, J. C. (2003). *Intervenções breves para uso de risco e nocivo de álcool: Manual para uso em atenção primária* (C. M. Corradi, Trad.). Ribeirão Preto, SP: PAI-PAD.

Babor, T. F., Higgins-Biddle, J. C., Saunders, J. B., & Monteiro, M. G. (2006). *AUDIT—Teste para identificação de problemas relacionados ao uso de álcool: Roteiro para uso em atenção primária.* Ribeirão Preto, SP: PAI-PAD.

Ballesteros, J., Duffy, J. C., Querejeta, I., Ariño, J., & González-Pinto, A. (2004). Efficacy of brief interventions for hazardous drinkers in primary care: Systematic review and meta-analyses. *Alcoholism, Clinical and Experimental Research, 28*(4), 608–618.

Barnett, N. P., Apodaca, T. R., Magill, M., Colby, S. M., Gwaltney, C., Rohsenow, D. J., et al. (2011). Moderators and mediators of two brief interventions for alcohol in the emergency department. *Addiction, 105*(3), 452–465.

Barnett, N. P., Murphy, J. G., Colby, S. M., & Monti, P. M. (2007). Efficacy of counselor vs. computer-delivered intervention with mandated college students. *Addictive Behaviors, 32*(11), 2529–2548.

Bernstein, J., Bernstein, E., Tassiopoulos, K., Heeren, T., Levenson, S., & Hingson, R. (2005). Brief motivational intervention at a clinic visit reduces cocaine and heroin use. *Drug and Alcohol Dependence, 77*(1), 49–59.

Bien, T. H . (1992). *Motivational Intervention with Alcohol Outpatients,* doctoral dissertation (University of New Mexico).

Bien, T. H., Miller, W. R., & Tonigan, J. S. (1993). Brief interventions for alcohol problems: A review. *Addiction, 88*(3), 315–336.

Bricker, J. B. (2015). Climbing above the forest and the trees: Three future directions in addiction treatment research. *Addiction, 110*(3), 414–415.

Brown, J. M., & Miller, W. R. (1993). Impact of motivational interviewing on participation and outcome in residential alcoholism treatment. *Psychology of addictive behaviors, 7*(4), 211.

Burke, B. L., Arkowitz, H., & Menchola, M. (2003). The efficacy of motivational interviewing: A meta-analysis of controlled clinical trials. *Journal of Consulting and Clinical Psychology, 71* (5), 843–861.

Carey, K. B., Carey, M. P., Maisto, S. A., & Henson, J. M. (2006). Brief motivational interventions for heavy college drinkers: A randomized controlled trial. *Journal of Consulting and Clinical Psychology, 74*(5), 943–954.

Carpenter, R. A., Lyons, C. A., & Miller, W. R. (1985). Peer-managed self-control program for prevention of alcohol abuse in American Indian high school students: A pilot evaluation study. *International Journal of the Addictions, 20*(2), 299–310.

Castro, L. A., & Laranjeira, R. (2009). Ensaio clínico duplo-cego randomizado e placebocon-trolado com naltrexona e intervenção breve no tratamento ambulatorial da dependência de álcool. *Jornal Brasileiro de Psiquiatria, 58*(2), 79–85.

Chapman, P. L. H., & Huygens, I. (1988). An Evaluation of Three Treatment Programmes for Alcoholism: an experimental study with 6-and 18-month follow-ups. *British journal of addiction, 83*(1), 67–81.

Chick, J., Lloyd, G., & Crombie, E. (1985). Counselling problem drinkers in medical wards: a controlled study. *Br Med J (Clin Res Ed), 290*(6473), 965–967.

Chick, J., Ritson, B., Connaughton, J., Stewart, A., & Chick, J. (1988). Advice versus extended treatment for alcoholism: A controlled study. *British Journal of Addiction, 83*(2), 159–170.

Connors, G. J., Carroll, K. M., DiClemente, C. C., Longabaugh, R., & Donovan, D. M. (1997). The therapeutic alliance and its relationship to alcoholism treatment participation and outcome. *Journal of Consulting and Clinical Psychology, 65*(4), 588–598.

Daniels, V., Somers, M., Orford, J., & Kirby, B. (1992). How can risk drinking amongst medical patients be modified? The effects of computer screening and advice and a self-help manual. *Behavioural Psychotherapy, 20*(1), 47–60.

De Micheli, D., Fisberg, M., & Formigoni, M. L. O. S. (2004). Estudo da efetividade da intervenção breve para o uso de álcool e outras drogas em adolescentes atendidos num serviço de assistência primaria a saúde. *Revista da Associação Médica Brasileira, 50*(3), 305–313.

DiClemente, C. C., Carbonari, J., Zweben, A., Morrel, T., & Lee, R. E. (2001). Motivation hypothesis causal chain analysis. In R. Longabaugh & P. W. Wirtz (Eds.), *Project MATCH hypotheses: Results and causal chain analyses* (pp. 206–222). Bethesda, MD: U.S. Department of Health and Human Services, National Institute on Alcohol Abuse and Alcoholism.

Dodge, K. A., Bates, J. E., & Pettit, G. S. (1990). Mechanisms in the cycle of violence. *Science, 250*(4988), 1678–1683.

Donovan, D. M., Bogenschutz, M. P., Perl, H., Forcehimes, A., Adinoff, B., Mandler, R., et al. (2012). Study design to examine the potential role of assessment reactivity in the Screening, Motivational Assessment, Referral, and Treatment in Emergency Departments (SMART-ED) protocol. *Addiction Science & Clinical Practice, 7*, 16.

Donovan, D. M., & Mattson, M. E. (Special Issue Editors) (1994). Alcoholism treatment matching research: Methodological and clinical approaches. *Journal of Studies on Alcohol Supplement, 12*, 5–171.

Drummond, D. C., Thom, B., Brown, C., Edwards, G., & Mullan, M. J. (1990). Specialist versus general practitioner treatment of problem drinkers. *The Lancet, 336*(8720), 915–918. doi:10.1016/0140-6736(90)92279-Q

Edwards, G. & Orford, J. (1977). A plain treatment for alcoholism. *Proceedings of the Royal Society of Medicine, 70,* pp. 344–348.

Elvy, G. A., Wells, J. E., & Baird, K. A. (1988). Attempted referral as intervention for problem drinking in the general hospital. *British journal of addiction, 83*(1), 83–89.

Finney, J. W., Noyes, C. A., Coutts, A. I., & Moos, R. H. (1998). Evaluating substance abuse treatment process models: I. Changes on proximal outcome variables during 12-step and cognitive-behavioral treatment. *Journal of Studies on Alcohol, 59*(4), 371–380.

Formigoni, M. L. O. S. (1992). *A Intervenção Breve na Dependência de Drogas: A Experiência Brasileira*. São Paulo: Contexto.

Fromme, K., & Corbin, W. (2004). Prevention of heavy drinking and associated negative consequences among mandated and voluntary college students. *Journal of Consulting and Clinical Psychology, 72*(6), 1038–1049.

Galbraith, I. G. (1989). Minimal interventions with problem drinkers—A pilot study of the effect of two interview styles on perceived self-efficacy. *Health Bulletin, 6,* 311–314.

Gilbert, P., & Leahy, R. L. (2007). *The therapeutic relationship in the cognitive behavioral psychotherapies*. Londres/Nova York: Routledge.

Gwaltney, C. J., Magill, M., Barnett, N. P., Apodaca, T. R., Colby, S. M., & Monti, P. M. (2011). Using daily drinking data to characterize the effects of a brief alcohol intervention in an emergency room. *Addictive behaviors, 36*(3), 248–250.

Harris, K. B., & Miller, W. R. (1990). Behavioral self-control training for problem drinkers: Components of efficacy. *Psychology of Addictive Behaviors, 4*(2), 82.

Heather, N., Whitton, B., & Robertson, I. (1986). Evaluation of a self-help manual for media-recruited problem drinkers: Six-month follow-up results. *British Journal of Clinical Psychology, 25*(1), 19–34.

Heather, N., Robertson, I., MacPherson, B., Allsop, S., & Fulton, A. (1987). Effectiveness of a controlled drinking self-help manual: One-year follow-up results. *British Journal of Clinical Psychology, 26*(4), 279–287.

Heather, N., Kissoon-Singh, J. E. A. N., & Fenton, G. W. (1990). Assisted natural recovery from alcohol problems: effects of a self-help manual with and without supplementary telephone contact. *British Journal of Addiction, 85*(9), 1177–1185.

Heather, N. (1995). Interpreting the evidence on brief interventions for excessive drinkers: The need for caution. *Alcohol and Alcoholism, 30*(3), 287–296.

Horvath, A. O., & Symonds, B. D. (1991). Relation between working alliance and outcome in psychotherapy: A meta-analysis. *Journal of Counseling Psychology, 38*(2), 139–149.

Kahan, M., Wilson, L., & Becker, L. (1995). Effectiveness of physician-based interventions with problem drinkers: A review. *CMAJ Canadian Medical Association Journal, 152*(6), 851.

Kaner, E. F., Beyer, F., Dickinson, H. O., Pienaar, E., Campbell, F., Schlesinger, C., Heather, N., et al. (2007). Effectiveness of brief alcohol interventions in primary care populations. *The Cochrane Database of Systematic Reviews (electronic resource), 18*(2), CD004148.

Kazdin, A. E., & Nock, M. K. (2003). Delineating mechanisms of change in child and adolescent therapy: Methodological issues and research recommendations. *Journal of Child Psychology and Psychiatry and Allied Disciplines, 44*(8), 1116–1129.

Kristenson, H., Öhlin, H., Hultén-Nosslin, M. B., Trell, E., & Hood, B. (1983). Identification and intervention of heavy drinking in middle-aged men: Results and follow-up of 24–60 months of long-term study with randomized controls. *Alcoholism: clinical and experimental research, 7*(2), 203–209.

Kuchipudi, V., Hobein, K., Flickinger, A., & Iber, F. L. (1990). Failure of a 2-hour motivational intervention to alter recurrent drinking behavior in alcoholics with gastrointestinal disease. *Journal of studies on alcohol, 51*(4), 356–360.

Lock, C. A., Kaner, E., Heather, N., Doughty, J., Crawshaw, A., McNamee, P., et al. (2006). Effectiveness of nurse-led brief alcohol intervention: A cluster randomized controlled trial. *Journal of Advanced Nursing, 54*(4), 426–494.

Longabaugh, R., & Magill, M. (2012). Recent advances in behavioral addiction treatments: focusing on mechanisms of change. *Current Psychiatry Reports, 13*(5), 382–389.

Longabaugh, R., & Wirtz, P. W. (2001). Substantive review and critique. In R. Longabaugh & P. W. Wirtz (Eds.), *Project MATCH Hypotheses: Results and causal chain analyses* (Vol. 8, pp. 305–325). Rockville, MD: National Institute on Alcohol Abuse and Alcoholism.

Longabaugh, R., Donovan, D. M., Karno, M. P., McCrady, B. S., Morgenstern, J., & Tonigan, J. S. (2005). Active ingredients: How and why evidence-based alcohol behavioral treatment interventions work. *Alcoholism, Clinical and Experimental Research, 29*(2), 235–247.

MacKinnon, D. P., Fairchild, A. J., & Fritz, M. S. (2007). Mediation analysis. *Annual Review of Psychology, 58*, 593–614.

Maheswaran, R., Beevers, M., & Beevers, D. G. (1992). Effectiveness of advice to reduce alcohol consumption in hypertensive patients. *Hypertension, 19*(1), 79–84.

Maisto, S. A., Roos, C. R., O'Sickey, A. J., Kirouac, M., Connors, G. J., Tonigan, J. S., et al. (2015). The indirect effect of the therapeutic alliance and alcohol abstinence self-efficacy on alcohol use and alcohol-related problems in Project MATCH. *Alcoholism, Clinical and Experimental Research, 39*(3), 504–513.

Magill, M., & Longabaugh, R. (2013). Efficacy combined with specified ingredients: A new direction for empirically supported addiction treatment. *Addiction, 108*(5), 874–881.

Marques, A. C. P. R., & Furtado, E. F. (2004). Intervenções breves para problemas relacionados ao álcool. *Revista Brasileira de Psiquiatria, 26*(Suppl 1), 28–32.

McCambridge, J. (2013). Brief intervention content matters [Editorial]. *Drug and Alcohol Review, 32*(4), 339–341.

McCambridge, J., & Day, M. (2008). Randomized controlled trial of the effects of completing the Alcohol Use Disorders Identification Test questionnaire on self-reported hazardous drinking. *Addiction, 103*(2), 241–248.

Meier, P. S., Barrowclough, C., & Donmall, M. C. (2005). The role of the therapeutic alliance in the treatment of substance misuse: A critical review of the literature. *Addiction, 100*(3), 304–316.

Miller, W. R., & Rollnick, S. (1991). Motivational interviewing: Preparing people to change their addictive behavior. *New York: Guilford*.

Miller, W. R., & Rollnick, S. (2001). *A entrevista motivacional*. Porto Alegre: Artmed.

Miller, W. R., & Sanchez, V. C. (1993). Motivating young adults for treatment and lifestyle change. In G. Howard (Ed.), *Issues in alcohol use and misuse by young adults* (pp. 55–82). Notre Dame: University of Notre Dame Press.

Miller, W. R., & Taylor, C. A. (1980). Relative effectiveness of bibliotherapy, individual and group self-control training in the treatment of problem drinkers. *Addictive Behaviors, 5*(1), 13–24.

Miller, W. R., Gribskov, C. J., & Mortell, R. L. (1981). Effectiveness of a self-control manual for problem drinkers with and without therapist contact. *International Journal of the Addictions, 16*(7), 1247–1254.

Miller, W. R., Sovereign, R. G., & Krege, B. (1988). Motivational interviewing with problem drinkers: II. The Drinker's Check-up as a preventive intervention. *Behavioural Psychotherapy, 16*(4), 251–268.

Miller, W. R., Taylor, C. A., & West, J. C. (1980). Focused versus broad-spectrum behavior therapy for problem drinkers. *Journal of consulting and clinical psychology, 48*(5), 590.

Monti, P. M., Barnett, N. P., Colby, S. M., Gwaltney, C. J., Spirito, A., Rohsenow, D. J., et al. (2007). Motivational interviewing versus feedback only in emergency care for young adult problem drinking. *Addiction, 102*(8), 1234–1243.

Moyer, A., Finney, J. W., Swearingen, C. E., & Vergun, P. (2002). Brief interventions for alcohol problems: A meta-analytic review of controlled investigations in treatment-seeking and non-treatment-seeking populations. *Addiction, 97*(3), 279–292.

Neal, D. J., Fromme, K., Boca, F. K., Parks, K. A., King, L. P., Pardi, A. M., et al. (2006). Capturing the moment: Innovative approaches to daily alcohol assessment. *Alcoholism, Clinical and Experimental Research, 30*(2), 282–291.

Nilsen, P., Kaner, E., & Babor, T. F. (2008). Brief intervention, three decades on. *Nordic Studies on Alcohol and Drugs, 25*(6), 453–468.

O'Donnell, A., Anderson, P., Newbury-Birch, D., Schulte, B., Schmidt, C., Reimer, J., et al. (2014). The impact of brief alcohol interventions in primary healthcare: A systematic review of reviews. *Alcohol and Alcoholism, 49*(1), 66–78.

Oliveira, M. S., Andretta, I., Rigoni, M. S., & Szupszynski, K. P. R. (2008). A entrevista motivacional com alcoolistas: um estudo longitudinal. *Psicologia: Reflexão e Crítica, 21*(2), 261–266.

Pengpid, S., Peltzer, K., Skaal, L., & Van der Heever, H. (2013). Screening and brief interventions for hazardous and harmful alcohol use among hospital outpatients in South Africa: Results from a randomized controlled trial. *BMC Public Health, 13*(1), 644.

Pereira, M. O., Anginoni, B. M., Ferreira, N. C., Oliveira, M. A. F., Vargas, D., & Colvero, L. A. (2013). Efetividade da intervenção breve para o uso abusivo de álcool na atenção primária: revisão sistemática. *Revista Brasileira de Enfermagem, 66*(3), 420–428.

Persson, J., & Magnusson, P. H. (1989). Early intervention in patients with excessive consumption of alcohol: a controlled study. *Alcohol, 6*(5), 403–408.

Prochaska, J. O., & DiClemente, C. (1992). Stages of change in the modification of problem behaviors. In M. Hersen, M. Eiser, & W. Miller (Eds.), *Progress in behavior modification* (pp. 184–214). Sycamore: Sycamore Press.

Project MATCH Research Group. (1998). Matching alcoholism treatments to client heterogeneity: Project MATCH three year drinking outcomes. *Alcoholism, Clinical and Experimental Research, 22*(6), 1300–1311.

Robertson, I., Heather, N., Dzialdowski, A., Crawford, J., & Winton, M. (1986). A comparison of minimal versus intensive controlled drinking treatment interventions for problem drinkers. *British Journal of Clinical Psychology, 25*(3), 185–194.

Rohsenow, D. J., Monti, P. M., Martin, R. A., Colby, S. M., Myers, M. G., Gulliver, S. B., et al. (2004). Motivational enhancement and coping skills training for cocaine abusers: Effects on substance use outcomes. *Addiction, 99*(7), 862–874.

Romelsjö, A., Andersson, L., BARRNER, H., Borg, S., Granstrand, C., Hultman, O., ... & Nyman, K. (1989). A randomized study of secondary prevention of early stage problem drinkers in primary health care. *British journal of addiction, 84*(11), 1319–1327.

Sales, C. M. B., & Figlie, N. B. (2009). Revisão de literatura sobre a aplicação da entrevista motivacional breve em usuários nocivos e dependentes de álcool. *Psicologia em Estudo, 14*(2), 333–340.

Sannibale, C. (1988). The differential effect of a set of brief interventions on the functioning of a group of "early-stage" problem drinkers. *Drug and Alcohol Review, 7*(2), 147–155. http://dx.doi.org/10.1080/09595238880000321.

Scott, E., & Anderson, P. (1990). Randomized controlled trial of general practitioner intervention in women with excessive alcohol consumption. *Drug and Alcohol Review, 10*(4), 313–321.

Skutle, A., & Berg, G. (1987). Training in controlled drinking for early-stage problem drinkers. *British Journal of Addiction, 82*(5), 493–501.

Thom, B., Herring, R., Luger, L., & Annand, F. (2014). Delivering Alcohol IBA: Broadening the base from health to non-health contexts. *Alcool Insights, 116*, 1–5.

U.S. Preventive Services Task Force. (2004). Screening and behavioral counseling interventions in primary care to reduce alcohol misuse: Recommendation statement. *Annals of Internal Medicine, 140*(7), 554–556.

Wallace, P., Cutler, S., & Haines, A. (1988). Randomised controlled trial of general practitioner intervention in patients with excessive alcohol consumption. *Bmj, 297*(6649), 663–668.

Whitlock, E. P., Polen, M. R., Green, C. A., Orleans, T., & Klein, J. (2004). Behavioral counseling interventions in primary care to reduce risky/harmful alcohol use by adults: A summary of the evidence for the US Preventive Services Task Force. *Annals of Internal Medicine, 140*(7), 557–568.

Wilk, A. I., Jensen, N. M., & Havighurst, T. C. (1997). Meta-analysis of randomized control trials addressing brief interventions in heavy alcohol drinkers. *Journal of General Internal Medicine, 12*(5), 274–283.

Zweben, A., Pearlman, S., & Li, S. (1988). A comparison of brief advice and conjoint therapy in the treatment of alcohol abuse: The results of the marital systems study. *British Journal of addiction, 83*(8), 899–916.

Chapter 9
Web-Based Interventions for Substance Abuse

Michael P. Schaub

Introduction

In recent times, the international literature has described treatment models targeting the general population and, besides supplying informative measures at the level of primary and secondary prevention, also offering Web-based self-help tools for problematic substance users in line with tertiary prevention (Blankers et al. 2011; Postel et al. 2010; Riper et al. 2008). So far, there is a good and constant evidence for Web-based self-help interventions for problematic drinking, but only a few studies have investigated the scientific effectiveness of such interventions for problematic stimulant drug use (Schaub et al. 2012). Some Web-based self-help studies exist for the reduction of cannabis use in problematic users so far divergent results.

The interventions' backgrounds are, however, more or less the same. They are based on classical therapy approaches from cognitive-behavioural therapy for substance abuse (e.g. Carroll 2005), motivational interviewing (McKee et al. 2007), principles of self-control (Sobell and Sobell 1993; Velicer et al. 1990) and the well-established relapse prevention model, that is often integrated in the corresponding cognitive-behavioural therapy. There are also numerous Web-based brief intervention studies that are mainly focusing on personalized individual feedback based on established addiction measurement instruments such as the Alcohol Use Disorders Identification Test (Babor et al. 2001). So far, there is also enough

M.P. Schaub (✉)
Swiss Research Institute for Public Health and Addiction ISGF,
Zurich University, Postfach, 8031 Zürich, Switzerland
e-mail: michael.schaub@isgf.uzh.ch

© Springer International Publishing Switzerland 2016
A.L.M. Andrade and D. De Micheli (eds.), *Innovations in the Treatment of Substance Addiction*, DOI 10.1007/978-3-319-43172-7_9

evidence for the effectiveness of these studies. The pooled effect sizes are smaller than in the more comprehensive Web-based therapy intervention mentioned before.

On the other hand, there is a growing number of Internet counselling services. Assuming many of them based on classical e-mail exchange, some on anonymous chat sessions and a few clinical case examples based on more intensive Internet exchange forms such as video sessions (e.g. with Skype or Google Hangouts). The overwhelming majority of these services and of these Internet communication modalities have not been scientifically tested for effectiveness in the field of substance abuse. In contrast, there are numerous studies on other mental health problems with the so-called guided Internet therapy interventions. There is increasing evidence that guided (e.g. by chat based or e-mail based) cognitive-behavioural therapy is boosting the effects previously found for Web-based self-help-only intervention for subclinical depression and anxiety disorders (Andersson and Cuijpers 2009; Spek et al. 2007). Moreover, there are investigations demonstrating that a sufficient therapeutic alliance can be reached by guided individual predominantly e-mail-based cognitive-behavioural treatment of depression, generalized anxiety and social anxiety disorders and PTSD (e.g. Andersson et al. 2012; Knaevelsrud and Maercker 2007; Preschl et al. 2011).

The present chapter aims at summarizing the current scientific evidence on the effectiveness of unguided and guided Web-based therapy interventions for substance use/abuse. Moreover, it aims at providing a theoretical background for these interventions, summarizing the therapeutic concepts applied, developing a suitable framework to arrange current scientific evidence and providing future research perspectives.

Theoretical Background

The perhaps strongest advantage of Internet addiction therapy is that it can be fully anonymous, place- and time-independent (e.g. Haug et al. 2011). Historically, Internet counselling and therapy emerged as an emergency solution in developed countries with partially very long distances to travel to reach, e.g. a family doctor or even further for an addiction specialist. These early developments started amongst others in Australia, Canada and the USA in the early 1990s. Some of them are known to the author more as non-professional self-help group or peer-to-peer exchange services in order to reach also isolated persons in need. In the last 10–15 years, these emergency solutions became more and more professional, more widespread and developed also into a special solution for persons with specific needs that are also very prominent in individual with substance abuse problems. These are help-seeking persons that explicitly do not wish to see a professional person or visit a service as of fear of stigmatization or a distinct need for anonymity (Kersting et al. 2009; Leuschner and Tossmann 2009). A third reason is that they do want to keep the personal distance to the counselling person or the therapist (Leuschner and Tossmann 2009). Addiction therapy and addiction counselling on

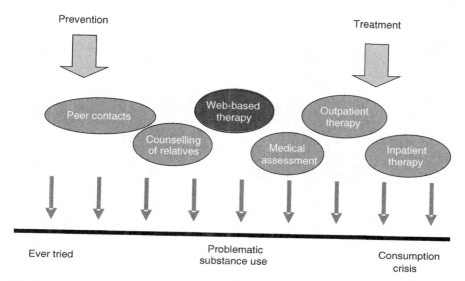

Fig. 9.1 Different forms of counselling and therapy between the two poles that addiction treatment and prevention services can cover

the Internet can be arranged in the middle field between the two poles "ever tried once a substance" and "inpatient treatment" (see Fig. 9.1).

In general, addiction therapy or addiction counselling is independent in their form of Internet communication. Doering (2003) stated in his media-economic framework model for the social psychology of the Internet that the choice of a communication medium is a conscious decision. This means for example that a person with a substance use problem will choose rather a user forum, a self-help intervention or a guided chat session depending on his/her need. Therefore, it is also obvious that a person will use different communication mediums depending on his/ her therapy process phase. A first contact could for instance be rather in a guided user forum while guided chat contacts are more considered in later therapy phases. Initial e-mail contacts can thus quite often end also in later face-to-face therapies. More frequently occur on the contrary single questions to distinct and limited questions to specific addiction-related problems..

The proximity and distance in a face-to-face therapy can be theorized as located on a continuum as it might be the case for single Internet communication medium. One issue that merits a specific note is the fact that there is in contrast a clear discrepancy between the proximity and distance for time-simultaneous and time-divergent communication mediums (see Fig. 9.2). While there is a gap of several hours and days between a question of a help-seeking person and the answer of his/her therapist in an e-mail-based addiction therapy, there is just a short break or even almost no break in a chat-based or a video-chat-based Internet therapy (e.g. with Skype and Google Hangouts). Self-help therapy approaches build the largest personal distance between the initial developer of the therapy interventions and the

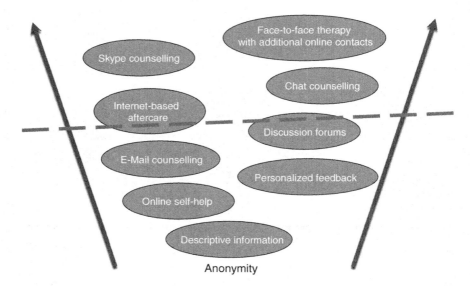

Fig. 9.2 Technical options for Web-based addiction counselling and therapy

help-seeking person. Completely anonymous is finally descriptive non-interactive information presented for example on an addiction information website.

Last but not least, it has to be mentioned that amongst the several advantages a Web-based guided or unguided addiction therapy intervention can have, there is certainly one disadvantage. The access to a computer with Internet connection is a requirement and—although to a lesser extent—sufficient computer and Internet literacy (Neale and Stevenson 2014; Redpath et al. 2006). Moreover, in the written communication modalities, the non-verbal communication (facial expression, gesture) is very difficult to be realized, and thus, the phenomenon of a substance use problem can hardly be captured in its whole complexity (e.g. Kersting et al. 2009). Preliminary findings however demonstrated that the quality of the therapeutic relationship can be—in the comprehension of Carl R. Rogers (empathy, congruence and appreciation)—at least in the longer term as good than in a face-to-face therapy (David et al. 2005). Thus, it can be assumed that it is rather a matter of intensity (number and frequency of contacts) until a good addiction therapist can reach sufficient therapeutic alliance for an as successful therapy as in a face-to-face condition. On the other hand, intimate topics such as unprotected sexual contacts or other behaviours that might result in unwanted sexual transmitted disease infections are often easier and earlier broached as an issue in an online compared to a face-to-face therapy.

Current Evidence for Web-Based Interventions Aimed at the Reduction or Cessation of Alcohol Use

So far, the best-investigated substance use field in terms of Web-based therapy interventions is the alcohol use field. Meta-analyses demonstrated effectiveness for Web-based personalized feedback interventions for the reduction of alcohol use post-intervention (Riper et al. 2009) with low-to-moderate effect sizes [$d = 0.22$ (95 % CI = 0.16, 0.29)] and for the reduction of grams of ethanol consumed in the longer term (Riper et al. 2011). A further meta-analyses that also included more thorough interventions yielded similar effect sizes for the reduction of alcohol use ($d = 0.22$ (95 % CI = 0.14, 0.29) and in comparison for the cessation of tobacco use ($d = 0.14$ (95 % CI = 0.06, 0.23); Rooke et al. 2010). One of the earlier studies found a higher effect for a comprehensive guided chat therapy in addition to self-help in comparison with self-help alone for the reduction of alcohol use 6 months post-intervention start (Blankers et al. 2011). Interestingly, this effect even increased in the long-term 12 months after intervention start. The question whether more comprehensive guided addiction counselling for the reduction of alcohol use in problematic alcohol users is more effective than (brief) self-help interventions is still unclear. A very recent meta-analysis did not find evidence to support such an obvious assumption (Riper et al. 2014). However, as the authors of this recent meta-analysis point out correctly, the number of guided studies for the reduction of alcohol consumption is currently low and most of these included subjects sought help for the first time. Studies with more severe cases with more pronounced alcohol consumption are rare. Not surprisingly, studies that aimed at the reduction of substance use in general yielded higher effect sizes that those aiming at abstinence (Rooke et al. 2010).

In the recent years, there is also a newer trend developing that combines Web-based self-help interventions or brief face-to-face interventions for the reduction of alcohol use with mobile phone technologies such as SMS. This has been shown to be especially promising in keeping youth and young adults in interventions aiming at the reduction of risky alcohol consumption (Haug et al. 2013) or as a kind of additional aftercare support in young adults after emergency department visits (Suffoletto et al. 2014) or in adults after outpatient treatment (Haug et al. 2015). On the other hand, it is somewhat surprising that there are no studies conducted so far, that combined face-to-face alcohol treatment with Web-based interventions and compared them with Web-based interventions alone. Finally, no study investigated the effectiveness of video-chat-based interventions.

Current Evidence for Web-Based Interventions Aimed at the Reduction of Stimulant Use

While there are over two dozens of Web-based studies that aimed at the reduction of alcohol use, there are only four studies so far, that focus on the reduction of stimulants. One is ongoing (Champion et al. 2013), two are published (Schaub et al. 2011, 2012; Tait et al. 2012, 2014), and a fourth just started.

The results of the first snow control study demonstrated the feasibility and initial effectiveness of an anonymous, fully automated, Web-based self-help intervention. Participants in this intervention group received interactive cognitive-behavioural modules and a consumption diary to reduce cocaine use, whereas participants in the control group received online psycho-educative information modules. The Web-based intervention attracted older and more educated participants than existing outpatient treatment programmes for which cocaine is the primary substance of abuse. Participants in the intervention group showed greater treatment retention compared with the control group. However, the response rates at the follow-up assessments were very low and restricted the explanatory power of the analyses. At the follow-up assessments, the severity of cocaine dependence did not differ between the intervention and control groups. Furthermore, there were no differences in cocaine craving, depression, or alcohol and other substance use. Using the consumption diaries, the average number of cocaine-free days per week did not change significantly, whereas the weekly quantity of cocaine used decreased equally in both groups. The snow control intervention is currently under revision, and a new three-arm randomized controlled trial will be conducted in order to test the effectiveness of this revised version with additional chat-counselling versus self-help alone versus a classical waiting list.

Another study called breaking the ice is evaluated in a randomized controlled trial the effect of an Internet intervention for amphetamine-type stimulant problems in 160 adult Australians compared with a wait list control group (Tait et al. 2012, 2014). Breaking the ice consists of three modules requiring an estimated total completion time of 90 min. The content of the modules was adapted from face-to-face clinical techniques based on cognitive-behavioural therapy and motivation enhancement. The result of the study was generally mixed. At 3 months, 43 % of intervention and 57 % of control participants provided follow-up data. In the intervention group, 63 % completed at least one module. The only significant group by time interaction was for days out of role. The pre-/post-change effect sizes showed small changes (range $d = 0.14$–0.40) favoring the intervention group for poly-drug use, distress, actual help seeking and days out of role. In contrast, the control group was favored by reductions in ATS use, improvements in quality of life and increases in help-seeking intentions (range $d = 0.09$–0.16).

Another ongoing study in Australia investigates within an already positively evaluated Internet school prevention programme for the prevention of alcohol and cannabis use the effectiveness of a programme to prevent from ecstasy use of 10- to 12-year-old students in a cluster randomized controlled trial (Champion et al. 2013).

No studies currently combine face-to-face stimulant treatment with Web-based interventions or investigate the effectiveness of video-chat-based interventions for stimulant users.

Current Evidence for Web-Based Interventions Aimed at the Reduction of Cannabis and Other Drug Use

Currently, there are only two specific Web-based programmes published that aimed at the reduction of cannabis use that have been investigated in randomized controlled trials, and these programmes employ different intervention approaches (Rooke et al. 2013; Tossmann et al. 2011). The German "Quit the Shit" programme (Tossmann et al. 2011) is based on principles of self-regulation and self-control and is a solution-focused approach. This programme is structured into weekly personalized feedback sessions based on participants' consumption diary entries, intake and termination chats, and the total allowed programme time is 50 days. Attrition in the German study of Tossmann et al. (2011) was high and higher in the intervention (11.6 %) condition than in the waiting list control condition (24.7 %). Nevertheless, these authors found significant effects on cannabis use reduction in their per-protocol and last-observation-carried-forward analyses. The Australian programme "Reduce Your Use: How to Break the Cannabis Habit" (Rooke et al. 2013) is a fully automated self-help intervention consisting of 6 modules for the amelioration of cannabis use disorders based on cognitive-behavioural therapy (CBT) approaches (Goldstein et al. 1989; Marlatt 1985), motivational interviewing (Miller and Rollnick 1991) and behavioural self-management (Copeland et al. 2001). This programme was tested for effectiveness in a randomized controlled trial and compared to a psycho-educative control condition also consisting of 6 modules. Study retention was higher in the intervention and the control condition after 6 weeks (66 vs. 64 %) and at a 3-month follow-up (54 vs. 52 %) than in the aforementioned German study (Tossmann et al. 2011). The frequency of cannabis use and the quantity of cannabis consumed were both more reduced in the intervention group than in the control group at 6 weeks and at the 3-month follow-up.

An ongoing Swiss study investigates the effectiveness of the combination of a fully automated self-help intervention for the reduction of cannabis use with additional individual chat sessions (Schaub et al. 2013). No studies conducted so far if face-to-face cannabis use disorder treatment combined with Web-based interventions is more effective than Web-based interventions alone. No study investigated the effectiveness of video-chat-based interventions for the reduction of cannabis use.

There is also a positively evaluated school prevention programme from Australia that involved 10-year-old students. The so-called Climate School Alcohol and Cannabis course successfully increased cannabis and alcohol-related knowledge, and decreased the average consumption of alcohol use and the frequency of cannabis use and binge drinking amongst young people (Newton et al. 2009, 2010). There is a first meta-analysis published that found a positive pooled effect size of $g = 0.16$ (95 % CI = 0.09, 0.22) for a total of 10 computer- and/or Internet-based interventions that aimed at the reduction of cannabis use frequency (Tait et al. 2013). However, this very preliminary meta-analysis mixed these two types of interventions and consequently yielded no effects on subgroup analyses.

Three new studies from the USA investigated Internet-based intervention in opioid substitution therapy. The first one investigated the effectiveness of a Web-based behavioural intervention that partially substituted for standard counselling in a community-based methadone substitution programme (Marsch et al. 2014). Replacing a portion of standard treatment with this intervention resulted in greater rates of objectively measured opioid abstinence. In a second study, participants of a buprenorphine substitution treatment programme received an Internet-based community reinforcement approach intervention plus contingency management (money for negative urine screenings) or contingency management alone (Christensen et al. 2014). Compared to those receiving contingency management alone, recipients of the combined intervention exhibited more of abstinence and had a reduced hazard of dropping out of treatment. The third study is the only one in the entire Internet-based substance use treatment field that tested the feasibility and acceptability of a video-chat-based intervention (King et al. 2014). Study participants in the video-chat condition showed lower study retention than those receiving classical face-to-face counselling. However, they had similar rates of counselling attendance and drug-positive urinalysis results, and reported similar and strong ratings of treatment satisfaction and therapeutic alliance.

Current Evidence for Cost-Effectiveness for Web-Based Interventions Aimed at the Reduction of Substance Use

The question of cost-effectiveness of Web-based interventions aimed at the reduction of substance use and especially its impact on a population level has been rarely addressed in scientific studies. Many practitioners take it already as a fact that the introduction and implementation of Web-based interventions can save money in the addiction care system. However, it is not that easy as those few available studies currently published show. There is only one study in the alcohol field from the Netherlands that compared the cost-effectiveness of Internet therapy with up to 10 chat sessions versus Internet self-help (Blankers et al. 2012). The effort of Internet therapy for the reduction of alcohol use in problematic alcohol user yielded a median incremental cost-effectiveness ratio of €3683 per additional treatment responder and €14,710 per quality-adjusted life-year (QALY) gained. At a willingness to pay €20,000 for one additional quality-adjusted life-year, Internet therapy for the reduction of alcohol use had a 60 % likelihood of being more cost-effective than Internet self-help.

Another study from the Netherlands—a country where health insurance companies nota bene partially pay Internet-based therapy—simulated costs and gains of quality-adjusted life-years on population level in case that half of the alcohol treatment services ranging from counselling for problematic drinking until inpatient alcohol treatment will be replaced by Internet-based addiction services. This study estimated that in the current health care system for alcohol addiction problems, every invested Euro results in a health gain of Euro 1.08. Under the new system, where 50 % would be replaced, every invested Euro will result in a health gain of Euro 1.64. The current system costs 233 Million Euro. However, the estimated costs to reach the new system are estimated 86 Million Euro. Therefore, in the Netherlands, much more persons with alcohol problems could be helped and this help would be much more successful. However, this would need an initial strong investment.

Another important message merits attention concerning cost-effectiveness. Classical face-to-face addiction treatments must at least partially be replaced by Internet-based addiction services to gain cost-effectiveness. To add simply new Internet-based service to existing face-to-face services per se ends up with higher costs, increases working loads of present therapists, and potentially could displease some of them.

Discussion

The present chapter provides a good update brief overview of the current evidence on Web-based interventions for problematic substance use and substance abuse. This field is currently very active, and it can be expected that there will be numerous studies in the coming years. For the reduction of alcohol use, there is already considerable evidence for effectiveness from meta-analyses for Web-based interventions that aim at reducing problematic alcohol use. Compared to Web-based interventions aiming at the reduction of other mental health problems than substance abuse problems, those aiming at the reduction or cessation of substance use have to deal with comparatively strong attrition problems. This is especially the case for interventions aiming at the reduction of stimulant use, less for interventions aiming at the reduction of cannabis or opioid use and the least for those for the reduction of alcohol use. New ways have to be found in the future in order to reduce these problems. Some of these problems could be solved in trying to tailor these Web-based interventions better for substance use specific subgroups and potentially also for their subpopulations, e.g. Web-based intervention for the reduction of cannabis use in male users aged 16–25, etc. Another approach might be the integration of modules aiming at the reduction of frequently observed comorbidity factors into the Web-based substance use interventions. There are initial findings that, e.g., those individuals with higher depression symptoms do stay longer in Web-based interventions for the reduction of cocaine use (Schaub et al. 2012). So why do we not offer also core modules from Web-based interventions aiming at the treatment of depression symptoms for those who might benefit from these? However, the evidence for Web-based interventions other than those aiming at the reduction of alcohol use has to be increased, and thus, more studies are needed in general.

Interestingly, studies on the effectiveness of the combination of face-to-face therapy with Web-based intervention have been rarely addressed. To my personal experience, there are sometimes concerns from addiction therapist that Web-based interventions aim at the reduction of treatment costs and of their work in the end. However, as long as between 10 and 20 % of those with addiction-related problems do not receive any treatment, these concerns appear to be unethical indeed. We must increase addiction treatment access and treatment provision by using Web-based interventions according to the principal of concurrent cover (i.e. non-invasive, low-cost interventions in which therapeutic intensity can be enhanced according to need). However, the introduction of Web-based services first needs additional investments before treatment access can be increased. This investment might be a rewarding investment for almost all countries worldwide as Internet access is even increasing in some Third-World countries now. However, Web-based interventions should, in order to keep investments and workloads low, not be in addition to already implemented face-to-face treatments; they should complete or partially replace them.

Whether Web-based interventions do reach the same effectiveness as face-to-face addiction treatments in 1 day—as it is currently the case for Web-based intervention that reduces depression symptoms when compared to depression treatment as usual—is a difficult question. Currently, we are not at this stage. However, the interventions are improving quickly, and we are approximating more and more this stage.

References

Andersson, G., & Cuijpers, P. (2009). Internet-based and other computerized psychological treatments for adult depression: A meta-analysis. *Cognitive Behaviour Therapy, 38*(4), 196–205. doi:10.1080/16506070903318960

Andersson, G., Paxling, B., Wiwe, M., Vernmark, K., Felix, C. B., Lundborg, L., et al. (2012). Therapeutic alliance in guided internet-delivered cognitive behavioural treatment of depression, generalized anxiety disorder and social anxiety disorder. *Behaviour Research and Therapy, 50*(9), 544–550. doi:10.1016/j.brat.2012.05.003

Babor, T. F., Higgins-Biddle, J. C., Saunders, J. B., & Monteiro, M. G. (2001). *AUDIT: The Alcohol Use Disorders Identification Test: Guidelines for use in primary care* (2nd Ed.). World Health Organization: Department of Mental Health and Substance Dependence.

Blankers, M., Koeter, M. W., & Schippers, G. M. (2011). Internet therapy versus internet self-help versus no treatment for problematic alcohol use: A randomized controlled trial. *Journal of Consulting and Clinical Psychology, 79*(3), 330–341. doi:10.1037/a0023498

Blankers, M., Nabitz, U., Smit, F., Koeter, M. W., & Schippers, G. M. (2012). Economic evaluation of internet-based interventions for harmful alcohol use alongside a pragmatic randomized controlled trial. *Journal of Medical Internet Research, 14*(5), 71–83. doi:10.2196/jmir.2052

Carroll, K. M. (2005). Recent advances in the psychotherapy of addictive disorders. *Current Psychiatry Reports, 7*(5), 329–336.

Champion, K. E., Teesson, M., & Newton, N. C. (2013). A cluster randomised controlled trial of the Climate Schools: Ecstasy and emerging drugs module in Australian secondary schools: Study protocol. *BMC Public Health, 13*, 1168. doi:10.1186/1471-2458-13-1168

Christensen, D. R., Landes, R. D., Jackson, L., Marsch, L. A., Mancino, M. J., Chopra, M. P., et al. (2014). Adding an internet-delivered treatment to an efficacious treatment package for opioid dependence. *Journal of Consulting and Clinical Psychology, 82*, 1–9. doi:10.1037/a0037496

Copeland, J., Swift, W., Roffman, R., & Stephens, R. (2001). A randomized controlled trial of brief cognitive-behavioral interventions for cannabis use disorder. *Journal of Substance Abuse Treatment, 21*(2), 55–64. doi:10.1016/S0740-5472(01)00179-9

David, N., Peter, D., Prudlo, U. (2005). *Zur therapeutischen Beziehung im virtuellen Raum (Internet)—Eine explorative Online-Studie.* Verfügbar unter: http://www.fob.uni-tuebingen.de/fachpublikum/forschung/feldstudie.php.

Doering, N. (2003). *Sozialpsychologie des Internets. Die Bedeutung des Internets für Kommunikationsprozesse, Identitäten, soziale Beziehungen und Gruppen.* Göttingen: Hogrefe. doi:10.1024//0044-3514.31.3.166

Goldstein, M. G., Niaura, R., Follick, M. J., & Abrams, D. B. (1989). Effects of behavioral skills training and schedule of nicotine gum administration on smoking cessation. *The American Journal of Psychiatry, 146*(1), 56–60.

Haug, S., Dymalski, A., & Schaub, M. P. (2011). *Webbasierte Tabakprävention: Evaluation vorhandener Angebote, allgemeiner Wirksamkeitsnachweis und Nutzeneinschätzung von Zielgruppen in der Schweiz. Syntheseberricht.* Zürich: ISGF.

Haug, S., Lucht, M. J., John, U., Meyer, C., & Schaub, M. P. (2015). A pilot study on the feasibility and effectiveness of text message-based aftercare among alcohol outpatients. *Alcohol and Alcoholism, 50*(2), 188–194.

Haug, S., Schaub, M. P., Venzin, V., Meyer, C., John, U., & Gmel, G. (2013). A pre-post study on the appropriateness and effectiveness of a web- and text messaging-based intervention to reduce problem drinking in emerging adults. *Journal of Medical Internet Research, 15*(9), 126–137. doi:10.2196/jmir.2755

Kersting, A., Schlicht, S., & Kroker, K. (2009). Internet therapy. Opportunities and boundaries. *Nervenarzt, 80*(7), 797–804. doi:10.1007/s00115-009-2721-5

King, V. L., Brooner, R. K., Peirce, J. M., Kolodner, K., & Kidorf, M. S. (2014). A randomized trial of web-based videoconferencing for substance abuse counseling. *Journal of Substance Abuse Treatment, 46*(1), 36–42. doi:10.1016/j.jsat.2013.08.009

Knaevelsrud, C., & Maercker, A. (2007). Internet-based treatment for PTSD reduces distress and facilitates the development of a strong therapeutic alliance: A randomized controlled clinical trial. *BMC Psychiatry, 7*, 13. doi:10.1186/1471-244X-7-13

Leuschner, F., & Tossmann, P. (2009). Internet-based drug treatment interventions. Insights, Issue 10 edited by EMCDDA, 07/2009; *European Monitoring Centre for Drugs and Drug Addiction (EMCDDA)*, Lisbon. ISBN: 978-92-9168-348-2

Marlatt, G. A. (1985). *Relapse prevention: Maintenance strategies in treatment of addictive behaviors.* New York: Guildford Press.

Marsch, L. A., Guarino, H., Acosta, M., Aponte-Melendez, Y., Cleland, C., Grabinski, M., et al. (2014). Web-based behavioral treatment for substance use disorders as a partial replacement of standard methadone maintenance treatment. *Journal of Substance Abuse Treatment, 46*(1), 43–51. doi:10.1016/j.jsat.2013.08.012

McKee, S. A., Carroll, K. M., Sinha, R., Robinson, J. E., Nich, C., Cavallo, D., et al. (2007). Enhancing brief cognitive-behavioral therapy with motivational enhancement techniques in cocaine users. *Drug and Alcohol Dependence, 91*(1), 97–101.

Miller, W. R., & Rollnick, S. (1991). *Motivational interviewing: Preparing people for change.* New York: Guilford Press.

Neale, J., & Stevenson, C. (2014). Homeless drug users and information technology: A qualitative study with potential implications for recovery from drug dependence. *Substance Use and Misuse, 49*(11), 1456–1472. doi:10.3109/10826084.2014.912231

Newton, N. C., Andrews, G., Teesson, M., & Vogl, L. E. (2009). Delivering prevention for alcohol and cannabis using the internet: A cluster randomised controlled trial. *Preventive Medicine: An International Journal Devoted to Practice and Theory, 48*(6), 579–584. doi:10.1016/j.ypmed.2009.04.009

Newton, N. C., Teesson, M., Vogl, L. E., & Andrews, G. (2010). Internet-based prevention for alcohol and cannabis use: Final results of the Climate Schools course. *Addiction, 105*(4), 749–759. doi:10.1111/j.1360-0443.2009.02853.x

Postel, M. G., de Haan, H. A., ter Huurne, E. D., Becker, E. S., & de Jong, C. A. J. (2010). Effectiveness of a web-based intervention for problem drinkers and reasons for dropout: Randomized controlled trial. *Journal of Medical Internet Research, 12*(4), 11–22. doi:10.2196/jmir.1642

Preschl, B., Maercker, A., & Wagner, B. (2011). The working alliance in a randomized controlled trial comparing online with face-to-face cognitive-behavioral therapy for depression. *BMC Psychiatry, 11*, 189. doi:10.1186/1471-244X-11-189

Redpath, D. P., Reynolds, G. L., Jaffe, A., Fisher, D. G., Edwards, J. W., & Deaugustine, N. (2006). Internet access and use among homeless and indigent drug users in Long Beach, California. *CyberPsychology & Behavior, 9*(5), 548–551. doi:10.1089/cpb.2006.9.548

Riper, H., Blankers, M., Hadiwijaya, H., Cunningham, J., Clarke, S., Wiers, R., et al. (2014). Effectiveness of guided and unguided low-intensity internet interventions for adult alcohol misuse: A meta-analysis. *PLoS ONE, 9*(6), e99912. doi:10.1371/journal.pone.0099912

Riper, H., Kramer, J., Smit, F., Conijn, B., Schippers, G., & Cuijpers, P. (2008). Web-based self-help for problem drinkers: A pragmatic randomized trial. *Addiction, 103*(2), 218–227. doi:10.1111/j.1360-0443.2007.02063.x

Riper, H., Spek, V., Boon, B., Conijn, B., Kramer, J., Martin-Abello, K., et al. (2011). Effectiveness of E-self-help interventions for curbing adult problem drinking: A meta-analysis. *Journal of Medical Internet Research, 13*(2), 44–56. doi:10.2196/jmir.1691

Riper, H., van Straten, A., Keuken, M., Smit, F., Schippers, G., & Cuijpers, P. (2009). Curbing problem drinking with personalized-feedback interventions: A meta-analysis. *American Journal of Preventive Medicine, 36*(3), 247–255. doi:10.1016/j.amepre.2008.10.016

Rooke, S., Copeland, J., Norberg, M., Hine, D., & McCambridge, J. (2013). Effectiveness of a self-guided web-based cannabis treatment program: Randomized controlled trial. *Journal of Medical Internet Research, 15*(2), 48–61. doi:10.2196/jmir.2256

Rooke, S., Thorsteinsson, E., Karpin, A., Copeland, J., & Allsop, D. (2010). Computer-delivered interventions for alcohol and tobacco use: A meta-analysis. *Addiction, 105*(8), 1381–1390. doi:10.1111/j.1360-0443.2010.02975.x

Schaub, M. P., Haug, S., Wenger, A., Berg, O., Sullivan, R., Beck, T., et al. (2013). Can reduce—The effects of chat-counseling and web-based self-help, web-based self-help alone and a waiting list control program on cannabis use in problematic cannabis users: A randomized controlled trial. *BMC Psychiatry, 13*, 305. doi:10.1186/1471-244X-13-305

Schaub, M., Sullivan, R., Haug, S., & Stark, L. (2012). Web-based cognitive behavioral self-help intervention to reduce cocaine consumption in problematic cocaine users: Randomized controlled trial. *Journal of Medical Internet Research, 14*(6), 47–60. doi:10.2196/jmir.2244

Schaub, M., Sullivan, R., & Stark, L. (2011). Snow control—An RCT protocol for a web-based self-help therapy to reduce cocaine consumption in problematic cocaine users. *BMC Psychiatry, 11*, 153. doi:10.1186/1471-244X-11-153

Sobell, M. B., & Sobell, L. C. (1993). Treatment for problem drinkers: A public health priority. In J. S. Baer, G. A. Marlatt, & R. J. McMahon (Eds.), *Addictive behaviors across the life span: Prevention, treatment, and policy issues* (pp. 138–157). Thousand Oaks, CA: Sage.

Spek, V., Cuijpers, P., Nyklíček, I., Riper, H., Keyzer, J., & Pop, V. (2007). Internet-based cognitive behaviour therapy for symptoms of depression and anxiety: A meta-analysis. *Psychological Medicine, 37*(3), 319–328. doi:10.1017/S0033291706008944

Suffoletto, B., Kristan, J., Callaway, C., Kim, K. H., Chung, T., Monti, P. M., et al. (2014). A text message alcohol intervention for young adult emergency department patients: A randomized clinical trial. *Annals of Emergency Medicine, 64*(6), 664.e4–674.e4. doi:10.1016/j. annemergmed.2014.06.010

Tait, R. J., McKetin, R., Kay-Lambkin, F., Bennett, K., Tam, A., Bennett, A., et al. (2012). Breakingtheice: A protocol for a randomised controlled trial of an internet-based intervention addressing amphetamine-type stimulant use. *BMC Psychiatry, 12*, 67. doi:10.1186/1471-244X-12-67

Tait, R. J., McKetin, R., Kay-Lambkin, F., Carron-Arthur, B., Bennett, A., Bennett, K., et al. (2014). A web-based intervention for users of amphetamine-type stimulants: 3-Month outcomes of a randomized controlled trial. *JMIR Mental Health, 1*, e1. doi:10.2196/mental. 3278

Tait, R. J., Spijkerman, R., & Riper, H. (2013). Internet and computer based interventions for cannabis use: A meta-analysis. *Drug and Alcohol Dependence, 133*(2), 295–304. doi:10.1016/j.drugalcdep.2013.05.012

Tossmann, H. P., Jonas, B., Tensil, M. D., Lang, P., & Strüber, E. (2011). A controlled trial of an internet-based intervention program for cannabis users. *Cyberpsychology, Behavior, and Social Networking, 14*(11), 673–679. doi:10.1089/cyber.2010.0506

Velicer, W. F., DiClemente, C. C., Rossi, J. S., & Prochaska, J. O. (1990). Relapse situations and self-efficacy: An integrative model. *Addictive Behaviors, 15*(3), 271–283. doi:10.1016/0306-4603(90)90070-E

Chapter 10
An Open Uncontrolled Pilot Trial of Online Cognitive-Behavioral Therapy for Insomnia for Ukrainian Alcohol-Dependent Patients

Olena Zhabenko, Nataliya Zhabenko, Deirdre A. Conroy, Oleg Chaban, Anna Oliinyk, Iryna Frankova, Alexander Mazur, Kirk J. Brower and Robert A. Zucker

Introduction

Heavy drinking patterns among adults are common in Ukraine (Webb et al. 2005). According to the WHO Global Information System on Alcohol and Health, the total recorded and unrecorded alcohol per capita consumption among adults (15+) in Ukraine was 14.3 (in liters of pure alcohol) in 2003–2005 which decreased to 13.9 in 2008–2010, with spirits being the main beverage group (48 % of all the alcohol) followed by beer (40 %) and wine (9 %). The 12-month prevalence of alcohol use disorders (including alcohol dependence and harmful use of alcohol) and alcohol dependence estimates (15+) among males were 9.3 and 4.2 % and

O. Chaban · I. Frankova
Bogomolets National Medical University, 8a Kotsubinskiy Str., Kyiv 01030, Ukraine
e-mail: ocs@ukr.net

I. Frankova
e-mail: iryna.frankova@gmail.com

O. Zhabenko (✉) · O. Chaban · A. Oliinyk
Department of Psychoneurology, Railway Clinical Hospital #1,
Station Kyiv, 8a Kotsubinskiy Str., Kyiv 01030, Ukraine
e-mail: olena.zhabenko@gmail.com

A. Oliinyk
e-mail: anna_ol@ukr.net

N. Zhabenko
Department of Psychiatry and Addiction Psychiatry, State Establishment "The Lugansk State Medical University", 50 Rokiv Oborony Luganska 1, Lugansk 91045, Ukraine
e-mail: zhabenkonataliya@gmail.com

© Springer International Publishing Switzerland 2016
A.L.M. Andrade and D. De Micheli (eds.), *Innovations in the Treatment of Substance Addiction*, DOI 10.1007/978-3-319-43172-7_10

females 1.1 and 0.5 %, respectively (WHO 2014). The same report found that the highest patterns of drinking score, i.e., the most risky patters of drinking, have been found in Russia and Ukraine.

Insomnia is a common symptom that may interfere with the efforts of patients with alcohol dependence to initiate and maintain sobriety (Krystal et al. 2008; Stein and Friedmann 2006). Across 12 studies with a range from 36 to 91 %, a mean of 58.4 % of 3294 alcohol-dependent patients endorsed symptoms of insomnia (Baekeland et al. 1974; Bokstrom and Balldin 1992; Brower et al. 2001, 2011; Caetano et al. 1998; Cohn et al. 2003; Escobar-Córdoba et al. 2009; Feuerlein 1974; Foster and Peters 1999; Mello and Mendelson 1970; Perney et al. 2012; Zhabenko et al. 2012). This varied range can be described by a number of issues, such as characteristics of the sample size and type (inpatients, outpatients, community sample, etc.), severity of alcohol dependence, time since last drink, the definition and assessment of insomnia, comorbidity, and geographical variation. Treatment of insomnia is important because of its role in relapse (Brower 2003; Brower and Perron 2010).

Brower and colleagues reported several predictors of insomnia and its severity based on analyses of two studies—one cross-sectional and one longitudinal with a sample size over 600 alcohol-dependent patients recruited from United States and Poland. The main findings of the longitudinal study performed in United States were that about one-half of patients near the time of treatment entry had symptoms of insomnia that occurred at least 15 days or more in the preceding month. These insomnia symptoms were independently associated with female gender and psychiatric symptom severity. Insomnia symptoms improved significantly over 6 months with either abstinence or reduction in drinking to moderate levels, whereas symptoms did not improve among patients who relapsed to heavy drinking. Insomnia symptoms also failed to improve in one-third of patients with baseline insomnia (i.e., one-half of patients with persistent insomnia) despite abstinence or moderate drinking levels, indicating that good drinking outcomes do not necessarily always ensure improvement in sleep (Brower et al. 2011). Another two analyses found that quantity of drinking was related to insomnia, and both depressive symptoms (Zhabenko et al. 2013a) and psychiatric severity (Zhabenko et al. 2013b)

D.A. Conroy · K.J. Brower · R.A. Zucker
Department of Psychiatry and Addiction Research Center, University of Michigan,
4250 Plymouth Road, Ann Arbor, MI 48109-2700, USA
e-mail: daconroy@umich.edu

K.J. Brower
e-mail: kbrower@med.umich.edu

R.A. Zucker
e-mail: zuckerra@med.umich.edu

A. Mazur
Department of Anatomy and Cell Biology, McGill University, 3640 University Street,
Montreal, QC H3A 0C7, Canada
e-mail: mtlru.com@gmail.com

mediated the effects of drinking on sleep. These findings have significant clinical implications—psychiatric symptoms and alcohol use must be treated concurrently in order to reduce insomnia.

Another Polish study found that mental and physical health status, severity of alcohol dependence, number of drinking days in the past 3 months, and childhood abuse were independent predictors of insomnia (Zhabenko et al. 2012). Perney and colleagues found that moderate anxiety and depression, patients living alone and higher gamma-glutamyltransferase (γ-GT) levels were significantly associated with high sleep disturbance (Perney et al. 2012), suggesting that other predisposing factors to insomnia, such as anxiety and depression, may play a role in future insomnia.

Thus, an untested hypothesis is that treatment of insomnia can facilitate abstinence when provided as an adjunct to alcoholism treatment (Brower 2003). To date, at least four studies have evaluated non-pharmacological approaches to insomnia complaints in subjects with AD early recovery (Arnedt et al. 2007, 2011; Currie et al. 2004; Greeff and Conradie 1998). Arnedt and colleagues found that cognitive-behavioral insomnia therapy may benefit recovering alcoholics with mild-to-moderate insomnia by improving sleep and daytime functioning in uncontrolled (Arnedt et al. 2007) and controlled studies (Arnedt et al. 2011). Another randomized controlled trial of brief cognitive-behavioral interventions for insomnia in recovering alcoholics found that treated participants were significantly more improved than control participants on diary measures of sleep quality, sleep efficiency, awakenings, and time to fall asleep (Currie et al. 2004). The fourth study of progressive relaxation training on insomnia illustrated improvement in the sleeping patterns of the treated group and did not find any changes in the sleeping patterns of the control group (Greeff and Conradie 1998). However, none of these studies were computer-based, and none were performed in Ukraine. Professor Ritterband and his team created and evaluated an Internet-based behavioral intervention for a non-alcoholic sample of adults with insomnia (http://shuti.bht.virginia.edu/modules/8?page=1). Intention-to-treat analyses showed that insomnia severity significantly improved, wake after sleep onset significantly decreased, and sleep efficiency increased for the Internet group. All these variables did not change for the control group (Ritterband et al. 2009).

Over the past few years, Internet CBT-I programs have expanded, particularly throughout North America (Beaulac et al. 2015; Cheng and Dizon 2012; Espie et al. 2014; Gosling et al. 2014; Hedman et al. 2013; Lancee et al. 2013; Thorndike et al. 2013; van Straten et al. 2014). An Internet CBT-I program may be a more convenient way for patients to receive care. These programs also show promise as an effective way for individuals with insomnia to receive CBT-I. This treatment is best delivered by individuals certified in Behavioral Sleep Medicine (BSM) and involves multiple follow-up visits. However, there are few providers certified in BSM and CBT-I outside of the USA, and it is not available to patients in many areas of the world such as Ukraine.

The aim of the current study was to develop and pilot the efficacy of a 6-week online computer-based CBT-I for Ukrainian patients in recovery from alcohol dependence. We hypothesized that CBT-I-AD would improve subjective sleep and daytime functioning and reduce the severity of drinking in AD patients with comorbid insomnia.

Survey design: This is a longitudinal study, with data collected via a web-based survey. Patients were recruited via advertisements and flyers in the places of Alcoholics Anonymous (AA) meetings, newspaper, personal e-mail for professionals, physician referrals, "Ukrainian young psychiatrists" Google group, and social networks (i.e., Facebook, Odnoklassniki, Vkontakte). Participants were provided the URL to complete the pre-assessment, post-assessment and online treatment.

Participants: The main inclusion criteria were as follows: (1) diagnosis for AD screened by the International Classification of Diseases and Related Health Problems 10th Revision (ICD-10) version for 2010 (World Health Organization); (2) diagnosis of insomnia according to ICD-10; (3) at least 3 weeks of continuous sobriety; (4) self-reported sleep problems ≥ 1 month; (4) high-speed Internet access and a home computer (for those who did not have a computer with Internet access, an onsite computer was provided); (5) 18–80 years old; and (6) an online informed consent for participation. The main exclusion criteria were as follows: (1) current diagnosis of psychosis, acute suicidality, bipolar affective disorder, schizophrenia, seizure disorder, untreated sleep apnea. The study was approved by the Lugansk Regional Clinical Psychoneurological Hospital Review Board.

A web-based platform (http://cbt-insomnia.com/) included psychoeducational information, five CBT-I sessions, and a battery of scales developed by the Ukrainian team to examine the effectiveness of the CBT-I package (Zhabenko O., Zhabenko N., Linskaya K., Oliinyk A. and Frankova I.). The package is based on Dr. Gregg Jacobs' 25 years of research and clinical practice (Jacobs 2000–2010) and incorporates additional material from the treatment manual (version 2.0) *Cognitive-behavioral therapy for insomnia for alcohol dependence* (with permission Arndt 2004). Both authors gave permission to develop the online project based on their treatment manuals.

Psychoeducational information on the Web site is divided into three sections: alcohol dependence, insomnia, and cognitive-behavioral therapy for insomnia (Fig. 10.1). The CBT-I-AD package consists of access to five sequential online audiovisual (multimedia) computer-based sessions (~ 45 min each) over 6 weeks.

Session 1: "Sleep Education and Cognitive Restructuring for Insomnia" consists of two parts. (1) *Sleep and insomnia basic concepts* define insomnia. This part describes the association of insomnia, alcohol, tobacco, and relapse, provides a rationale for a CBT approach to treating insomnia, and explains the sleep and wakefulness systems. (2) *Cognitive restructuring* provides an introductory explanation about thoughts and the effects of these thoughts on the body and sleep. The user learns that the hallmark of insomnia is negative, inaccurate thoughts about sleep at bedtime or during the night, that negative sleep thoughts cause negative emotions, and that negative sleep thoughts can occur upon awakening and during the day. The goal of cognitive restructuring is to recognize, challenge, and replace

Online computer-based cognitive-behavior therapy for insomnia program for alcohol-dependent patients

Alcohol dependence	Insomnia	CBT-I
• Alcohol use in Ukraine • Signs of alcohol dependence • Codependency • Comorbidity of alcohol dependence • Abstinence • Tips for craving • Useful links	• Insomnia • Symptoms of insomnia • Prevalence of insomnia among alcohol dependent individuals • Comorbidity of insomnia • Biology of sleep • Insomnia treatment • Sleep hygiene • Predictor of insomnia • Useful links	• CBT • CBT-I • CBT-I for alcohol-dependent patients • Useful links

Fig. 10.1 Psychoeducational information on the Web site

negative sleep thoughts with more accurate and adaptive positive sleep thoughts. This section also explores some of the research regarding the effects of insomnia on health, daytime functioning, subjective estimates of sleep, mood and alcohol consumption as well as the effects of drinking on insomnia (Fig. 10.2).

Session 2: "Sleep Medication Withdrawal and Sleep Scheduling Techniques" discusses sleep stages and body temperature. Additionally, information about *sleep medications* (types, side effects, a significant placebo effect of sleep medications) is provided. *Sleep scheduling and restriction techniques* consists of an introduction to the concepts of prior wakefulness and sleep efficiency, the importance of a regular arising time, reducing time allotted for sleep, and reviews tips for reducing time allotted for sleep (Fig. 10.3).

Session 3: "Stimulus Control (SC) Techniques" the use of the bed for sleep and sex only, so it does not become associated with other stimulating activities. The goal of SC is to learn to associate the bed with drowsiness and sleep (Fig. 10.4).

Session 4: "The Relaxation Response" (RR) leads the patient through a 10-min *RR exercise*. Session 4 reviews the stress response, RR, and mini-relaxations. This session also reviews the use of the RR at bedtime or after nighttime awakening (Fig. 10.5).

Session 5: "Sleep Hygiene Techniques" reviews the effects of alcohol, tobacco, caffeine, exercise, temperature and baths, bright light, food, noise, and sleep. This session also reviews relapse prevention (Fig. 10.6).

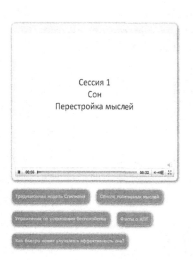

Session 1
Sleep Education and
Cognitive Restructuring for Insomnia
Duration: 58 min 32 sec
Additional materials:
- Spielman Model
- Facts about CBT
- Positive Sleep Thoughts
- Constructive Worry Worksheet
- Sleep Efficiency

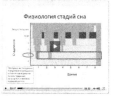
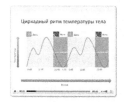

Fig. 10.2 Session 1 "Sleep Education and Cognitive Restructuring for Insomnia"

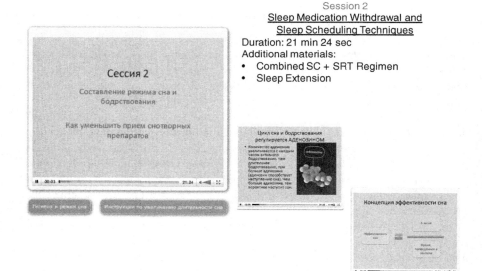

Session 2
Sleep Medication Withdrawal and
Sleep Scheduling Techniques
Duration: 21 min 24 sec
Additional materials:
- Combined SC + SRT Regimen
- Sleep Extension

Fig. 10.3 Session 2 "Sleep Medication Withdrawal and Sleep Scheduling Techniques." *Note SC* stimulus control, *SRT* scheduling regime technics

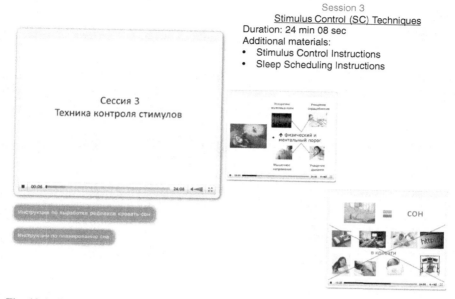

Fig. 10.4 Session 3 "Stimulus Control (SC) Techniques"

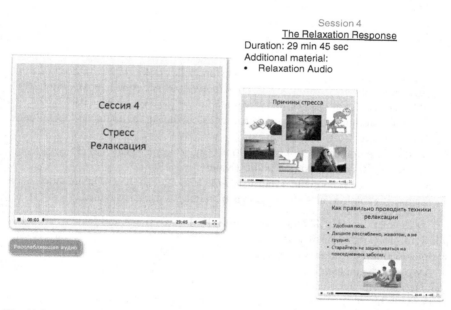

Fig. 10.5 Session 4 "The Relaxation Response"

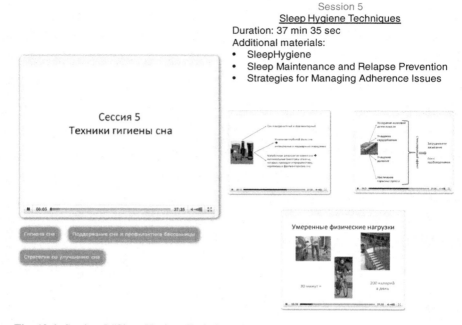

Fig. 10.6 Session 5 "Sleep Hygiene Techniques"

Each session has its own additional resources for homework:

- Session 1: Spielman Model (Spielman and Glovinsky 1991), list of positive sleep thoughts, facts about CBT, constructive worry worksheet (Harvey 2002, 2005; Harvey et al. 2007), and sleep efficiency (Spielman et al. 1987).
- Session 2: combined stimulus control with scheduling regimens and techniques, and sleep extension instructions;
- Session 3: stimulus control instructions (Bootzin and Perlis 1992);
- Session 4: 20-min relaxation audio (Kahn et al. 1968);
- Session 5: sleep hygiene (Hauri 1977) (Fig. 10.7), sleep maintenance with relapse prevention, and strategies for managing adherence issues.

Treatment sessions 1, 2 and 3 are weekly, while sessions 4 and 5 are biweekly to allow for consolidation of learning (thus, the program is a total of 6 weeks). The various techniques are taught in order of clinical efficacy and importance.

Assessment measures: Socio-demographic variables included age, gender, satisfaction with income, education level, ethnicity, marital status, employment, work with Internet, smoking status and childhood sexual/physical abuse which were measured at baseline.

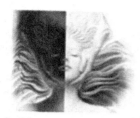

Гигиена Сна
(Arnedt J.T., Conroy D.A., Brower K.J., 2007)

1. Отходите ко сну в одно и то же время каждый день, в том числе в выходные дни.
2. Не употребляйте алкоголь, для того чтобы улучшить засыпание.
3. Исключите употребление кофеинсодержащих напитков и продуктов (кофе, чай, сода, шоколад) в вечернее время.
4. Помните, что курение и другие наркотические средства нарушают сон.
5. Принимайте пищу регулярно. Не ложитесь на голодный желудок – съедайте углеводный бутерброд.
6. За один час до сна занимайтесь «спокойными» делами.
7. Ограничьте прием жидкости вечером.
8. Избегайте дремоты днем.
9. Занимайтесь физическими упражнениями регулярно, но не позже, чем за 3 часа до сна.
10. Убедитесь, что Ваша кровать комфортна.
11. Проконтролируйте температуру Вашей спальной комнаты, она должна быть прохладной (18°C).
12. Убедитесь, что Ваша спальня темная и тихая.
13. Каждый день проводите время на улице (при естественном освещении).

(Perlis M.L., Jungquist C., Smith M.T., Posner D., 2005)

1. Принимайте теплую ванную за 1,5-2 часа до сна.
2. Не берите свои проблемы «в кровать».
3. Не пытайтесь заставить себя уснуть.
4. Ставьте часы так, чтобы их не видеть (под кровать или циферблатом от себя).

Fig. 10.7 Example of additional material

At baseline, at the end of the study, and at 6- and 12-week follow-up, patients reported substance use and related clinical variables, daytime functioning measures, and sleep variables.

Alcohol and tobacco use. The Alcohol Use Disorders Identification Test (AUDIT) has been developed by the World Health Organization as a screening tool to assess the early signs of hazardous and harmful drinking. The AUDIT includes 3 main domains: questions 1, 2 and 3 represent hazardous alcohol consumption, questions 4, 5 and 6 measure an alcohol dependence syndrome, and questions 7, 8, 9 and 10 represent adverse reactions and alcohol-related problems (Saunders et al. 1993). On the basis of the research, it is suggested that the following interpretation be given to AUDIT scores: Scores between 8 and 15 are most appropriate for simple advice focused on the reduction of hazardous drinking; scores between

16 and 19 suggest brief counseling and continued monitoring; scores of 20 or above clearly warrant further diagnostic evaluation for alcohol dependence (Babor et al. 2002). The Fagerstrom Test for Nicotine Dependence (FTND) was used to recognize severity of nicotine dependence at baseline. It is a highly reliable, self-administered, 6-item questionnaire, with a range of scores from 0 to 10, with higher scores specifying more dependence. FTND has been correlated with biochemical measures of nicotine dependence including exhaled carbon monoxide, salivary cotinine, and salivary nicotine (Heatherton et al. 1991).

Daytime functioning measures. The Depression Anxiety Stress Scale (DASS 21) consists of three self-reported scales and was used for quantitative measurement of the negative emotional states of depression, anxiety and stress. Each item was scored from 0 to 3, with 0 representing "did not apply to me at all," 1—"applied to me to some degree, or some of the time," 2—"applied to me to a considerable degree, or a good part of time," 3—"applied to me very much, or most of the time." All items of each subscale were summed with higher scores indicating greater levels of depression, anxiety, and stress (Lovibond and Lovibond 1995, 1996). The Epworth Sleepiness Scale (ESS) measured sleepiness during the day. For each of eight situations, the following ratings were used: 0—"would never fall asleep in that situation," 1—"there is a slight chance of falling asleep in that situation," 2—"there is a medium chance of falling asleep in that situation," 3—"there is a high chance of falling asleep in that situation." A total score of up to 10 is regarded as normal, whereas a score of 11 to 12 is borderline, and 13 to 24 points indicates an unusual level of sleepiness (Johns 1991).

Sleep variables. To assess insomnia, subjects completed the Sleep Problems Questionnaire (SPQ) during the course of the study. Its four items asked, "How often in the past month did you..." (1) "have trouble falling asleep?"; (2) "wake up several times per night?"; (3) "have trouble staying asleep (including waking far too early)?"; and (4) "wake up after your usual amount of sleep feeling tired and worn out?" Each item was scored from 0 to 5, with 0 representing 0 days, $1 = 1$–3 days, $2 = 4$–7 days, $3 = 8$–14 days, $4 = 15$–21 days, and $5 = 22$–31 days per month. The four items were summed with total possible scores ranging from 0 to 20 with higher scores indicating greater insomnia (Jenkins et al. 1988). The STOP Questionnaire was used to screen for obstructive sleep apnea (OSA). The four-item STOP questionnaire is a self-reported, forced-choice (yes/no) scale. It consists of the following four questions: S—"Do you snore loudly (louder than talking or loud enough to be heard through closed doors?" T—"Do you often feel tired, fatigued, or sleepy during daytime?" O—"Has anyone observed you stop breathing during your sleep?" P—"Do you have or are you being treated for high blood pressure?" The four items were summed, indicating high risk—"yes" to two or more questions" and low risk—"yes" to less than two questions (Chung et al. 2008).

Statistical analyses: All statistical analyses were performed using SPSS version 20.0 for Mac (IBM Corporation, New York, NY).

Results: Eight participants were Ukrainians, mostly middle-aged (44 ± 11.97), predominantly females, two were mainly satisfied and the other two were not satisfied with their income. Five out of seven got a university degree. Mainly,

Table 10.2 Alcohol, sleep and daytime symptom outcomes [mean (±SD)] at baseline and post-treatment time points

Variable	Baseline	End of the study	6-week follow-up	12-week follow-up
Alcohol and tobacco use				
AUDIT	29.2 ± 2.39	10 ± 2.82	7.5 ± 10.6	–
Fagestrom test for nicotine dependence	5.75 ± 4.65	–	–	–
Daytime functioning measures				
DASS 21				
Depression	21.33 ± 12.04	15 ± 21.21	25 ± 12.72	15 ± 9.9
Anxiety	21.0 ± 11.91	14.0 ± 16.97	19.0 ± 12.73	19.0 ± 18.38
Stress	27.0 ± 11.36	24.0 ± 22.63	31.0 ± 15.56	26.0 ± 16.97
Epworth sleepiness scale	13.0 ± 3.46	7.5 ± 9.19	–	7.0 ± 9.9
Sleep				
SPQ	17.17 ± 3.19	10 ± 14.14	7.5 ± 10.6	9.5 ± 13.44
STOP	2.3 ± 1.26	–	–	1.5 ± 2.12

participants were unmarried (57.1 %), and unemployed (42.9 %) or retired (28.6 %). All participants used their own computers; one individual came to the clinic to participate in the study. The majority of them smoked cigarettes (71.4 %). One participants experienced childhood sexual abuse before 18 years (14.3 %), one participant experienced childhood physical abuse before 18 years (14.3 %) and two after 18 years (28.6 %) (Table 10.1).

Mean (±SD) total AUDIT scores at baseline and at the 6-week follow-up of the study were 29.2 ± 2.39 and 7.5 ± 10.6, respectively. The mean FTND score was 5.75. Depression, anxiety, and stress subscales of the DASS, ESS, and STOP were decreased from baseline to the 12-week follow-up. Depression scores fell from severe to moderate levels. All individuals were categorized if having insomnia if they endorsed any one SPQ item with a 4 or 5. Mean (±SD) total SPQ scores at baseline and at 12-week follow-up of the study were 17.17 ± 3.19 and 9.5 ± 13.44, respectively (Table 10.2).

Discussion: The main finding of the current study was its effective demonstration of the viability of a new 6-week online computer-based cognitive-behavior therapy for insomnia for Ukrainian alcohol-dependent patients in recovery from alcohol dependence. This uncontrolled study found that self-reported sleep, alcohol, and daytime measures improved in sober alcoholics followed by a five-session online, non-pharmacological insomnia treatment. Subjective improvements of those variables were clinically significant. Conclusions regarding the impact of the intervention on relapses to alcohol are difficult to know because of short follow-up.

These results need replication and require to be interpreted cautiously given the small sample size, lack of control group, absence of objective or verified measures of sleep and drinking, and follow-up assessments.

Clinical significance: Insomnia and alcoholism are significantly associated; moreover, there is evidence to suggest that sleep is a universal risk factor for relapse (Brower and Perron 2010). Cognitive-behavioral therapy (CBT) is the most scientifically proven non-drug insomnia. Three Internet-based studies for adults who met DSM-IV-TR criteria for primary insomnia resulted in significant improvements in insomnia severity, general fatigue, and sleep quality (Ritterband et al. 2009; Ström et al. 2004; Vincent and Lewycky 2009). An open-label, uncontrolled trial of cognitive-behavioral treatment for insomnia comorbid with alcohol dependence by Arnedt et al. (2007) found that subjectively reported sleep continuity and some collateral measures of daytime impairment improved in recovery alcoholics with mild-to-moderate insomnia following an eight-session individual non-pharmacological insomnia treatment. A randomized controlled study performed by Arnedt et al. (2011) showed that CBT-I-AD participants demonstrated greater improvements on one of the primary sleep diary outcomes (sleep efficiency) and select daytime symptoms (ratings of insomnia severity and fatigue) and were more likely to be classified as sleep treatment responders than behavioral placebo treatment. The knowledge about effectiveness of CBT-I-AD could help psychiatrists and addiction psychiatrists to improve treatment outcomes of alcohol-dependent patients. Another randomized controlled trial of CBT-I for AD patients found self-reported improvement on diary measures of sleep quality, sleep efficiency, awakenings, and time to fall asleep, which were corroborated by clinician and spousal ratings (Currie et al. 2004).

Benefits of participation include free five sessions of CBT-I-AD treatment. However, benefits are primary to future patients in treatment settings who may benefit from CBT-I-AD Internet computer-delivered interventions that are developed as the result of this research. Self-help manuals and Internet computer-based programs have potential as a cost-effective treatment that can be more widely disseminated to people in recovery than face-to-face intervention.

Innovation: This Internet computer-based CBT-I-AD intervention is the first computer-based intervention in the Ukrainian population.

Limitations of the study design: (1) A potential barrier for some was the absence of home Internet access. Therefore, computers at treatment sites were provided for subjects without this access. (2) The subjects did not undergo polysomnography and therefore it is possible that insomnia symptoms may have been associated with sleep apnea or another primary sleep disorder. (3) Absence of biological markers of alcohol dependence. Self-reported methods offer a reliable and valid approach to measuring alcohol consumption (Del Boca and Darkes 2003). (4) Small sample size limits the ability to generalize to a large population of outpatients with AD. (5) The study required insomnia symptoms to be present for only 1 month. This is no longer consistent with current guidelines. Insomnia disorder in the Diagnostic and Statistical Manual of Mental Disorders, Fifth Edition (DSM-5) and the International Classification of Sleep Disorders, Third Edition (ICSD-3) guidances requires symptoms to be present for at least 3 months.

Strengths of the study design (1) The study had four time points for assessment and five treatment sessions. (2) Exploring the effect of an Internet computer-based CBT intervention on insomnia among alcohol-dependent patients. (3) Exploring characteristics of people seeking Internet computer-based intervention among Ukrainian population. (4) Its demonstration that Internet computer-based interventions may lower some of the barriers associated with traditional face-to-face treatments. However, telephone consultations and face-to-face meeting from therapists were provided. (5) The community-recruited, media-recruited participants, and physician-referred participants involved access to a population of alcohol-dependent individuals with sleep problems who might not otherwise be willing to enter into treatment.

Acknowledgement This research was supported in part by the University of Michigan Addiction Research Center, through funding from the National Institutes of Health Fogarty International Center and the National Institute on Drug Abuse.

Declaration of Interest The authors report no conflict of interest. The authors alone are responsible for the content and writing of the article.

Contributors Olena Zhabenko, Nataliya Zhabenko, Kirk J. Brower, and Robert A. Zucker designed the study and wrote the protocol. Alexander Mazur designed the Web site. Olena Zhabenko, Nataliya Zhabenko, Oleg Chaban, Anna Oliinyk, Iryna Frankova, Alexander Mazur, Deirdre A. Conroy, Kirk J. Brower, and Robert A. Zucker conducted literature review, directed the statistical analyses, and wrote presented article. All authors contributed to and approved the final manuscript.

References

Arnedt, J. T. (2004). *Cognitive behavioral therapy for insomnia for alcohol dependence (CBT-I for AD). Treatment Manual (Version 2.0).* Ann Arbor, MI.

Arnedt, J. T., Conroy, D., Rutt, J., Aloia, M. S., Brower, K. J., & Armitage, R. (2007). An open trial of cognitive-behavioral treatment for insomnia comorbid with alcohol dependence. *Sleep Medicine, 8*(2), 176–180.

Arnedt, J. T., Conroy, D. A., Armitage, R., & Brower, K. J. (2011). Cognitive-behavioral therapy for insomnia in alcohol dependent patients: A randomized controlled pilot trial. *Behaviour Research and Therapy, 49*(4), 227–233.

Babor, T. F., Higgins-Biddle, J. C., Saunders, J. B., & Monteiro, M. G. (2002). *The alcohol use disorders identification test. Guidelines for use in primary care* (2nd Ed.). World Health Organization. Department of Mental Health and Substance Dependence.

Baekeland, F., Lundwall, L., Shanahan, T. J., & Kissin, B. (1974). Clinical correlates of reported sleep disturbance in alcoholics. *Quarterly Journal of Studies on Alcohol, 35*(4 Pt A), 1230–1241.

Beaulac, J., Vincent, N., & Walsh, K. (2015). Dissemination of an Internet-based treatment for chronic insomnia into primary care. *Behavioral Sleep Medicine, 13*(2), 124–139.

Bokstrom, K., & Balldin, J. (1992). A rating scale for assessment of alcohol withdrawal psychopathology (AWIP). *Alcoholism, Clinical and Experimental Research, 16*(2), 241–249.

Bootzin, R. R., & Perlis, M. L. (1992). Nonpharmacologic treatments of insomnia [Review]. *The Journal of clinical psychiatry, 53*(Suppl), 37–41.

Brower, K. J. (2003). Insomnia, alcoholism and relapse. *Sleep Medicine Reviews, 7*(6), 523–539.

Brower, K. J., Aldrich, M. S., Robinson, E. A. R., Zucker, R. A., & Greden, J. F. (2001). Insomnia, self-medication, and relapse to alcoholism. *American Journal of Psychiatry, 158*(3), 399–404.

Brower, K. J., Krentzman, A., & Robinson, E. A. R. (2011). Persistent insomnia, abstinence, and moderate drinking in alcohol-dependent individuals. *The American Journal on Addictions, 20*(5), 435–440.

Brower, K. J., & Perron, B. E. (2010). Sleep disturbance as a universal risk factor for relapse in addictions to psychoactive substances. *Medical Hypotheses, 74*(5), 928–933.

Caetano, R., Clark, C., & Greenfield, T. (1998). Prevalence, trends, and incidence of alcohol withdrawal symptoms. *Alcohol Health & Research World, 22*, 73–79.

Cheng, S. K., & Dizon, J. (2012). Computerised cognitive behavioural therapy for insomnia: A systematic review and meta-analysis. *Psychotherapy and Psychosomatics, 81*(4), 206–216.

Chung, F., Yegneswaran, B., Liao, P., Chung, S. A., Vairavanathan, S., Islam, S., et al. (2008). STOP questionnaire: A tool to screen patients for obstructive sleep apnea. *Anesthesiology, 108*(5), 812–821.

Cohn, T., Foster, J., & Peters, T. (2003). Sequential studies of sleep disturbance and quality of life in abstaining alcoholics. *Addiction Biology, 8*(4), 455–462.

Currie, S. R., Clark, S., Hodgins, D. C., & El Guebaly, N. (2004). Randomized controlled trial of brief cognitive–behavioural interventions for insomnia in recovering alcoholics. *Addiction, 99*(9), 1121–1132.

Del Boca, F. K., & Darkes, J. (2003). The validity of self reports of alcohol consumption: State of the science and challenges for research. *Addiction, 98*, 1–12.

Escobar-Córdoba, F., Ávila-Cadavid, J. D., & Cote-Menendez, M. (2009). Complaints of insomnia in hospitalized alcoholics. *Revista Brasileira de Psiquiatria, 31*, 261–264.

Espie, C. A., Kyle, S. D., Miller, C. B., Ong, J., Hames, P., & Fleming, L. (2014). Attribution, cognition and psychopathology in persistent insomnia disorder: Outcome and mediation analysis from a randomized placebo-controlled trial of online cognitive behavioural therapy. *Sleep Medicine, 15*(8), 913–917.

Feuerlein, W. (1974). The acute alcohol withdrawal syndrome: Findings and problems. *British Journal of Addiction to Alcohol & Other Drugs, 69*(2), 141–148.

Foster, J. H., & Peters, T. J. (1999). Impaired sleep in alcohol misusers and dependent alcoholics and the impact upon outcome. *Alcoholism, Clinical and Experimental Research, 23*(6), 1044–1051.

Gosling, J. A., Glozier, N., Griffiths, K., Ritterband, L., Thorndike, F., Mackinnon, A., et al. (2014). The GoodNight study-online CBT for insomnia for the indicated prevention of depression: Study protocol for a randomised controlled trial. *Trials, 15*, 56.

Greeff, A. P., & Conradie, W. S. (1998). Use of progressive relaxation training for chronic alcoholics with insomnia. *Psychological Reports, 82*(2), 407–412.

Harvey, A. (2002). A cognitive model of insomnia. *Behaviour Research and Therapy, 40*, 869–893.

Harvey, A. (2005). A cognitive theory for chronic insomnia. *Journal of Cognitive Psychotherapy, 19*, 41.

Harvey, A., Sharpley, A. L., Ree, M., Stinsond, K., & Clark, D. (2007). An open trial of cognitive therapy for chronic insomnia. *Behaviour Research and Therapy, 45*, 2491–2501.

Hauri, P. (1977). *The sleep disorders. Current concepts.* Kalamazoo, MI: Scope Publications, Upjohn.

Heatherton, T. F., Kozlowski, L. T., Frecker, R. C., & Fagerstrom, K. O. (1991). The Fagerstrom test for nicotine dependence: A revision of the Fagerstrom Tolerance Questionnaire. *British Journal of Addiction, 86*(9), 1119–1127.

Hedman, E., Ljotsson, B., Blom, K., El Alaoui, S., Kraepelien, M., Ruck, C., et al. (2013). Telephone versus internet administration of self-report measures of social anxiety, depressive symptoms, and insomnia: Psychometric evaluation of a method to reduce the impact of missing data. *Journal of medical Internet research, 15*(10), e229.

Jacobs, G. D. (2000–2010). *Clinical training manual for a CBT-i insomnia program.*

Jenkins, C. D., Stanton, B. A., Niemcryk, S. J., & Rose, R. M. (1988). A scale for the estimation of sleep problems in clinical research. *Journal of Clinical Epidemiology, 41*(4), 313–321.

Johns, M. W. (1991). A new method for measuring daytime sleepiness: The Epworth sleepiness scale. *Sleep, 14*(6), 540–545.

Kahn, M., Baker, B. L., & Weiss, J. M. (1968). Treatment of insomnia by relaxation training. *Journal of Abnormal Psychology, 73*(6), 556–558.

Krystal, A. D., Thakur, M., & Roth, T. (2008). Sleep disturbance in psychiatric disorders: Effects on function and quality of life in mood disorders, alcoholism, and schizophrenia. *Annals of Clinical Psychiatry, 20*(1), 39–46.

Lancee, J., van den Bout, J., Sorbi, M. J., & van Straten, A. (2013). Motivational support provided via email improves the effectiveness of internet-delivered self-help treatment for insomnia: A randomized trial. *Behaviour Research and Therapy, 51*(12), 797–805.

Lovibond, P. F., & Lovibond, S. H. (1995). The structure of negative emotional states: Comparison of the Depression Anxiety Stress Scales (DASS) with the Beck Depression and Anxiety Inventories. *Behaviour Research and Therapy, 33*(3), 335–343.

Lovibond, S., & Lovibond, P. F. (1996). *Manual for the depression anxiety stress scales.* Sydney: Psychology Foundation of Australia.

Mello, N. K., & Mendelson, J. H. (1970). Behavioral studies of sleep patterns in alcoholics during intoxication and withdrawal. *Journal of Pharmacology and Experimental Therapeutics, 175*(1), 94–112.

Morin, C. M. (2000). The nature of insomnia and the need to refine our diagnostic criteria. *Psychosomatic Medicine, 62*(4), 483–485.

Perney, P., Lehert, P., & Mason, J. (2012). Sleep disturbance in alcoholism: Proposal of a simple measurement, and results from a 24-week randomized controlled study of alcohol-dependent patients assessing Acamprosate efficacy. *Alcohol and Alcoholism, 47*(2), 133–139.

Reite, M., Buysse, D., Reynolds, C., & Mendelson, W. (1995). The use of polysomnography in the evaluation of insomnia. *Sleep, 18*(01), 58–70.

Ritterband, L. M., Thorndike, F. P., Gonder-Frederick, L. A., Magee, J. C., Bailey, E. T., Saylor, D. K., et al. (2009). Efficacy of an Internet-based behavioral intervention for adults with insomnia. *Archives of General Psychiatry, 66*(7), 692.

Saunders, J. B., Aasland, O. G., Babor, T. F., Fuente, J. R., & Grant, M. (1993). Development of the alcohol use disorders identification test (AUDIT): WHO collaborative project on early detection of persons with harmful alcohol consumption II. *Addiction, 88*(6), 791–804.

Spielman, A., & Glovinsky, P. (1991). The varied nature of insomnia. In P. Hauri (Ed.), *Case studies in insomnia.* New York: Plenum Publishing Corporation.

Spielman, A. J., Saskin, P., & Thorpy, M. J. (1987). Treatment of chronic insomnia by restriction of time in bed. *Sleep, 10*(1), 45–56.

Stein, M. D., & Friedmann, P. D. (2006). Disturbed sleep and its relationship to alcohol use. *Substance Abuse, 26*(1), 1–13.

Ström, L., Pettersson, R., & Andersson, G. (2004). Internet-based treatment for insomnia: A controlled evaluation. *Journal of Consulting and Clinical Psychology, 72*(1), 113.

Thorndike, F. P., Ritterband, L. M., Gonder-Frederick, L. A., Lord, H. R., Ingersoll, K. S., & Morin, C. M. (2013). A randomized controlled trial of an internet intervention for adults with insomnia: Effects on comorbid psychological and fatigue symptoms. *Journal of Clinical Psychology, 69*(10), 1078–1093.

van Straten, A., Emmelkamp, J., de Wit, J., Lancee, J., Andersson, G., van Someren, E. J., et al. (2014). Guided Internet-delivered cognitive behavioural treatment for insomnia: A randomized trial. *Psychological Medicine, 44*(7), 1521–1532.

Vincent, N., & Lewycky, S. (2009). Logging on for better sleep: RCT of the effectiveness of online treatment for insomnia. *Sleep, 32*(6), 807.

Webb, C. P. M., Bromet, E. J., Gluzman, S., Tintle, N. L., Schwartz, J. E., Kostyuchenko, S., et al. (2005). Epidemiology of heavy alcohol use in Ukraine: Findings from the world mental health survey. *Alcohol and Alcoholism, 40*(4), 327.

WHO. (2014). *Global status report on alcohol and health 2014*. Country profile, from http://www.who.int/substance_abuse/publications/global_alcohol_report/msb_gsr_2014_2.pdf?ua=1. Accessed 16 August 2014.

World Health Organization. (1993). *The ICD-10 classification on mental and behavioral disorders: Diagnostic criteria for research*. Geneva: World Health Organization.

Zhabenko, N., Wojnar, M., & Brower, K. J. (2012). Prevalence and correlates of insomnia in a Polish sample of alcohol-dependent patients. *Alcoholism, Clinical and Experimental Research, 36*(9), 1600–1607.

Zhabenko, O., Krentzman, A. R., Robinson, E. A., & Brower, K. J. (2013a). A longitudinal study of drinking and depression as predictors of insomnia in alcohol-dependent individuals. *Substance Use and Misuse, 48*(7), 495–505. doi:10.3109/10826084.2013.781182

Zhabenko, O., Krentzman, A. R., Robinson, E. A. R., & Brower, K. J. (2013b). Prediction of insomnia severity among alcohol-dependent patients using a lagged mediational analysis. *Psychiatria et Neurologia Japonica, 115*, SS441–SS451.

Author Biographies

Olena Zhabenko, MD, PhD, Psychiatrist, certified by the International Society of Addiction Medicine. She has been a Fogarty Research Fellow at the University of Michigan Addiction Research Center (2010–2011). Her interests focus on alcoholism, insomnia, cognitive-behavior therapy for insomnia and Internet intervention.

Nataliya Zhabenko, MD, PhD, Practicing Clinical Psychiatrist (Ukraine, Germany). She has been a Fogarty Research Fellow at the University of Michigan Addiction Research Center (2010–2011). Her interests focus on alcohol dependence, insomnia and non-pharmacological treatment of insomnia.

Deirdre A. Conroy, PhD, Clinical Associate Professor at the University of Michigan, Department of Psychiatry. She is a Clinical Director of the Behavioral Sleep Medicine Program. Her clinical interests are sleep disorders, behavioral sleep medicine, cognitive behavioral therapy for insomnia. Her research focuses on relationship between sleep disturbances and substance use disorders, childhood sleep problems and early onset of substance use.

Oleg Chaban, MD, PhD, Professor of Psychiatry and Chair of the Psychosomatic Medicine and Psychotherapy Department at the Bogomolets National Medical University. Vice President of Ukrainian Association of Psychotherapists and Psychoanalytics, and Academician of the Ukrainian Academy of Sciences of High School.

Anna Oliinyk, MS, Practicing psychologist at the Railway Clinical Hospital #1, Station Kyiv. She is a mental health provider specializes on cognitive behavioral therapy. She is a member of Ukrainian Association of Cognitive Behavior Therapy and Ukrainian Association of Psychotherapists.

Iryna Frankova, MD, Assistant at the Bogomolets National Medical University. She is a licensed mental health provider, works as a clinical psychologist at Psychosomatic Medicine and Psychotherapy Department and specializes in anxiety disorders, psychological trauma and related disorders. She is a member of Ukrainian Association of Psychotherapists and Psychoanalysts.

Alexander Mazur, PhD, Research associate at the McGill University and Genome Quebec Innovation Center. His research interest focuses on bioinformatics and biomedical data analysis, clinical proteomics, SNV detection in Proteomics, ProteoGenomics, NextGen sequencing, Software development, data warehousing and data cleaning, E-business, web application development.

Kirk J. Brower, MD is a Professor of Psychiatry at the University of Michigan (UM). He graduated from medical school at the University of California (UC) in Irvine and completed his residency in psychiatry at UC Los Angeles (UCLA). Board-certified in addiction psychiatry, he is Executive Director of UM Addiction Treatment Services and training director for the UM Addiction Psychiatry Fellowship Program.

Rober A. Zucker, PhD, ABPP, Professor of Psychiatry at the University of Michigan Medical School, and Professor, Department of Psychology, University of Michigan, and Director Emeritus, University of Michigan Addiction Research Center. He is a Principal Investigator or Coinvestigator on 77 grants from the NIH, NIAAA, NIDA and MICHR. His research focuses on multi-level etiology and course of alcohol and other drug use disorders, neural circuitry and genetics associated with substance use disorders and lifespan developments. He is a Consulting Editor/Associate Editor of the Drug and Alcohol Dependence, Alcoholism: Clinical and Experimental Research (Field Editor), Development and Psychopathology, Current Drug Abuse Reviews and Ukrainskiy Visnyk Psykhonevrologiyi (Ukrainian Bulletin of Psychoneurology) (Member, Editorial Council).

Chapter 11
The Effect of Laying-on of Hands on the Substance Abuse

Ricardo Monezi, Adriana Scatena and André Luiz Monezi Andrade

Introduction

Among the many resources available for the therapeutic handling of patients under treatment for the use of psychoactive substances, there are several Integrative and Complementary Health Practices (ICHP) such as meditation, music therapy, and many techniques of laying-on of hands that have been gaining more and more prominence in this specialized area of care.

Laying-on of Hands: A Tradition in Caring

Care interventions based on the laying-on of hands, related to a possible transmission of energies not supported by the current physics, have been described across history. There are records that Hippocrates of Kos himself (460 BC–400 BC) already suggested the probable existence of a bioenergetic field present in living beings (Jain and Mills 2010; Ventegodt et al. 2004).

It is believed that techniques of laying-on of hands and transmission of energy, present in many cultures as in China, Tibet, Japan, Africa, India, and the native

R. Monezi (✉)
Departamento de Saúde Coletiva, Universidade Federal de São Paulo, Rua Botucatu, 740 - 4° Andar, São Paulo, SP 04023-062, Brazil
e-mail: ricardomonezi@gmail.com

A. Scatena · A.L.M. Andrade
Departamento de Psicobiologia, Universidade Federal de São Paulo, Rua Botucatu, 862 - 1° Andar, Edifício de Ciências Biomédicas, São Paulo, SP 04023-062, Brazil
e-mail: adriana.scatena7@gmail.com

A.L.M. Andrade
e-mail: andremonezi@gmail.com

© Springer International Publishing Switzerland 2016
A.L.M. Andrade and D. De Micheli (eds.), *Innovations in the Treatment of Substance Addiction*, DOI 10.1007/978-3-319-43172-7_11

North American peoples, might have therapeutic properties. Various of those cultures believe that illnesses originate from the blockage in the flow of energetic biofield (Vandervaart et al. 2009).

Various reports on the application of those techniques in countless medical areas as a complementary resource to conventional therapies have demonstrated promising results, mainly in the recovery of patients with chronic diseases, such as oncologic patients, both pediatric and adult (Coakley and Barron 2012), AIDS patients (Mills et al. 2005), obstetric patients during pregnancy (Rakestraw 2009), and patients with nervous system diseases that can affect behavior, as in the case of epilepsy (A; Kumar and Kurup 2003), dementia (Woods et al. 2009), and Alzheimer's disease (Crawford et al. 2006). Studies also report positive effects of that kind of treatment in the rehabilitation of drug users (Blacher and Rundio 2014; Brooks et al. 2006; Hagemaster 2000; Larden et al. 2004; Li et al. 2002; Shamsalina et al. 2014).

Studies in the medical literature carried out with humans identified alterations resulting from treatment by various practices of laying-on of hands as, for instance, activation and increase of functions of the body defense system (immune system) in bereaved individuals going through that difficult situation (Quinn and Strelkauskas 1993). Moreover, there are reports according to which practices of laying-on of hands might act positively on the heart health (Friedman et al. 2010) and the blood vessels (Macintyre et al. 2008), preventing cardiac diseases and hypertension (Diaz-Rodriguez et al. 2011).

In addition to the benefits to the organs and systems that compose the human body, treatments based on the laying-on of hands have proved effective in the reduction of pain and stress-related psychological symptoms (Winstead-Fry and Kijek 1999), as well as positive alterations as to behavioral patterns, mainly regarding levels of consciousness, leading users of those therapeutic techniques to the perception and better understanding of a state of harmony and well-being (Ring 2009). There are scientific descriptions that the use of laying-on of hands, along with classic psychological treatments, might promote a strong feeling of encouragement in their users, which in turn leads them to feel responsible for and willing to actively work for their integral health (Latorre 2005). Other studies report decrease of fatigue in patients under chemotherapy (Post-White et al. 2003), improvement in the quality of life in patients under radiotherapy (Cook et al. 2004), and decrease in the stress levels of pregnant women with substance dependence (Larden et al. 2004).

The diversity of promising results yielded by laying-on of hands as a complementary therapy to treat several diseases and clinical conditions has been published by professionals of different academic backgrounds in the area of health, such as biologists, psychologists, nurses, physical therapists, and physicians, which shows a multidisciplinary interest in the issue.

Studies point out some factors that might contribute to the acceptance of laying-on of hands techniques in hospitals and health services, namely the growing interest of the public and the number of health professionals, from various sectors, who learn the techniques and apply them integrated with conventional care, and their low cost and risk (Hart 2012; Wardell and Engebretson 2001).

Among the various techniques that use laying-on of hands, we can mention therapeutic touch (Monzillo and Gronowicz 2011), Qi Gong (Chu et al. 2004), Johrei (Canter et al. 2006), and Reiki (Miles and True 2003).

Therapeutic Touch, Qi Gong, Johrei, and Reiki: Different Names that Preserve the Essence of Care by the Laying-on of Hands

The therapeutic touch (TT), or the Krieger–Kunz method, was described in the early 1970's by Dolores Krieger, from the Nursing Division of New York University. According to the authors, it is a method in which the hands are used to modulate human energies. Its practitioners claim that the therapist can detect the "energetic fields" of the patient and intentionally manipulate them (Coppa 2008).

As reported by its creator herself, "TT does not have any religious basis and does not depend on faith or belief from the one receiving it or the one practicing it to be effective. Its application requires, however, conscious intention on the part of the practitioner with the intent to re-pattern the energetic human field" (Krieger 1976).

Qi Gong is considered a millenarian Chinese technique of laying-on of hands. "Qi" means energy, and "Gong" is the union of the emotional, mental, and physiological conditions of the practitioner. It aims at working with, harmonizing and applying the "energy flow" in the body. Practitioners believe that the practice of Qi Gong exercises opens the energy entry points, absorbing the energy of nature (Jahnke et al. 2010; Zhang et al. 1998).

Johrei is a technique of laying-on of hands described by Mokiti Okada in Japan, and associated with the Messianic Church. Its practitioners believe that through the laying-on of the hands over a person's body, "divine universal energies" can cause alterations in the physical, emotional, social, and spiritual dimensions of the human being (Naito et al. 2003; Oschman 2000).

Reiki is a technique of laying-on of hands defined in Japan in the middle of the nineteenth century. The word Reiki is of Japanese origin and means "Energy of the vital force of the universe." Asian traditional medicine and its practitioners believe this energy can be transmitted to the body of another person (Bullock 1997; Tattam 1994; Vandervaart et al. 2009; Vitale and O'Connor 2006; Wardell and Engebretson 2001). Reiki is now classified as a modality of energetic medicine by the National Center for Complementary and Integrative Health (NCCIH) (Vandervaart 2011), being officially recommended by the National Health Service Trusts (NHST 2006) and the Prince of Wales's Foundation for Integrated Health (TPWFIH 2005). Data of the Brazilian Ministry of Health point Reiki as one of the most specialized ICHPs in the country (MS-BR 2006). Corroborating this fact, we can see a growing interest in this practice, which can bring countless benefits to its practitioners, in many research centers the world over. However, just as in the other laying-on of hands techniques, science does not fully understand its mechanism of action.

The principle of laying-on of hands therapies, independently of their denomination, is to take care of the individual as a whole rather than provide relief of the symptoms. Hence, laying-on of hands can be considered an integral health care by acting on the biological, psychological, social, and spiritual dimensions of the individual (Ring 2009; Vandervaart et al. 2009).

Since the 1990s, science has been discussing evidence which suggests that many of the results achieved by treatments with laying-on of hands techniques are a consequence of changes related to spirituality (Wardell and Engebretson 2001), conceptualized as an orientation directed to or aimed at feelings, at wishing to be connected to something bigger than oneself, a search for the sacred in one's life (Labbe and Fobes 2010).

Researches propose that spiritualized individuals are more involved in the search and promotion of healthy lifestyles and social support. They are more optimistic and persistent in the face of life challenges (Labbe and Fobes 2010; Manning 2013; Strout and Howard 2012), resisting the urge to go back to substance use, thus ensuring the effectiveness of the rehabilitation treatment (Shamsalina et al. 2014). Corroborating those data, a study published in 2007 by the Division of Alcoholism and Drug Abuse at New York University highlights the fact that spirituality is considered an extremely important aspect in the recovery of participants in Alcoholics Anonymous groups (Galanter 2007).

Another common factor among the treatments by the different laying-on of hands techniques is the promotion of a relaxation state that helps reduce the perception of tension and enhances the perception of well-being, leading to higher indices of quality of life (Bowden et al. 2011).

Examples of Effects of Laying-on of Hands Interventions on the Treatment of Drug Users

Substance abuse-related disorders often become chronic and repetitive, leading to a significant worsening of the biological, psychological, and social aspects of the user, even compromising their spirituality. In spite of the development of medications aimed at the treatment of those disorders, such as *Baclofen* or *Ondansetron*, conventional therapies are often unable to change the outcome (Behere et al. 2009). Therefore, a need arises to look back at the use of alternative and complementary care, as laying-on of hands, that might prove a valuable resource in the rehabilitation of a human being integrality at a moment of extreme vulnerability due to drug use and abuse.

With a view to examine the effectiveness of therapeutic touch as a treatment intervention that could lengthen the abstinence period related to the abusive use of alcohol and other drugs, the University of Kansas (USA) carried out a study in 2000 that involved substance dependents who received therapeutic touch once a week for eight weeks. At the end of the research, the volunteers who had received laying-on of hands presented decrease in depression symptoms, frequency of search for, and use of alcohol and other drugs, in addition to improvement of family and social relations. The sensations most often reported by the volunteers were warmth, relaxation, energy, and "feeling like laughing or crying" during and immediately after the treatment session. Many of them reported feeling capable and not seeing why they should resort to alcohol and other drugs anymore. One man stated that, in addition to all those things, now he could handle his wife's criticism, which was used to be the excuse that led him to the abusive use of alcohol. Those results taken together led to the conclusion that therapeutic touch can be very effective in lengthening the periods of withdrawal from alcohol and other substance dependences in two ways: first, by the reduction of the depression levels of participants, which in turn improved mood, thus facilitating abstinence maintenance; second, by the improvement of social relations as a result of longer periods of sobriety (Hagemaster 2000).

A study published in 2002 described the therapeutic action of 10 days of Qi Gong on heroin users in rehabilitation. The results showed that as of the fifth day of intervention there was a significant reduction in the levels of anxiety among the volunteers who received the Qi Gong treatment, and suggest that this laying-on of hands might be an effective alternative for heroin detoxification without side effects (Li et al. 2002).

In order to assess the effects of Johrei on patients in home treatment for the recovery from substance abuse, a preliminary study was carried out in 2006 with 22 volunteers divided into two groups: 12 volunteers who received three 20-minute sessions of Johrei a week for 35 days, and 10 volunteers who were in a waiting list. All the participants continued their conventional rehabilitation treatments across the research. The participants who received the Johrei exhibited significant reductions in their levels of depression, stress, and physical pain, in addition to enhancement of spirituality, energy, optimism, and general well-being. Consequently, the study concluded that Johrei might be a promising adjuvant treatment in the process of recovery from substance abuse (Brooks et al. 2006).

Reiki has yielded promising results as well. A study carried out in 2011 with HIV patients over 50 years of age and with a history of substance dependence revealed a significant decrease in the search for the substance after the Reiki treatment, and a greater acceptance of and search for psychological support treatments (Mehl-Madrona et al. 2011).

Conclusions About the Use of Laying-on of Hands Techniques for the Treatment of Substance Use and Abuse

Scientific evidence suggests that the use of laying-on of hands techniques for the treatment of substance abuse promotes reduction of stress, anxiety symptoms, depression, and perception of tension, followed by enhanced feeling of well-being, improved quality of life, and spirituality, in addition to physiological alterations that indicate a relaxation state. Such results might be triggering elements of a possible restructuring of paradigms, thoughts, and mainly behaviors that lead the substance user to the understanding that his recovery and integral health care is literally at hand.

References

Behere, R. V., Muralidharan, K., & Benegal, V. (2009). Complementary and alternative medicine in the treatment of substance use disorders—a review of the evidence. *Drug and Alcohol Review, 28*(3), 292–300. doi:10.1111/j.1465-3362.2009.00028.x. ISSN 1465-3362.

Blacher, S., Rundio, A. (2014). Complementary and integrative modalities in addiction treatment. *Journal of Addictions Nursing, 25*(4), 165–166. Available in: http://journals.lww.com/jan/Fulltext/2014/10000/Complementary_and_Integrative_Modalities_in.2.aspx. ISSN 1088-4602.

Bowden, D., Goddard, L., Gruzelier, J. (2011). A randomised controlled single-blind trial of the efficacy of Reiki at benefitting mood and well-being. *Evidence-Based Complementary and Alternative Medicine*, 381862. ISSN 1741-4288 (Electronic), 1741-427X (Linking). Available in: http://www.ncbi.nlm.nih.gov/pubmed/21584234

Brooks, A. J., et al. (2006). The effect of Johrei healing on substance abuse recovery: A pilot study. *Journal of Alternative and Complementary Medicine, 12*(7), 625–631. 1075-5535 (Print), 1075-5535 (Linking). Available in: http://www.ncbi.nlm.nih.gov/pubmed/16970532

Bullock, M. (1997). Reiki: A complementary therapy for life. *American Journal of Hospice and Palliative Medicine, 14*(1), 31–33. 1049-9091 (Print), 1049-9091 (Linking). Available in: http://www.ncbi.nlm.nih.gov/pubmed/9069762

Canter, P. H., et al. (2006). Johrei family healing: A pilot study. *Evidence-Based Complementary and Alternative Medicine, 3*(4), 533–540. 1741-427X (Print), 1747-427X (Linking). Available in: http://www.ncbi.nlm.nih.gov/pubmed/17173118

Chu, D. A., Chi, T., Gong, Q., & Reiki (2004). *Physical Medicine and Rehabilitation Clinics of North America, 15*(4), 773–781, vi. ISSN 1047-9651 (Print), 1047-9651 (Linking). Available in: http://www.ncbi.nlm.nih.gov/pubmed/15458751

Coakley, A. B., & Barron, A. M. (2012). Energy therapies in oncology nursing. *Seminars in Oncology Nursing, 28*(1), 55–63. ISSN 1878-3449 (Electronic), 0749-2081 (Linking). Available in: http://www.ncbi.nlm.nih.gov/pubmed/22281310

Cook, C. A., Guerrerio, J. F., & Slater, V. E. (2004). Healing touch and quality of life in women receiving radiation treatment for cancer: A randomized controlled trial. *Alternative Therapies in Health and Medicine, 10*(3), 34–41. ISSN 1078-6791 (Print), 1078-6791 (Linking). Available in: http://www.ncbi.nlm.nih.gov/pubmed/15154151

Coppa, D. (2008). The internal process of therapeutic touch. *Journal of Holistic Nursing, 26*(1), 17–24. ISSN 0898-0101 (Print), 0898-0101 (Linking). Available in: http://www.ncbi.nlm.nih.gov/pubmed/18332355

Crawford, S. E., Leaver, V. W., & Mahoney, S. D. (2006). Using Reiki to decrease memory and behavior problems in mild cognitive impairment and mild Alzheimer's disease. *Journal of Alternative and Complementary Medicine, 12*(9), 911–913. ISSN 1075-5535 (Print), 1075-5535 (Linking). Available in: http://www.ncbi.nlm.nih.gov/pubmed/17109583

Diaz-Rodriguez, L., et al. (2011). The application of Reiki in nurses diagnosed with Burnout Syndrome has beneficial effects on concentration of salivary IgA and blood pressure. *Revista Latino-Americana de Enfermagem, 19*(5), 1132–1138. ISSN 0104-1169 (Print), 0104-1169 (Linking). Available in: http://www.ncbi.nlm.nih.gov/pubmed/22030577

Friedman, R. S., et al. (2010). Effects of Reiki on autonomic activity early after acute coronary syndrome. *Journal of the American College of Cardiology, 56*(12), 995–996. ISSN 1558-3597 (Electronic), 0735-1097 (Linking). Available in: http://www.ncbi.nlm.nih.gov/pubmed/20828654

Galanter, M., et al. (2007). Assessment of spirituality and its relevance to addiction treatment. *Journal of Substance Abuse Treatment, 33*(3), 257–264. ISSN 0740-5472. Available in: http://www.sciencedirect.com/science/article/pii/S0740547206002066

Hagemaster, J. (2000). Use of therapeutic touch in treatment of drug addictions. *Holistic Nursing Practice, 14*(3), 14–20. ISSN 0887-9311 (Print), 0887-9311 (Linking). Available in: http://www.ncbi.nlm.nih.gov/pubmed/12119624

Hart, J. (2012). Healing touch, therapeutic touch, and Reiki: Energy medicine advances in the medical community. *Alternative and Complementary Therapies, 18*(6), 309–313. ISSN 1076-2809, 1557-9085.

Jahnke, R., et al. (2010). A comprehensive review of health benefits of qigong and tai chi. *American Journal of Health Promotion, 24*(6), e1–e25. ISSN 0890-1171 (Print), 0890-1171 (Linking). Available in: http://www.ncbi.nlm.nih.gov/pubmed/20594090

Jain, S., & Mills, P. J. (2010). Biofield therapies: Helpful or full of hype? A best evidence synthesis. *International Journal of Behavioral Medicine, 17*(1), 1–16. ISSN 1532-7558 (Electronic), 1070-5503 (Linking). Available in: http://www.ncbi.nlm.nih.gov/pubmed/19856109

Krieger, D. (1976). Healing by the laying-on of hands as a facilitator of bioenergetic exchange: The response of in vivo human hemoglobin. *International Journal for Psychoenergetic, 2,* 121–129.

Kumar, R. A., & Kurup, P. A. (2003). Changes in the isoprenoid pathway with transcendental meditation and Reiki healing practices in seizure disorder. *Neurology India, 51*(2), 211–214. ISSN 0028-3886, 0028-3886 (Linking). Available in: http://www.ncbi.nlm.nih.gov/pubmed/14571006

Labbe, E. E., & Fobes, A. (2010). Evaluating the interplay between spirituality, personality and stress. *Applied Psychophysiology and Biofeedback, 35*(2), 141–146. ISSN 1573-3270 (Electronic), 1090-0586 (Linking). Available in: http://www.ncbi.nlm.nih.gov/pubmed/19847641

Larden, C. N., Palmer, M. L., & Janssen, P. (2004). Efficacy of therapeutic touch in treating pregnant inpatients who have a chemical dependency. *Journal of Holistic Nursing, 22*(4), 320–332. ISSN 0898-0101 (Print), 0898-0101 (Linking). Available in: http://www.ncbi.nlm.nih.gov/pubmed/15486152

Latorre, M. A. (2005). The use of Reiki in psychotherapy. *Perspectives in Psychiatric Care, 41*(4), 184–187. ISSN 0031-5990 (Print), 0031-5990 (Linking). Available in: http://www.ncbi.nlm.nih.gov/pubmed/16297024

Li, M., Chen, K., Mo, Z. (2002). Use of qigong therapy in the detoxification of heroin addicts. *Alternative Therapies in Health And Medicine, 8*(1), 50–54, 56–59. ISSN 1078-6791 (Print), 1078-6791 (Linking). Available in: http://www.ncbi.nlm.nih.gov/pubmed/11795622

MS-BR. (2006). Política nacional de práticas integrativas e complementares no SUS—Atitude de ampliação de acesso. MINISTÉRIO DA SAÚDE, B. Brasília: Ministério da Saúde: 92 pp.

Macintyre, B., et al. (2008). The efficacy of healing touch in coronary artery bypass surgery recovery: A randomized clinical trial. *Alternative Therapies in Health and Medicine, 14*(4), 24–32. ISSN 1078-6791 (Print), 1078-6791 (Linking). Available in: http://www.ncbi.nlm.nih.gov/pubmed/18616066

Manning, L. K. (2013). Navigating hardships in old age: Exploring the relationship between spirituality and resilience in later life. *Qualitative Health Research, 23*(4), 568–575. ISSN 1049-7323 (Print), 1049-7323 (Linking). Available in: http://www.ncbi.nlm.nih.gov/pubmed/23282796

Mehl-Madrona, L., Renfrew, N. M., & Mainguy, B. (2011). Qualitative assessment of the impact of implementing reiki training in a supported residence for people older than 50 years with HIV/AIDS. *The Permanente Journal, 15*(3), 43–50. ISSN 1552-5775 (Electronic), 1552-5767 (Linking). Available in: http://www.ncbi.nlm.nih.gov/pubmed/22058669

Miles, P., & True, G. (2003). Reiki—review of a biofield therapy history, theory, practice, and research. *Alternative Therapies in Health and Medicine, 9*(2), 62–72. ISSN 1078-6791 (Print), 1078-6791 (Linking). Available in: http://www.ncbi.nlm.nih.gov/pubmed/12652885

Mills, E., Wu, P., & Ernst, E. (2005). Complementary therapies for the treatment of HIV: In search of the evidence. *International Journal of STD and AIDS, 16*(6), 395–403. ISSN 0956-4624 (Print), 0956-4624 (Linking). Available in: http://www.ncbi.nlm.nih.gov/pubmed/15969772

Monzillo, E., & Gronowicz, G. (2011). New insights on therapeutic touch: A discussion of experimental methodology and design that resulted in significant effects on normal human cells and osteosarcoma. *Explore (NY), 7*(1), 44–51. ISSN 1878-7541 (Electronic), 1550-8307 (Linking). Available in: http://www.ncbi.nlm.nih.gov/pubmed/21194672

NHST. (2006). *The NHS new guide to healthy living.* London: The NHS Trusts Association.

Naito, A., et al. (2003). The impact of self-hypnosis and Johrei on lymphocyte subpopulations at exam time: A controlled study. *Brain Research Bulletin, 62*(3), 241–253. ISSN 0361-9230 (Print), 0361-9230 (Linking). Available in: http://www.ncbi.nlm.nih.gov/pubmed/14698357

Oschman, J. L. (2000). *Energy medicine—The scientific basis* (p. 275). London: Churchill Livingstone.

Post-White, J., et al. (2003). Therapeutic massage and healing touch improve symptoms in cancer. *Integrative Cancer Therapies, 2*(4), 332–344. ISSN 1534-7354 (Print), 1534-7354 (Linking). Available in: http://www.ncbi.nlm.nih.gov/pubmed/14713325

Quinn, J. F., & Strelkauskas, A. J. (1993). Psychoimmunologic effects of therapeutic touch on practitioners and recently bereaved recipients: A pilot study. *ANS Advances in Nursing Science, 15*(4), 13–26. ISSN 0161-9268 (Print), 0161-9268 (Linking). Available in: http://www.ncbi.nlm.nih.gov/pubmed/8512301

Rakestraw, T. (2009). Reiki: The energy doula. *Midwifery Today International Midwife, 92*, 16–17. ISSN 1551-8892 (Print), 1551-8892 (Linking). Available in: http://www.ncbi.nlm.nih.gov/pubmed/20092137

Ring, M. E. (2009). Reiki and changes in pattern manifestations. *Nursing Science Quarterly, 22* (3), 250–258. ISSN 0894-3184 (Print), 0894-3184 (Linking). Available in: http://www.ncbi.nlm.nih.gov/pubmed/19567731

Shamsalina, A., et al. (2014). Recovery based on spirituality in substance abusers in Iran. *Global Journal of Health Science, 6*(6), 154–162. ISSN 1916-9736 (Print), 1916-9736 (Linking). Available in: http://www.ncbi.nlm.nih.gov/pubmed/25363097

Strout, K. A., & Howard, E. P. (2012). The six dimensions of wellness and cognition in aging adults. *Journal of Holistic Nursing, 30*(3), 195–204. ISSN 1552-5724 (Electronic), 0898-0101 (Linking). Available in: http://www.ncbi.nlm.nih.gov/pubmed/22713605

TPWFIH. (2005). *Complementary health care: A guide for patients.* London: The Prince of Wales's Foundation for Integrated Health.

Tattam, A. (1994). Reiki–healing and dealing. *Australian Journal of Advanced Nursing, 2*(2), 3, 52. ISSN 1320-3185 (Print), 1320-3185 (Linking). Available in: http://www.ncbi.nlm.nih.gov/pubmed/7849997

Vandervaart, S., et al. (2009). A systematic review of the therapeutic effects of Reiki. *Journal of Alternative and Complementary Medicine, 15*(11), 1157–1169. ISSN 1557-7708 (Electronic).

Vandervaart, S., et al. (2011). The effect of distant Reiki on pain in women after elective Caesarean section: A double-blinded randomised controlled trial. *BMJ Open, 1*(1):e000021. ISSN 2044-6055 (Electronic). Available in: http://www.ncbi.nlm.nih.gov/pubmed/22021729, 1075-5535 (Linking). Available in: http://www.ncbi.nlm.nih.gov/pubmed/19922247

Ventegodt, S., Morad, M., & Merrick, J. (2004). Clinical holistic medicine: Classic art of healing or the therapeutic touch. *Scientific World Journal, 4*, 134–147. ISSN 1537-744X (Electronic), 1537-744X (Linking). Available in: http://www.ncbi.nlm.nih.gov/pubmed/15010568

Vitale, A. T., & O'Connor, P. C. (2006). The effect of Reiki on pain and anxiety in women with abdominal hysterectomies: A quasi-experimental pilot study. *Holistic Nursing Practice, 20*(6), 263–272; quiz 273–274. ISSN 0887-9311 (Print), 0887-9311 (Linking). Available in: http://www.ncbi.nlm.nih.gov/pubmed/17099413

Wardell, D. W., & Engebretson, J. (2001). Biological correlates of Reiki Touch(sm) healing. *Journal of Advanced Nursing, 33*(4), 439–445. ISSN 0309-2402 (Print), 0309-2402 (Linking). Available in: http://www.ncbi.nlm.nih.gov/pubmed/11251731

Winstead-Fry, P., & Kijek, J. (1999). An integrative review and meta-analysis of therapeutic touch research. *Alternative Therapies in Health and Medicine, 5*(6), 58–67. ISSN 1078-6791 (Print), 1078-6791 (Linking). Available in: http://www.ncbi.nlm.nih.gov/pubmed/10550906

Woods, D. L., Beck, C., & Sinha, K. (2009). The effect of therapeutic touch on behavioral symptoms and cortisol in persons with dementia. *Forsch Komplementmed, 16*(3), 181–189. ISSN 1661-4127 (Electronic), 1661-4119 (Linking). Available in: http://www.ncbi.nlm.nih.gov/pubmed/19657203

Zhang, W. B., Yu, W. L., & Yang, Y. J. (1998). Absence of an analgesic effect of qigong "external qi" in rats. *American Journal of Chinese Medicine, 26*(1), 39–46. ISSN 0192-415X (Print), 0192-415X (Linking). Available in: http://www.ncbi.nlm.nih.gov/pubmed/9592592

Chapter 12
The Effects of Yoga on Substance Abuse

Rui Ferreira Afonso

Introduction

Excused one time to a more philosophical and theoretical approach to understand Yoga in its original context and not mistaken with exercise.

Yoga originated in remote India, but the date of his birth is a mystery. We know it is very old, some millennia before the Christian era. Yoga is reported already in the early books of mankind, the Vedas, which date back more than 3500 BC. The word Yoga comes from the Sanskrit, a language that was spoken in India, and means union, united, join. Also has the meaning of work and application. Well, with this, we can start to define Yoga. Because it is a tradition based on psychospiritual transformation of the human being, Yoga aims to unite the individual being (you) with the all, the divine, the sacred, etc. So it is not far from the original meaning of religions whose goal was to "*religare*" (Latin)—etymological origin of the word religion that means reconnection. But to be possible, this unite or "rewiring" a work is required, an application or a specific set of techniques. These techniques also are called Yoga. Thus, Yoga means both, the end (the state unite) and the means (the tools) that leads practitioner to the unite. More recently, the contemporary and pragmatic man realized that the ancient techniques of Yoga can be used for therapeutic purposes and quality of life. However, what is behind the techniques, (teachings to life, values, behavior, and conduct) should also be practiced because Yoga can be seen as a "philosophy of life." Thus, in addition to developing physical health, Yoga has the ability to transform the psyche, character, and soul (Taimini 1961).

R.F. Afonso (✉)
Neurociências, Hospital Israelita Albert Einstein, Av. Albert Einstein,
627/701-Bloco A-2o Subsolo (Sala de Pesquisadores), São Paulo
SP 05601-901, Brazil
e-mail: ruiafonsobr@yahoo.com.br

© Springer International Publishing Switzerland 2016
A.L.M. Andrade and D. De Micheli (eds.), *Innovations in the Treatment of Substance Addiction*, DOI 10.1007/978-3-319-43172-7_12

193

So far, we talked very generally about Yoga. But how to practice it? The first "manual" of Yoga arose about 200–400 BC and based on this manual almost all of the schools or different forms of Yoga we know today were developed. In a very brief little book of only 196 sutras (or phrases), the author, Patañjali, wrote the Yoga Sutra or the Yoga Aphorisms. Right at the beginning of this text, Patañjali defines Yoga:

"Yoga is the inhibition of the modifications of the mind," or, to make it easier for the layman to understand: Yoga is not the identification of being (individual) with the different roles and characters that he/she represents. If you ask me who am I, my answer can vary greatly. If this question is asked in the condominium meeting, I say: I am the resident of apartment 12. If the same question is asked in a professional environment, I say I am Yoga teacher. If the same question is asked in my child's school meeting, the answer will be different and so on. Did you realize we represent various roles? But what is the relationship of that in the context of drug addiction? In the case of addiction, it is very common to hear: I'm dependent; I am anxious; I am user of substance; I'm a failure; I am... In these examples, the subject took part for the whole. The individual may have symptoms of anxiety or any other problem, but it does not define anyone. According to Yoga, this guy who says I'm anxious is identified with some physical or mental sensations and it takes so much importance that it becomes unable to get rid of these thoughts and realize that he or she is not this feeling, this symptom, or this thought and therefore cannot inhibit the modifications of the mind as defined at the beginning of the Yoga Sutra text. What Patanjali teaches is that we can see our true nature which is free from limitations, happy and full of bliss, and not limited by small settings. For this, he reveals a path with 8 steps: self-restraints (*yama*), fixed observances (*niyama*), posture (*asana*), regulation of breath (*pranayama*), abstraction (*pratyahara*), concentration (*dharana*), meditation (*dhyana*), and contemplation (s*amadhy*) (Kupfer 2001).

The first two steps, yama and niyama, are a moral and behavioral code of conduct. The yama are nonviolence, truthfulness, nonstealing, continence, non-possessiveness. The niyama are purity, contentment, self-discipline, self-study, surrender. These first two steps serve to harmonize the individual with society and himself. If observed, the yama and niyama will be a deep inner peace, which helps a lot in practice whose aim is to calm the mind.

Asanas and pranayama are the third and fourth steps, those best known by laymen. The asana are psychophysical postures—psychophysical because it is through the body that reached internal states of higher consciousness. The body takes many forms during a practice. Bends, stretches, twists, compressions, and many other bodily actions are made. This step can be confused with physical exercise, gymnastics, or stretching. However, the goal is not the development of physical performance but calm the body and its movements, thus calming the mind. The postures are held for a period of time, seeking comfort and stability moment by moment. In the pause of the movement, which takes place during the asana, the practitioner may experience various sensations, developing body awareness and consequently a better understanding of yourself, something very important to the user of the substance. The pranayama are breathing exercises. Most of the time, breathing happens automatically, that is, we don't think to breathe. But the breath can also be controlled by our will. We are not able to control organs like the heart, for example. We did not make the heart to obey our will and so with all the other organs. However, we have enough control over the respiratory movement. We are able to speed up the breath, we can pause the breath, we can control the volume of air entering in the lungs, etc. Because breathing is both, autonomous and voluntary nervous system, we can influence the various systems in our body through breathing, such as calming the heartbeat, help reducing blood pressure, increase or decrease brain activity in certain areas of brain, and many others. This becomes especially important when the patient is affected by some physical symptoms, such as anxiety, for example, that increases the heart rate. Through the respiratory control, we are able to reduce heart rate and thus reduce anxiety. Then, the pranayama are very useful for use acutely in the various situations and challenges faced by the patient.

From the moment that the body and its agitation is controlled, the breath and the various systems of the body come into balance, then it's time to deal with the five sense organs or Pratyahara—withdrawal of the senses. The mind is projected out through the senses: We are distracted by the sounds, the smells, different textures of objects, shapes, and colors of the environment. You may not realize it, but much of the agitation of the mind is due to the need to stay in the "outside world" through the senses and the consequent difficulty to contact the "inner world," where the senses are dispensable. In the context of substance abuse, many environmental factors can be triggers of harmful behaviors because mind is conditioned to smells, places, people, etc. Often relapse occurs because of a smell, for example, and thus arises the necessity of having greater control over the "voracity" of the senses.

In the last three steps of Yoga, one is the evolution of the other. Dharana is what we call concentration. At this time, the mind still has its distractions, but far less than a untrained mind. When we master mind and its distractions, we entered in Dhyana or meditation, then we are one step closer to Samadhi or "enlightenment." I will not dwell too much because this book there is one chapter on meditation (Feuerstein 2002).

For the individual whose conditioning makes him or her always repeat the same things, Yoga is a path that can help him to observe awareness and thus leave the conditioning cycle that imprisons us.

Nowadays, most of the types of Yoga are derived from an old school called Hatha Yoga. Hatha means balance between the energy of the sun and moon, meaning the balance between opposites. The ancient practitioners of Yoga noted that the body is influenced by opposing energies: relaxation and contraction; sleep and wakefulness; inhalation and exhalation; state of excitement and calm state; and many others. Making a parallel with Western science, we realize that these pairs of opposites coincide with the actions of the sympathetic nervous system (the one "active") and parasympathetic (one that "calm"). Therefore, this type of Yoga develops the balance between the sympathetic nervous system and the parasympathetic nervous system. For us, this is very interesting, because many symptoms of withdrawal and craving are caused by an imbalance in the autonomic nervous system, better understood in the following topic.

Yoga, Drug Addiction, and Research

Thus far, Yoga was approached in a theoretical and conceptual way. Now, I will talk about the experiences of Yoga as a complementary therapy in the treatment of chemical dependency. There are many scientific studies that use Yoga as a resource for the treatment of substance users. There are some clinics, especially outside Brazil, which offer this modality in addition to other treatments, with interesting results and good acceptance by the inmates.

Stress is one of the most common problems in modern society. In its chronic form, stress can generate a series physical, psychological, and social damage. The stress causes or aggravates most diseases: psychiatric disorders, immune diseases, neoplasias, cardiovascular diseases, and many others. In the context of substance abuse, the user faces painfully this problem, especially abstinence. Many people, not only dependent, resort to the use of these substances because they are very stressed and want to "relax." It is the false idea that a glass of alcoholic drink will help you relax and better address the problems. In Yoga practices, we learn to be observers of ourselves impartially. Basically, many use the excuse of "relax" to the use of substances with less guilt. Knowing how to identify this saboteur thought a real necessity is fundamental, and Yoga provides us this possibility through its contemplative practices. Yoga makes us more aware, in addition to reducing the symptoms of stress. Moreover, practitioners have reported the importance of Yoga in reduction of stress, and we observe in some scientific papers decreases in cortisol levels, a hormone related to stress. There is a neuroendocrine stress axis (HPA—hypothalamus, pituitary gland, and adrenal). The activation of this axis begins in the perception of stressor stimuli and the consequent release of hormones such as cortisol. In chronic states of stress, this axis is hyper-reactive. Several scientific studies conclude that Yoga can reduce the activation of this pathway. There were made some studies in populations with high levels of stress: cancer patients, war veterans, caregivers of Alzheimer's patients, etc., and in most studies that examined cortisol samples, this hormone greatly reduced in volunteers who practiced Yoga, thereby being an interesting contribution to the reduction of stress. In other studies, when the symptoms of stress were evaluated, there was a reduction of most of these symptoms such as blood pressure, irregular breathing, muscle aches, headache, irritability, physical and mental fatigue, and loss of concentration. Most of these symptoms are caused by an imbalance in autonomic nervous system, with increased tone in sympathetic nervous system (the one that "activate"), which is related to most of the symptoms of stress and craving, for example. As one of the proposals of Yoga is "to balance the opposites," it is offered to practitioner the ability to return to equilibrium and homeostasis. There is scientific evidence of reduction in sympathetic tone and increase in parasympathetic tone in Yoga practitioners, thus reducing stress via autonomic nervous system, in addition to those, HPA axis, already mentioned (Brown and Gerberg 2005).

Stress increases much in abstinence and craving, along with anxiety. Anxiety is a disorder that can be accompanied by very unpleasant physical and psychological symptoms such as angst, muscle tension, headaches, sleep problems, difficulty in concentrating and relaxation, and muscle pain. For a long time, Yoga has been used complementary treatment to anxiety. The report of the practitioners on its calming effect is almost unanimity. This can be verified in many research using anxiety symptom questionnaires to evaluate the effect of Yoga. In most of these studies, the practice of Yoga was effective in reducing anxiety levels. Moreover, there is an inhibitory neurotransmitter in the central nervous system called gamma aminobutyric acid or simply GABA. Low GABA levels are associated with anxiety and much of the effects of benzodiazepines (antianxiety drugs) are due to this neurotransmitter, so vital to the well-being physical and psychical. Researchers at Boston University in the United States conducted an experiment in which GABA concentrations were analyzed in certain brain regions of subjects that started a Yoga program, and these subjects were compared with a walking group (Streeter et al. 2007). After 12 weeks, there was an increase in GABA levels in those who practiced Yoga. There was also improvement in mood levels and stress, which was correlated with an increase in GABA concentrations of practitioners. Similar results had been found in a previous work done by the same group, in which they compared experienced Yoga practitioners with normal subjects. Initially, they did a epectroscopia MRI in both groups. After examination, Yoga practitioners did 60 min of practice while the other volunteers did 60 min of reading, supposedly languid and tranquilizer. At the end of this time, the same test was repeated in volunteers. In the group that practiced Yoga was a 27 % increase in GABA concentrations in certain brain areas, which did not happen in reading group. Thus, Yoga can greatly help chronic and acutely the patient in moments of anxiety or craving. Specific symptoms of anxiety such as pain and muscle tension are also relieved with some techniques such as relaxation called yoganidra and postures, asana. At this point, the practitioner learns to access a deep and conscious relaxation of each part of the body and develops body awareness and better understanding of contraction and relaxation states. Volunteers with chronic pain complaints (such as arthritis, arthrosis, and low back pain) and muscle tension stretch the muscles, align body, relieve the overload of joints, and greatly improve their complaints through Yoga techniques (Javnbakht et al. 2009).

Complaints such as insomnia can also be associated with addiction and its complications. Sometimes insomnia itself leads the individual to become dependent on benzodiazepines or other drugs. In my master's, I studied post-menopausal women with insomnia complaints (Afonso et al. 2012). Certainly they had no substance abuse problem, but shared many things with dependents such as anxiety, stress, and insomnia. In addition, these women had many menopausal symptoms and could not make use of any medication to relieve insomnia nor such menopausal symptoms and therefore a very difficult group. At the end of some sessions, they have reported improvements, but the evidence came at the end of study where tests showed that Yoga practice had reduced menopausal symptoms. In this study, there were not made melatonin dosages, a hormone related to sleep and wellness. However, researchers in Delhi, India, submitted a group of soldiers to a Yoga and meditation program and after 3 months of daily practice observed an increase in melatonin in military who practiced Yoga and also improvements in psychological profile of this group (Harinath et al. 2004).

Such changes, both physical and psychological, do not happen singly. There are several systems in the body acting together and, most of the time, a research measures only some of these variables, as those mentioned previously. We know that changes in mood and well-being are related to neurotransmitters like serotonin. A group of researchers at Defence Institute of Physiology and Allied Sciences in Delhi, India, measured some variables including serotonin, in a group of volunteers undergoing a Yoga program. Three months after the start of the program, there was an increase in serotonin levels in Yoga group. Much of antidepressant drugs act on the serotonin system, increasing levels of this neurotransmitter into synapses. Since there are positive moods and well-being, there are improvements in general health and quality of life. Several studies have been developed with all kinds of volunteers, susceptible to mood disorders such as cancer patients, elderly, chronic pain patients, victims of violence, and also primary depression (Bock et al. 2010). Yoga appears as a very efficient alternative to improvement in depression symptoms. Until then, we observed several symptoms that may be present in substance users. In terms of research, most part of studies which were applied Yoga as a complementary resource to treatment had positive results. Some studies have applied a specific technique of Yoga, such as breathing exercises, relaxation, or meditation. Other studies have made use of a complete Yoga program. A very interesting study was done in London, England. The researchers asked a group of smokers to stop smoking in order to investigate the acute withdrawal (Bock at al. 2014). A group of volunteers learned a particular breathing exercise (pranayama). From there, the volunteers could make use of this technique whenever necessary. At the end of 36 h of abstinence, the volunteers who have made the use of breathing exercise reduced the craving for cigarettes. When relaxation technique (yoganidra) was applied to another group of smokers, the results were similar, reducing craving, withdrawal symptoms, and reducing the systolic blood pressure (Elibero et al. 2011). In most programs developed for chemical dependent, interventions are another resource to help the patient to face, especially the withdrawal symptoms. After a one-week program of detoxification, alcoholic volunteers were divided into two groups in which Yoga practices were made by one of these groups. After two weeks, individuals who practice Yoga had greater reduction in depression symptoms and reduction in cortisol and ACTH levels (stress-related hormones and some psychiatric disorders). Improvement in depression symptoms is important not only for the patient's overall health, but also as an aspect of motivation to face the difficulties that will arise during the journey to become free of dependence, as many drop out. Regarding adherence to treatment, a program for women to stop smoking, the adherence rate to Yoga sessions was higher than the rate for a group of health and wellness (Bock et al. 2012). This study compared two groups: Yoga group and health and well-being group. There was a higher withdrawal rate in women in Yoga group. Also in this group, after 8 weeks of practices, women reported reduced temptation per cigarette, anxiety reduction, improved mood, and increased sense of well-being. In terms of Yoga and substance abuse, we should consider not only the treatment, but also prevention means to drug abuse and relapse prevention. People with PTSD have higher risk for developing dependence, for example. Results of a study suggest that the practice of Yoga in addition to alleviating symptoms of post-traumatic stress reduces the risk for alcohol and drugs, therefore a way of prevention (Reddy et al. 2014). Thus, the practice of Yoga is demonstrated as a viable complementary treatment for chemical substance user.

References

Afonso, R. F., Hachul, H., Kozasa, E. H., et al. (2012). Yoga decreases insomnia in postmenopausal women: A randomized clinical trial. *Menopause, 19*, 186–193. http://www.yoga.pro.brSiteforYogatexts

Bock, B. C., Fava, J. L., Gaskins, R., Morrow, K. M., Williams, D. M., et al. (2012). Yoga as a complementary treatment for smoking cessation in women. *Health (Larchmt), 21*(2), 240–248.

Bock, B. C., Morrow, K. M., Becker, B. M., Williams, D. M., Tremont, G., et al. (2010). Yoga as a complementary treatment for smoking cessation: Rationale, study design and participant characteristics of the Quitting-in-Balance study. *BMC Complementary and Alternative Medicine, 10*, 14.

Bock, B. C., Rosen, R. K., Fava, J. L., Gaskins, R. B., Jennings, E., et al. (2014). Testing the efficacy of yoga as a complementary therapy for smoking cessation: Design and methods of the BreathEasy trial. *Contemporary Clinical Trials, 38*(2), 321–332.

Brown, R. P., & Gerbarg, P. L. (2005). Sudarshan Kriya Yogic breathing in the treatment of stress, anxiety, and depression. Part IIV clinical applications and guidelines. *Journal of Alternative and Complementary Medicine, 11*, 711–717.

Elibero, A., Janse Van Rensburg, K., & Drobes, D. J. (2011). Acute effects of aerobic exercise and Hatha yoga on craving to smoke. *Nicotine & Tobacco Research, 13*(11), 1140–1148.

Feuerstein, G. (2002). *The yoga tradition* (3rd ed.). Prescott, AZ: Hohm Press.

Harinath, K., Malhotra, A. S., Pal, K., et al. (2004). Effects of Hatha yoga and Omkar meditation on cardiorespiratory performance, psychologic profile, and melatonin secretion. *Journal of Alternative and Complementary Medicine, 10*, 261–268.

Javnbakht, M., Hejazi Kenari, R., & Ghasemi, M. (2009). Effects of yoga on depression and anxiety of women. *Complementary Therapies in Clinical Practice, 15*, 102–104.

Kupfer, P. (2001). Yoga prático 3ª Dharma Florianópolis.

Reddy, S., Dick, A. M., Gerber, M. R., & Mitchell, K. (2014). The effect of a yoga intervention on alcohol and drug abuse risk in veteran and civilian women with posttraumatic stress disorder. *Journal of Alternative and Complementary Medicine, 20*(10), 750–756.

Streeter, C. C., Jensen, J. E., Perlmutter, R. M., et al. (2007). Yoga Asana sessions increase brain GABA levels: a pilot study. *Journal of Alternative and Complementary Medicine, 13*, 419–426.

Taimini, I. K. (1961). *The science of yoga*. Adyar: Theosophical Publishing House.

Author Biography

Rui Ferreira Afonso Rui Afonso is a practitioner and Yoga teacher. He studies scientifically the effects of Yoga practice in Brain Institute of Hospital Israelita Albert Einstein.

Chapter 13
Physical Exercise and Treatment of Addiction

Andrea Maculano Esteves, Paulo Daubian Rubini dos Santos Nosé and Marco Tulio de Mello

Physical Activity × Physical Exercise

The difference between physical activity (with no planning) and physical exercise (with planning) is well described in the literature. Physical activity regards any body movement produced by muscles, which results in higher energy expenditure. Physical exercise, on the other hand, is planned, structured, repetitive and purposeful physical exercise (Mcardle et al. 1988; Caspersen et al. 1985).

Therefore, we may refer to exercise in two ways: general effect exercise (GEE), which recruits over 1/7 to 1/6 of the body muscles, and local effect exercise (LEE), which recruits less than 1/7 to 1/6 of the body muscles. From this concept, we can classify GEE and LEE into aerobic and anaerobic. According to Barbanti (2011), aerobic exercise is a planned sequence of movements performed with energy from the aerobic metabolism, while resistance exercise (anaerobic) is a sequence of movements to which a resistance (load) is added as an additional demand to the muscle, aiming at increasing strength.

A.M. Esteves (✉) · P.D.R. dos Santos Nosé
Faculdade de Ciências Aplicadas, Curso de Ciências Do Esporte,
Universidade Estadual de Campinas, R. Pedro Zaccaria N.1300,
Jardim Santa Luiza, Limeira, SP 13484-350, Brazil
e-mail: andrea.esteves@fca.unicamp.br

M.T. de Mello
Escola de Educação Física, Universidade Federal de Minas Gerais,
Avenida Presidente Carlos Luz—de 3003/3004, Pampulha,
Belo Horizonte, MG 31310-250, Brazil
e-mail: tmello@demello.net.br

© Springer International Publishing Switzerland 2016
A.L.M. Andrade and D. De Micheli (eds.), *Innovations in the Treatment of Substance Addiction*, DOI 10.1007/978-3-319-43172-7_13

Importance of Physical Exercise

The benefits of physical exercise to health, quality of life, esthetics, performance, and rehabilitation are widely recognized. It also has several properties, among which we can highlight protection of the circulatory system, improvement of blood cholesterol levels, regulation of blood glucose, and increase in the response of the parasympathetic nervous system (not during exercise, but along the rest of the day), which reduces heart rate and blood pressure at rest, reduces inflammatory markers, and contributes to the prevention of and the fight against obesity (Tortora and Grabowski 2008).

Physical exercise acts in a multisystemic way, as follows:

1—Skeletal System;
2—Articular System;
3—Muscular System;
4—Circulatory System;
5—Respiratory System;
6—Immune System;
7—Nervous System.

Skeletal System

All of us are daily exposed to risks involving our bone health (such as stumbling on a footstep and falling, or a shock practicing some practicing some sports modality). According to Divasta and Gordon (2013), the bone is a dynamic tissue that responds to both internal stimuli and external environmental stimuli, including factors such as lifestyle during the course of life. The greatest proportion of bone health mediators is intrinsic, immutable factors that comprehend gender, ethnicity, and family history. Lifestyle and choices are among the few mutable factors that might lead to alterations in the structure or density of the bone. The bone connective tissue accounts for approximately 10 % of the body mass of young healthy individuals (Ahmed et al. 2005). Taken together, the bone mass and geometry determine the bone resistance, hence the resistance to fractures (Divasta and Gordon 2013).

Regular physical exercise is closely related to a wide range of health benefits that comprise improvement in bone inflammation, density, and metabolism (Marques et al. 2013). Women generally have a lower body mass as a result of hormonal differences between genders; therefore, physical exercise might play an important role in reducing the risk of osteoporosis (Bielemann et al. 2013). According to DiVasta and Gordon (2013), it is fundamental to characterize the types of physical activity associated with the most positive results, as well as make a longitudinal evaluation of the duration of those changes.

Articular System

Marchetti et al. (2007) define articulation as a set of elements through which two or more bones or cartilages are joined. They may be movable between each other or not. The synovial articulation has several key components that contribute to its general structure and function. The articular capsules, tendons, and ligaments of the synovial articulation are made of fibrous connective tissue, which provides stability and strength to the articulation (Ahmed et al. 2005).

Articular problems may arise throughout life; hence, we should prevent them for a better articular health and quality of life. Osteoarthritis (OA) is a common chronic disease that usually affects the articulations of the knees, hip, and hands (Bennell et al. 2014). According to the review of Hunter and Eckstein (2009), physical exercise plays a fundamental role in the pathogenesis and management of osteoarthritis.

Muscular System

The muscular system can be divided into three categories of muscles: cardiac, lean, and skeletal, each one with special characteristics and defined functions. Still according to Marchetti et al. (2007), muscles carry out a mechanic work and can be classified from two perspectives: dynamic (locomotion and movement of segments) and static (body posture and segmental support). Over 400 muscles comprise the human body, with the muscular tissue representing, on average, 30–50 % of the body mass (Ahmed et al. 2005; Marchetti et al. 2007; Tortora and Grabowski 2008). The skeletal muscle mass is largely dependent on the muscle protein synthesis (MPS), and the protein kinase, called the mammalian target of rapamycin (mTOR), is widely recognized as a key regulator in the muscular growth (Joy et al. 2014).

One of the properties of physical exercise is to enlarge the muscular functional state (enhancing intramuscular and intermuscular coordination), thus promoting hypertrophy (sarcoplasmatic and/or myofibrillar), and a number of other myopositive adaptations.

Circulatory System

As stated by Barbanti (2011), circulatory system is the system that transports necessary material into all the cells of an animal body and transports waste out of them. Physical exercise has proved beneficial to the heart as regards both GEE and LEE parameters.

High blood pressure is a severe public health issue the world over (Mobasseri et al. 2015). As reported by Rovere and Pinna (2014), regular physical activity is indicated to prevent or even improve disorders related to the age of the cardiac autonomic function. Physical training (with and without decreases in the sedentary time) improves VO_2 max, body composition, total body fat, and systolic blood (Keadle et al. 2014). Resistance exercise reduces blood glucose levels, restores the endothelial function, and reduces blood pressure (Mota et al. 2014), while aerobic exercise brings chronic benefits to cardiovascular complications (Mobasseri et al. 2015).

Respiratory System

Barbanti (2011) states that the respiratory system encompasses all the body components that contribute to the gas exchange between the external environment and the blood. Physiopathological determinants of respiratory dysfunction include obstruction of airways, lung hyperinflation, and undernourishment (Dassios 2015). Evidence also points to debilitated inhalation and exhalation functions (as a direct result of obesity), even in the absence of interstitial pulmonary disease (Arena and Cahalin 2014).

Adrianopoulos et al. (2014) suggest walking, resistance training, periodized exercise (nonlinear) and tai chi as effective alternatives for subgroups of patients with pulmonary disease.

Immune System

It is a complex system of interactions that protect the body from organisms that cause disease and other alien invaders, including humoral responses, mainly those that involve B cells and the production of antibodies, and the cell mediator responses, involving T cells and the activation of specific leukocytes (Barbanti 2011). It is known that infections, such as the flu and herpes zoster, are associated with the immunity of the human body and that individuals who have a substantial decrease in immune functions are more susceptible to infectious diseases (Rainbow et al. 2013).

Several studies in the literature associate physical exercise and immunological profile. Exercise entails a number of individual changes in the immune profile, varying according to the type, intensity, and duration of the activity during life course (Morro-García et al. 2014). Gholamnezhad et al. (2014) report that moderate exercise has a positive effect on the immunological function and the decrease in the susceptibility to viral infection.

Nervous System

The nervous system promotes the communication between the brain and the different parts of the body. Anatomically, it can be divided into central (encephalon and spinal cord) and peripheral (sensory and motor nerves). Functionally, it can be classified regarding its voluntary and involuntary control (Marchetti et al. 2007).

Physical exercise is a rational approach for the development of neuroprotective and neurorestorative treatments, increasing the production of mitochondrial energy, stimulating antioxidant defenses, reducing inflammations, and causing adaptations as angiogenesis and synaptogenesis (Zigmond and Smeyne 2014).

New evidence suggests that physical exercise can promote beneficial cortical adaptations. Plasticity of the motor cortex, for instance, is among the main objectives of rehabilitation programs to treat brain lesions, and much attention has been devoted to the ability of physical exercise to act as the first potential to changes of subsequent specific tasks in the cortical excitability associated with learning-based rehabilitation (Singh et al. 2014).

Physical exercise influences the dopaminergic, noradrenergic, and serotoninergic systems. In spite of the marked discrepancy among experimental protocols, results point to evidence in favor of alterations in the synthesis and metabolism of monoamines during physical exercise (Meeusen and De Meirleir 1985).

Evidence of Physical Exercise as an Adjuvant in the Treatment of Drug-Dependent Individuals

In addition to the benefits that physical exercise provides to mental and physical health, it also acts as a potential non-pharmacological treatment of dependence. Physical exercise acts in both phases of the dependence process (early and late), also entailing secondary health benefits, as the prevention of obesity and secondary diseases such as (Lynch et al. 2013).

Drugs of abuse, including psychostimulants, alcohol, nicotine, hallucinogenics, cannabinoids, and opiates, increase the level of dopamine in the *nucleus accumbens* (known as the reward pathway). Physical exercise acts by activating the same pathway of drugs of abuse through the increase in the concentrations of dopamine (Greenwood et al. 2011).

Therefore, keeping in mind that physical exercise is becoming more and more regarded as a potential treatment for dependence, and since it is a relatively easy practice to be implemented, and freely available, it is important to identify the conditions under which physical exercise produces beneficial effects and those that might lead to harmful effects (Lynch et al. 2013).

In this context, it is crucial to discuss the evidence for the efficacy of physical exercise in the different phases of the addiction process that includes first use, transition to dependence, withdrawal, and relapse.

Terry-Mc Elrath and O'Malley (2011) demonstrated that an increase in the adolescent participation in physical exercise programs predicts a decrease in the rates of tobacco, marijuana, and other illicit drugs use in adulthood (Terry-Mc Elrath and O'Malley 2011). In the same line, Korhonen et al. (2009) carried out a study with twins (who provide a better control of environmental factors) and showed that the most active twin as regards the practice of physical activity presented a lower risk of smoking and using illicit drugs in adult life compared to the less active twin (Korhonen et al. 2009).

However, not all researches show this negative association between the level of physical activity and the use of alcohol and drugs, reporting a variation according to gender and the type of exercise individuals practice (Martinsen and Sundgot-Borgen 2014; Peretti-Watel et al. 2003).

Those findings show that the kind of exercise and/or psychosocial interactions associated with certain sports/exercise modalities may also influence the onset of drug use. Participation in teams can also have an influence, since the levels of physical activity may vary enormously among sports and individuals (Lynch et al. 2013). Kulig et al. (2003) showed, in a sample of 15.349 American high school students, that almost one fourth of the individuals who participated in team sports were not vigorously more active, suggesting that participation in that type of sport may not be a useful measure of the level of physical activity or exercise (Kulig et al. 2003).

Barbosa Filho et al. (2012), in a recent review on the use of alcohol and tobacco among Brazilian adolescents, showed that the use of alcohol ranged from 23.0 to 67.7 %, with a mean prevalence of 34.9 %. The use of tobacco ranged from 2.4 to 22.0 %, mean prevalence of 9.3 %. They also showed that the Brazilian literature has highlighted environmental factors (religiosity, working conditions, and the use of substance among family members and friends) and psychosocial factors (conflict with parents, negative feelings, and loneliness) in association with the use of alcohol and tobacco among adolescents.

Neurobiological Basis for the Efficacy of Physical Exercise on Dependence

Exercise may work as an alternative of reward that competes with the drug and reduces the odds of it being used. This process takes place due to the effects of physical exercise on the signaling of the dopaminergic reward pathway, given the fundamental role dopamine plays in this phase of the dependence process.

Sutoo and Akiyama (1996) identified the ability of physical exercise to work as a reward factor due to the similarity of the process in the dopaminergic pathway. They observed that rats which performed forced running increased the transport of calcium to the brain, which in turn increased the synthesis of dopamine by means of a calmodulin-dependent system (Sutoo and Akiyama 1996).

Chronic exercise can also lead to a positive regulation of the dopamine D1 receptor, another marker of vulnerability to dependence (Lynch et al. 2007; Worsley et al. 2000; Zhang et al. 2006). These results are important as they suggest even though moderate levels of physical exercise produce alterations in the reward pathway that can initially protect against the use of drugs, later on the high levels of chronic physical exercise, as in chronic exposure to drugs of abuse, might sensitize the reward pathway. This idea is supported by studies which show that unlimited access to a running wheel increases the subsequent vulnerability to the acquisition of methamphetamine by self-administration and to the development of preference to an environment associated with the drug (Eisenstein and Holmes 2007; Mustroph et al. 2011; Smith et al. 2008; Engelmann et al. 2013). In humans, evidence indicates that excessive physical exercise produces many of the same behavioral changes, as well as neurochemical alterations in the brain, as the ones observed in the chronic exposure to drugs of abuse (Berczik et al. 2012).

The neurobiological basis for the efficacy of physical exercise during drug withdrawal is guided by the importance of exercise in normalizing the hypofunctioning of the mesolimbic system that happens after chronic exposure to drugs. This idea is reinforced by recent discoveries that show its efficacy in normalizing the global neuronal activity in the reward pathway. The withdrawal from chronic exposure to ethanol, for instance, is associated with the positive regulation of the excitatory glutamatergic neurotransmission (Bauer et al. 2013), since physical exercise normalizes high levels of glutamate. However, although the withdrawal from other drugs of abuse, including psychostimulants and opioids, is also associated with a positive regulation of the glutamatergic signaling, those effects are usually observed after prolonged withdrawal, (Fischer-Smith et al. 2012), as opposed to what happens in the initial withdrawal periods (Baker et al. 2003; Ben-Shahar et al. 2012). Consequently, physical exercise might produce different effects during the early versus the late withdrawal of psychostimulants and opioids. In this context, these results suggest that physical exercise might potentially serve as an intervention during withdrawal due to its capacity of upregulation of the dopaminergic signaling and normalization of the glutamatergic signaling (perhaps particularly in the case of alcohol) (Lynch et al. 2013).

Physical exercise has also been proposed as a treatment that might reduce the risk of relapse by reducing craving.

In a systematized review of 14 studies, Taylor et al. (2007) demonstrated that one single session of physical exercise may be recommended as an aid to smoking cessation, as it regulates craving, withdrawal syndrome and negative effects, as well as the necessity to drink alcohol patients in detoxification phase have (Ussher et al. 2004). Longer periods of physical exercise lead to the reduction in the level of craving among *cannabis*-dependent individuals (Buchowski et al. 2011). Similarly, physical exercise enhances the results of treatment among alcohol and illicit drug-dependent individuals when used as a complement to interventions. Brown et al. (2010) evaluated the viability of aerobic physical exercise as a complement in the treatment for substance abuse among drug-dependent patients. The patients in the study participated in a 12-week program of aerobic exercise of moderate intensity and achieved a significant increase in the abstinent days both from alcohol and drugs by the end of treatment. Those who attended at least 75 % of the physical exercise sessions obtained significantly better results than those who did not. Moreover, the participants showed a significant improvement in their cardiorespiratory capacity until the end of treatment.

Barbanti (2006) investigated changes in the quality of life of 141 substance-dependent (SD) (e.g., Alcohol, Tobacco, Drugs,) and depressive patients (DP) who participated in programs of physical exercise. The alterations in their quality of life were measured by the SF-36 questionnaire of quality of life. The results showed improvement in the quality of life after two and four months in those individuals who performed physical exercises.

A review carried out by Ferreira et al. (2001) indicated activities and intensity of performance for individuals in recovery from the use of psychotropic substances, presented in Table 13.1.

Finally, it is crucial to keep in mind that the effects of physical exercise depend on the underlying neurobiology that varies according to the phase of the dependence process; the age and gender of the individual; and the type of drug and the type of physical exercise (Volkow et al. 2011). Specifically, it is proposed that physical exercise during the beginning of drug use has the capacity to facilitate the

Table 13.1 Indication of activities and intensity of performance for individuals in recovery from the use of psychotropic substances

Activity	Intensity	Duration	Justification
Running	Initial: 60 % VO_2 max Progression up to 90 % VO_2 max	30 min (3 times/week)	↑ DA motor circuit (↓ progressive after 20′); ↑NA (during: ↓sympathetic activity, afterward: ↓↓); ↑5-HT and β-endorphin (improved mood) Upregulation of D1; downregulation of D2 and β;
Swimming	Initial: 60 % VO_2 max Progression up to 90 % VO_2 max	40 min (3 times/week)	Practically the same adaptations in running General conditioning
Body building	Initial: R.M.L. Resistance and strength training	90 min (2 times/week)	Muscle resistance and strength, lower myocardial demand for the effort
Dance	Moderate	90 min (2 times/week)	Socialization, improvement of motor coordination, and attention
Basketball	Moderate	60 min (2 times/week)	Motor coordination, socialization, and general conditioning
Stretching	Moderate	30 min	Stretching, flexibility, and relaxation

Ferreira et al. (2001)

dopaminergic neurotransmission, which in turn may stop the drug use, serving as an alternative reinforcement. Additionally, it produces persistent adaptations in the dopaminergic signaling, and such effects may alter the vulnerability of an individual to a subsequent substance use. Moderate levels of physical exercise can also be understood as a protective factor. Intense levels, on the other hand, might mimic the effects of drug abuse and hence increase vulnerability.

References

Adrianopoulos, V., Klijn, P., Franssen, F. M. E., & Spruit, M. A. (2014). Exercise training in pulmonary rehabilitation. *Clinics in Chest Medicine, 35*, 313–322.

Ahmed, M. S., Matsumura, B., & Cristian, A. (2005). Age-related changes in muscles and joints. *Physical Medicine and Rehabilitation Clinics of North America, 16*, 19–39.

Arena, R., & Cahalin, L. P. (2014). Evaluation of cardiorespiratory fitness and respiratory muscle function in the obese population. *Progress in Cardiovascular Diseases, 56*, 457–464.

Baker, D. A., McFarland, K., Lake, R. W., Shen, H., Tang, X. C., Toda, S., et al. (2003). Neuroadaptations in cystine-glutamate exchange underlie cocaine relapse. *Nature Neuroscience, 6*, 743–749.

Barbanti, E. J. (2006). Efeito da atividade física na qualidade de vida Em pacientes com depressão e dependência química. *Revista Brasileira de Atividade Física & Saúde, 11*, 37–45.

Barbanti, V. (2011). *Dicionário de Educação Física e Esporte* (3rd ed.). Barueri: Editora Manole.

Barbosa Filho, V. C., Campos, W., & Lopes, A. S. (2012). Prevalence of alcohol and tobacco use among Brazilian adolescents: A systematic review. *Rev Saúde Pública, 46*, 901–917.

Bauer, J., Pedersen, A., Scherbaum, N., Bening, J., Patschke, J., Kugel, H., et al. (2013). Craving in alcohol-dependent patients after detoxification is related to glutamatergic dysfunction in the nucleus accumbens and the anterior cingulate cortex. *Neuropsychopharmacology, 38*, 1401–1408.

Bennell, K. L., Dobson, F., & Hinman, R. S. (2014). Exercise in osteoarthritis: Moving from prescription to adherence. *Best Practice & Research Clinical Rheumatology, 28*, 93–117.

Ben-Shahar, O. M., Szumlinski, K. K., Lominac, K. D., Cohen, A., Gordon, E., Ploense, K. L., et al. (2012). Extended access to cocaine self-administration results in reduced glutamate function within the medial prefrontal cortex. *Addiction Biology, 4*, 746–757.

Berczik, K., Szabo, A., Griffiths, M. D., Kurimay, T., Kun, B., Urban, R., et al. (2012). Exercise addiction: symptoms, diagnosis, epidemiology, and etiology. *Substance Use and Misuse, 47*, 403–417.

Bielemann, R.M., Martinez-Mesa, J., & Gigante, D.P. (2013). Physical activity during life course and bone mass: a systematic review of methods and findings from cohort studies with young adults, vol. 14, p 77. http://www.biomedcentral.com

Brown, R. A., Abrantes, A. M., Read, J. P., Marcus, B. H., Jakicic, J., Strong, D. R., et al. (2010). A pilot study of aerobic exercise as an adjunctive treatment for drug dependence. *Mental Health and Physical Activity, 3*, 27–34.

Buchowski, M. S., Meade, N. N., Charboneau, E., Park, S., Dietrich, M. S., Cowan, R. L., & Martin, P. R. (2011). Aerobic exercise training reduces cannabis craving and use in non-treatment seeking cannabis-dependent adults. *PLoS One, 6*(3), e17465.

Caspersen, C. J., Powell, K. E., & Christenson, G. M. (1985). Physical activity, exercise and physical fitness: Definition and distinctions for health related research. *Public Health Reports, 100*, 126–131.

Dassios, T. (2015). Determinants of respiratory pump function in patients with cystic fibrosis. *Paediatric Respiratory Reviews, 16*(1), 75–79.

Divasta, A. D., & Gordon, C. M. (2013). Exercise and bone: Where do we stand? *Metabolism, Clinical and Experimental, 62*, 1714–1717.

Eisenstein, S. A., & Holmes, P. V. (2007). Chronic and voluntary exercise enhances learning of conditioned place preference to morphine in rats. *Pharmacology, Biochemistry and Behavior, 86*, 607–615.

Engelmann, A. J., Aparicio, M. B., Kim, A., Sobieraj, J. C., Yuan, C. J., Grant, Y., et al. (2013). Chronic wheel running reduces maladaptive patterns of methamphetamine intake: Regulation by attenuation of methamphetamine-induced neuronal nitric oxide synthase. *Brain Structure and Function, 219*, 657–672.

Ferreira, S. E., Tufik, S., & de Mello, M. T. (2001). Neuroadaptação: uma proposta alternativa de atividade física para usuários de drogas em recuperação. *Revista Brasileira de Ciência e Movimento, 9*, 31–39.

Fischer-Smith, K. D., Houston, A. C., & Rebec, G. V. (2012). Differential effects of cocaine access and withdrawal on glutamate type 1 transporter expression in rat nucleus accumbens core and shell. *Neuroscience, 210*, 333–339.

Gholamnezhad, Z., Boskabady, M. H., Hosseini, M., Sankian, M., & Rad, A. K. (2014). Evaluation of immune response after moderate and overtraining exercise in wistar rat. *Iranian Journal of Basic Medical Sciences, 17*, 1–8.

Greenwood, B. N., Foley, T. E., Le, T. V., Strong, P. V., Loughridge, A. B., Day, H. E., & Fleshner, M. (2011). Long-term voluntary wheel running is rewarding and produces plasticity in the mesolimbic reward pathway. *Behavioural Brain Research, 217*(2), 354–362.

Hunter, D. J., & Eckstein, F. (2009). Exercise and osteoarthritis. *Journal of Anatomy, 214*, 197–207.

Joy, J. M., Gundermann, D. M., Lowery, R. P., Jäger, R., Mccleary, S. A., Purpura, M., et al. (2014). Phosphatidic acid enhances mTOR signaling and resistance exercise, induced hypertrophy. *Nutrition & Metabolism, 11*, 29.

Keadle, S. K., Lyden, K., Staudenmayer, J., Hickey, A., Viskochil, R., Braun, B., et al. (2014). The independent and combined effects of exercise training and reducing sedentary behavior on cardiometabolic risk factors. *Applied Physiology, Nutrition and Metabolism, 39*, 770–780.

Korhonen, T., Kujala, U. M., Rose, R. J., & Kaprio, J. (2009). Physical activity in adolescence as a predictor of alcohol and illicit drug use in early adulthood: A longitudinal population-based twin study. *Twin Research and Human Genetics, 12*, 261–268.

Kulig, K., Brener, N. D., & McManus, T. (2003). Sexual activity and substance use among adolescents by category of physical activity plus team sports participation. *Archives of Pediatrics and Adolescent Medicine, 157*, 905–912.

Lynch, W. J., Kiraly, D. D., Caldarone, B. J., Picciotto, M. R., & Taylor, J. R. (2007). Effect of cocaine self-administration on striatal PKA-regulated signaling in male and female rats. *Psychopharmacology (Berlin), 191*(2), 263–271.

Lynch, W. J., Peterson, A. B., Sanchez, V., Abel, J., & Smith, M. A. (2013). Exercise as novel treatment for drug addiction: A neurobiological and stage-dependent hypothesis. *Neuroscience and Biobehavioral Reviews, 37*, 1622–1644.

Marchetti, P., Calheiros, R., & Charro, M. (2007). *Biomecânica Aplicada: Uma Abordagem para o Treinamento de Força*. São Paulo: Editora Phorte.

Marques, E. A., Mota, J., Viana, J. L., Tuna, D., Figueiredo, P., Guimarães, J. T., et al. (2013). Response of bone mineral density, inflammatory cytokines, and biochemical bone markers to a 32-week combined loading exercise programme in older men and women. *Archives of Gerontology and Geriatrics, 57*, 226–233.

Martinsen, M., & Sundgot-Borgen, J. (2014). Adolescent elite athletes' cigarette smoking, use of snus, and alcohol. *Scandinavian Journal of Medicine and Science in Sports, 24*, 439–446.

Mcardle, W. D., Katch, F. I., & Katch, V. L. (1988). *Fisiologia do Exercício: Energia, Nutrição e Desempenho Humano* (4th ed.). Rio de Janeiro: Editora Guanabara Koogan.

Meeusen, R., & De Meirleir, K. (1985). Exercise and brain neurotransmission. *Sports Medicine (Auckland, N. Z.), 20*, 160–188.

Mobasseri, M., Iavari, A., Najafipoor, F., Aliasgarzadeh, A., & Niafar, M. (2015). The effect of a long-term regular physical activity with hypertension and body mass index in type 2 diabetes patients. *The Journal of Sports Medicine and Physical Fitness, 55*(1–2), 84–90.

Morro-García, M. A., Fernandez-García, B., Echeverría, A., Rodríguez-Alonso, M., Suárez-García, F. M., Solano-Jaurrieta, J. J., et al. (2014). Frequent participation in high volume exercise throughout life is associated with a more differentiated adaptive immune response. *Brain, Behavior, and Immunity, 39*, 61–74.

Mota, M. M., Silva, T. L. T. B., Fontes, M. T., Barreto, A. S., Araújo, J. E. S., Oliveira, A. C. C., et al. (2014). Resistance exercise restores endothelial function and reduces blood pressure in type 1 diabetic rats. *Arquivos Brasileiros de Cardiologia, 103*, 25–32.

Mustroph, M. L., Stobaugh, D. J., Miller, D. S., DeYoung, E. K., & Rhodes, J. S. (2011). Wheel running can accelerate or delay extinction of conditioned place preference for cocaine in male C57BL/6 J mice, depending on timing of wheel access. *European Journal of Neuroscience, 34*, 1161–1169.

Peretti-Watel, P., Guagliardo, V., Verger, P., Pruvost, J., Mignon, P., & Obadia, Y. (2003). Sporting activity and drug use: Alcohol, cigarette and cannabis use among elite student athletes. *Addiction, 98*, 1249–1256.

Rainbow, T. H., Wang, C. W., Siu-Man, N. G., Andy, H. Y., Ziea, E. T. C., Wong, V. T., et al. (2013). The effect of T'ai chi exercise on immunity and infections: A systematic review of controlled trials. *The Journal of Alternative and Complementary Medicine, 5*, 389–396.

Rovere, M. T. L., & Pinna, G. D. (2014). Beneficial effects of physical activity on baroreflex control in the elderly. *Annals of Noninvasive Electrocardiology, 19*, 303–310.

Singh, A. M., Duncan, R. E., Neva, J. L., & Staines, W. R. (2014). Aerobic exercise modulates intracortical inhibition and facilitation in a nonexercised upper limb muscle. *BMC Sports Science, Medicine, and Rehabilitation, 6*, 23.

Smith, M. A., Schmidt, K. T., Iordanou, J. C., & Mustroph, M. L. (2008). Aerobic exercise decreases the positive-reinforcing effects of cocaine. *Drug and Alcohol Dependence, 98*, 129–135.

Sutoo, D., & Akiyama, K. (1996). The mechanism by which exercise modifies brain function. *Physiology & Behavior, 60*, 177–181.

Taylor, A. H., Ussher, M. H., & Faulkner, G. (2007). The acute effects of exercise on cigarette cravings, withdrawal symptoms, affect and smoking behaviour: A systematic review. *Addiction, 102*, 534–543.

Terry-Mc Elrath, Y. M., & O'Malley, P. M. (2011). Substance use and exercise participation among young adults: Parallel trajectories in a national cohort-sequential study. *Addiction, 106*, 1855–1865.

Tortora, G. J., & Grabowski, S. R. (2008). *Corpo humano: Fundamentos de Anatomia e Fisiologia* (6th ed.). Porto Alegre: Artmed.

Ussher, M., Sampuran, A. K., Doshi, R., West, R., & Drummond, D. C. (2004). Acute effect of a brief bout of exercise on alcohol urges. *Addiction, 99*, 1542–1547.

Volkow, N. D., Wang, G. J., Fowler, J. S., Tomasi, D., & Telang, F. (2011). Addiction: Beyond dopamine reward circuitry. *Proceedings of the National Academy of Sciences of the United States of America, 108*, 15037–15042.

Worsley, J. N., Moszczynska, A., Falardeau, P., Kalasinsky, K. S., Schmunk, G., Guttman, M., et al. (2000). Dopamine D1 receptor protein is elevated in nucleus accumbens of human, chronic methamphetamine users. *Molecular Psychiatry, 5*, 664–672.

Zhang, Y., Svenningsson, P., Picetti, R., Schlussman, S. D., Nairn, A. C., Ho, A., et al. (2006). Cocaine self-administration in mice is inversely related to phosphorylation at Thr34 (protein kinase A site) and Ser130 (kinase CK1 site) of DARPP-32. *Journal of Neuroscience, 26*, 2645–2651.

Zigmond, M. J., & Smeyne, R. J. (2014). Exercise: Is it a neuroprotective and if so, how does it work?. *Parkinsonism and Related Disorders, 20S1*, 123–127.

Chapter 14
Neurofeedback and Substance Abuse Disorder

Fateme Dehghani-Arani

What Is Neurofeedback

A person's different mental states are under the control of the brainwaves which occur at various frequencies and can be measured in cycles per second or hertz (Hz) by electroencephalography (EEG) techniques (Hammond 2011). These EEG bands are delta, theta, alpha, beta, and gamma. Gamma is a very fast EEG activity above 30 Hz. This activity is associated with intensely focused attention and in assisting the brain to process and bind together information from different areas of the brain. Beta is small, relatively fast brainwave (above 13–30 Hz) associated with a state of mental, intellectual activity and outwardly focused concentration. This is basically a "bright-eyed, bushy-tailed" state of alertness. Activity in the lower end of this frequency band (e.g., the sensorimotor rhythm or SMR) is associated with relaxed attentiveness. Alpha brainwave is slower and larger (8–12 Hz). It is generally associated with a state of relaxation. Activity in the lower half of this range represents to a considerable degree the brain shifting into an idling gear, relaxed and a bit disengaged, waiting to respond when needed. In closed eyes state and picturing something peaceful, alpha brainwaves start to increase. This is especially large in the back third of the head. Theta (4–8 Hz) activity generally represents a daydream-like and spacey state of mind that is associated with mental inefficiency. At very slow levels, theta brainwave activity is a very relaxed state, representing the twilight zone between waking and sleep. Delta is very slow, high-amplitude (0.5–3.5 Hz) brainwave that occur when areas of the brain go "off-line" to take up nourishment or in deep sleep, drowsy (with slower theta) or inattentive and wandering (with more theta) state. Delta is also associated with learning disabilities.

F. Dehghani-Arani (✉)
Department of Psychology, University of Tehran, Dr Kardan Street, Nasr Bridge, Jalal al Ahmad Street, Chamran Highway, Tehran 1445983861, Iran
e-mail: f.dehghani.a@ut.ac.ir

© Springer International Publishing Switzerland 2016
A.L.M. Andrade and D. De Micheli (eds.), *Innovations in the Treatment of Substance Addiction*, DOI 10.1007/978-3-319-43172-7_14

Generally, there is homogeneity in the EEG patterns and different diagnostic conditions. For instance, in exceptionally anxious and tense states, an excessively high frequency of beta brainwaves may be present in different parts of the brain, but this may be associated with an excess of inefficient alpha activity in frontal areas that are associated with emotional control. Persons with attention-deficit/hyperactivity disorder (AD/HD), head injuries, stroke, epilepsy, developmental disabilities, and often chronic fatigue syndrome and fibromyalgia tend to have excessive slow waves (usually theta and sometimes excess alpha) present. When an excessive amount of slow waves are present in the frontal parts of the brain, it becomes difficult to control attention, behavior, and emotions. Such persons generally have problems with concentration, memory, controlling their impulses and moods, or hyperactivity. They have problems with focusing and exhibiting diminished intellectual efficiency.

In the late 1970s, studies have shown that it is possible to recondition and retrain brainwave patterns and it may be possible to train individuals to control localized brain activation using real-time neuroimaging feedback (Johnson et al. 2012; Kamiya 2011; Sterman et al. 2010). These works began with training to increase the alpha brainwave activity for the purpose of increasing relaxation, whereas other work originating at University of California, Los Angeles, focused first on animal and then human research on assisting uncontrolled epilepsy. This brainwave training is called EEG biofeedback or neurofeedback (NFB). NFB is an operant conditioning technique that trains brainwaves to act in a more optimal way in order to improve the emotional, cognitive, behavioral, and physical experiences. It can be used to turn abnormal brainwaves' rhythms and frequencies into relatively normal rhythms and frequencies and subsequently turn abnormal psychological states into normal ones (Scott et al. 2005; Simkin et al. 2014).

During a NFB session, one or more electrodes are placed on the scalp and one or two are usually put on the earlobes. Then, high-tech electronic equipment provides real-time, instantaneous feedback (usually auditory and visual) about brainwave activity. The electrodes allow us to measure the electrical patterns coming from the brain—like a physician listens to the heart from the surface of the skin. No electrical current is put into the brain. The brain's electrical activity is relayed to the computer and then recorded. Ordinarily, people cannot reliably influence their brainwave patterns because they lack awareness of them. However, when they can see their brainwaves on a computer screen, it gives them the ability to influence and gradually change them. The mechanism of action is generally considered to be operant conditioning that is literally reconditioning and retraining the brain. With continuing feedback, coaching, and practice, healthier brainwave patterns can usually be retrained. The process is a little like exercising or doing physical therapy with the brain, enhancing cognitive flexibility and control. To facilitate peak performance in normal individuals and improve different symptoms such as ADHD, learning disability, stroke, head injury, deficits following neurosurgery, uncontrolled epilepsy, cognitive dysfunction associated with aging, depression, anxiety, obsessive–compulsive disorder, and autism, NFB offers additional opportunities for rehabilitation through directly retraining the electrical activity patterns in the brain.

Scientific Evidences of Neurofeedback

NFB studies have documented findings about cognitive and memory enhancement in normal individuals (Boulay et al. 2011; Keizer et al. 2010; Zoefel et al. 2010). In clinical fields, ADHD is the first and most cited disorder which has been studied in NFB researches. Most of the studies in this field demonstrated that NFB produced comparable improvements to Ritalin (Rossiter 2005). As the first randomized controlled study, Levesque et al. (2006) documented the positive changes in brain function and behavioral changes in ADHD children following NFB treatment. Also, Leins et al. (2007)'s and Gevensleben et al. (2009)'s randomized controlled studies and deBeus and Kaiser (2011)'s and Lansbergen et al. (2011)'s double-blind placebo-controlled studies have documented the effectiveness of NFB with ADHD. About lasting the NFB outcomes, Lubar (1995) published 10-year follow-ups on cases and found that in about 80 % of clients, NFB can substantially improve the symptoms of ADD and ADHD and that these changes are maintained. Also, behavior and attention improvements were found to be stable on 6-month follow-up in research studies reported by Strehl et al. (2006) and Gevensleben et al. (2010). A 2-year follow-up (Gani et al. 2008) research found that not only were improvements in attention and behavior stable but also that some parent ratings had shown continued improvement during the 2 years. These follow-up evaluations provide strong support that improvements from NFB with ADHD should be enduring.

With regard to learning disabilities, placebo-controlled studies (Breteler et al. 2010; Walker 2010a) and follow-up (Becerra et al. 2006) demonstrated that NFB could be an effective treatment and the improvements were sustained. In epilepsy, studies found that NFB on average produces a 70 % of reduction (Hammond 2011) with the average length of 4–6 seizure-free years in the follow-ups (Walker 2010b). NFB has been used as a therapeutic method to cure other types of disorders such as depression (Choi et al. 2011), anxiety disorders (Kleber et al. 2008), fibromyalgia (Muller et al. 2001), obsessive–compulsive disorder (Surmeli et al. 2011), autism and Asperger's syndrome (Knezevic et al. 2010), insomnia (Cortoos et al. 2010; Hammer et al. 2011), tinnitus (Crocetti et al. 2011), pain (Ibric and Dragomirescu 2009), and headaches and migraine (Stokes and Lappin 2010; Walker 2011). About TBI and stroke further high-quality research on NFB needs to be done (Hammond 2011).

Main Findings in Substance Abuse Disorder

Neuropsychophysiological abnormalities in substance abuse disorder (SAD) underline the need for complementary therapeutic methods for this disorder, which contain long-lasting effects and minimal side effects (Trudeau et al. 2009; Unterrainer et al. 2014). NFB appears to be one of these promising complementary therapeutic methods. The first NFB protocol employed in SAD was alpha training by Passini et al. (1977), who showed the effects of alpha NFB training in reducing anxiety and improvement in the personality measuring scales in SAD patients. Goldberg et al. (1976) also pointed out that the alpha conditioning program reduced drug use and increased self-control in 4 addicted patients. Afterward, the NFB method has been used as a therapeutic method for SAD and as the literature reported its use has been associated with reformed negative neuropsychological consequences of substance abuse, reduced drug-seeking symptoms, improved psychological and neurophysiological variables, and longer abstinence (Burkett et al. 2005; Dehghani-Arani et al. 2010, 2013; Kaiser et al. 1999; Peniston and Kulkosky 1989; Peniston and Saxby 1995; Rostami and Dehghani-Arani 2015; Sokhadze et al. 2008; Unterrainer et al. 2014). Alpha–theta protocol is the most important NFB program which has been commonly emphasized in all these studies. It has become known as Peniston protocol, as has been specified for SAD treatment by Eugene Peniston (Peniston and Kulkosky 1989).

The Peniston Protocol (Alpha-Theta Feedback)

Alpha–theta NFB was first described by Elmer Green and colleagues (Green et al. 1974) based on Green's observations of EEG single during meditative states. He noticed that when the feedback of alpha and theta signal was applied to subjects, states of profound relaxation occurred. The method could be seen as a use of brainwave signal feedback to enable a subject to maintain a state of consciousness similar to a psychotherapy insight in a meditative or hypnotic relaxed state. The first reported use of alpha–theta feedback in SAD was in an integrated program started in 1973 at Topeka. It included group and individual therapies in which daily 20-min NFB sessions (integrated with EMG biofeedback and temperature control biofeedback) were done over 6 weeks. Patients discussed their insights and experiences associated with NFB in group therapy sessions (Goslinga 1975; Twemlow and Bowen 1976, 1977). These initial studies showed the utility of alpha–theta NFB protocol in promoting insight and attitude change in alcoholics, with the assumptions that these changes are associated with heightened awareness and suggestibility, and that this heightened awareness and suggestibility would enhance recovery. But in these studies, outcome data regarding abstinence were not reported (Trudeau et al. 2009).

Thereafter, the first reported randomized and controlled study of addictive disorders by NFB was popularized by the work of Peniston (Peniston and Kulkosky 1989) in which Peniston introduced two additions to last studies protocols: temperature training and script. In this study, 10 alcoholic patients underwent approximately 15 occipital alpha–theta brainwave training sessions. They showed significant positive changes in brainwave activity and depression in comparison with the control group. In a further report on the same control and experimental subjects, Peniston and Kulkosky (1990) described significant changes in personality test (the Millon clinical multi-axial and 16-PF personality inventories) results in the experimental group as compared to the controls. Also, 80 % of them remained generally abstinent at least 3 years after NFB treatment.

Fahrion, Walters, Coyne, and Allen repeated these results in 1992 in a controlled case study. The same results were achieved in studies conducted by Bodehnamer and Callaway (2004) and Burkett et al. (2005) on crack cocaine abusers. They found that the addition of Peniston alpha/theta protocol to crack cocaine treatment regimens may promise to be an effective intervention for treating crack cocaine abuse and increasing treatment retention. In another study by Raymond et al. (2005), subjects who received alpha–theta training showed significant improvement in mood and Minnesota multiphase personality inventory-2 (MMPI-2) scores. Follow-up studies also reported consistent treatment outcomes in alcohol- or drug-addicted clients who completed an alpha/theta NFB protocol (Callaway and Bodenhamer-Davis 2008; Kelley 1997; Trudeau 2009). Trudeau (2005a, b) showed the same results on the effectiveness of NFB in adolescents with SAD.

In Peniston protocol, patients first employed autogenic phrases and were taught deep relaxation during five sessions of temperature feedback. They then are instructed in NFB and, in an eyes-closed and relaxed condition, receive auditory signals from EEG apparatus which receive brainwave signals from an electrode in left occipital site of the scalp (O1). At the same time, a standard induction script with suggestions to relax and "sink down" is read for the patient (Sokhadze et al. 2007; White and Richards 2009). Here is an example of such a script modified after Peniston that was used in the NFB lab at Minneapolis VA:

> With your eyes closed—allow yourself to relax completely—as you listen to the tones—tell your brain to make more alpha waves—allow yourself to sink down into a mentally alert and relaxed state—imagine what your brain looks like—imagine the subconscious part of your brain—tell the subconscious part of your brain to guide you—see yourself in a drug/alcohol using situation with the people you have used with—see yourself being offered drugs/alcohol—see yourself rejecting drugs and alcohol by getting up and saying "no thanks" and leaving the situation and your using friends behind—ask your subconscious brain to mellow out your personality—sink down into a reverie state letting your thoughts flow—completely relaxed—do it (Trudeau et al. 2009).

When alpha (8–12 Hz) brainwaves exceed a preset threshold, a pleasant tone is heard. By learning to voluntarily produce this tone, the subject becomes progressively relaxed. When theta brainwaves (4–8 Hz) are produced at high amplitude, a second tone is heard and the subject becomes more relaxed. It can enter a hypnagogic state of free reverie and high suggestibility. Following the session, with the patient in a relaxed and suggestible state, a therapy session is conducted between patients and therapist where the contents of the imagery experienced are explored (Saxby and Peniston 1995). According to this instruction, White (2008) believed that the power of the Peniston's alpha–theta protocol is based on what is carried within it: a combination of the procedure, the therapist's empathic involvement, the intention toward a positive and healthy outcome, and an ambiance of safety and support. She mentioned that the core element of the effectiveness of the Peniston protocol is the alteration of unconscious process (both the clearing of early trauma effects and dropping in a new program of behavior) which leads to profound changes in attitude and behavior. These outcomes frequently reduce to eliminate the patient's need to medicate by means of a substance. It seems to represent a technology which contains elements of the five senses and designed for the induction of higher states of consciousness and insight, helping to alter ones relationship to self and the world as the result of what is seen and understood in the higher states.

The technique involves the simultaneous measurement of occipital alpha (8–13 Hz) and theta (4–8 Hz), and feedback by separate auditory tones for each frequency representing amplitudes greater than the preset thresholds. The participant is encouraged to relax and increase the amount of time that signal is heard. It would increase the amount of time that amplitude of each defined bandwidth exceeds the threshold (Trudeau et al. 2009).

The Scott–Kaiser Modification of the Peniston Protocol

In 2005, Scott et al. extended the Pension's traditional alpha–theta NFB protocol to treat patients with mixed SAD, rich in stimulant abusers. Chronic EEG abnormalities and high incidence of preexisting ADHD in stimulant abusers suggest that they may be less able to engage in the hypnagogic and autosuggestive Peniston protocol. Furthermore, eyes-closed alpha feedback as a starting protocol may be deleterious in stimulant abusers because their most common QEEG abnormality is excess frontal alpha (Scott et al. 2005; Simkin et al. 2014; Trudeau et al. 2009). According to this explanation, in Scott et al. (2005) study, patients who had abused stimulants were treated using attention-deficit-type NFB protocols (beta and/or SMR augmentation with theta suppression), followed by the Peniston protocol. The beta and/or SMR protocol used to normalize attention, and then, the standard Peniston protocol without temperature training applied. This treatment approach is now widely known as the Scott–Kaiser modifications of the Peniston protocol (Sokhadze et al. 2008). In their study, Scott et al. (2005) found that this protocol doubled the recovery rate for drug dependence. They documented the significant improvements in psychological functioning and the ability of the experimental group to focus their thoughts and to process information. In addition, findings revealed substantial improvement in long-term abstinence rates in these patients. After only 45 days of treatment, almost one-third of the control group had dropped out of treatment residential facility compared with only 6 % of the experimental group.

The Scott–Kaiser modification of the Peniston protocol is dedicated for a population of subjects with a history of stimulant abuse. Based on this protocol, the NFB training protocols in the first 10 sessions were bipolar sensory motor rhythm (SMR) training protocols in the C_4 (the central brain cortex) and Pz (the central parietal cortex) areas, and bipolar beta training protocols in the C_3 (the left central cortex) and FPz (the central fronto-parietal cortex) areas, with each protocol lasting 25 min. After these beginning sessions, we decreased the time of SMR and beta training protocols and added 20 min of monopolar alpha/theta training protocols in the Pz (the central parietal brain cortex) area and continued to increase the time of this protocol until the final sessions. All these protocols were performed using the Thought Technology ProComp 2 system, a single-subject EEG used for self-training, research, and for working with others. The Thought Technology ProComp 2 system displayed the brain's electrical activity (via electrodes placed on the patient's scalp) on a monitor in the form of an audio/visual exercise. The feedback informed the patients of his success in making changes. The training was introduced as a computer game in which patients could score points using their brain. Subjects were advised to be attentive to the feedback and to find the most successful mental strategy to get as many points as possible; they received no other specific instructions.

In the SMR and beta training protocols, the feedback was audio/visual. Active electrodes were placed at the C_4 and C_3 areas and referenced with the Pz and FPz areas. A ground electrode was placed on the left ear. In this program, the reinforcement band was composed of SMR (12–15 Hz) and beta (15–18 Hz) frequency bands in each protocol, and the suppressed bands were delta (2–5 Hz), theta (5–8 Hz), and high beta (18–30 Hz) frequency bands in both protocols. Thresholds were adjusted such that when subjects maintained the reinforcement band above the threshold for 80 % of the time during at least 0.5 s, and the suppressed band below the threshold for 20 % of the time, the feedback was received. When the subjects were able to maintain the reinforcement band above the threshold for 90 % of the time during two continuous trials, the threshold was changed automatically so that it was closer to the optimal threshold (Scott et al. 2005).

Feedback in the alpha/theta training protocol on the Pz area was only in the audio format. In this protocol, the subjects closed their eyes and only listened to the sound being played to them. Three pathways connected with this protocol were dedicated to the theta (5–8 Hz), alpha (8–12 Hz), and beta (15–18 Hz) frequency bands, while an additional pathway was used to control the delta (2–5 Hz) frequency band. The initial sessions were used to train patients to decrease alpha levels that were ≥ 12 mV (peak to peak), while augmenting theta levels, until there was "crossover." This was defined as the point at which the alpha amplitude dropped below the theta level. After achieving the first crossover, both alpha and theta frequencies were augmented and the delta frequency range was inhibited. This was intended to discourage the sleep transition during low-arousal states. Each alpha/theta session began with the subject sitting in a chair with eyes closed. The active electrode was placed at the Pz area with a left-ear reference (A1) and right-ear ground (A2). Two distinct tones were employed for alpha and theta reinforcement, with the higher pitched sound used to index the higher frequency alpha band. At the start of each session, the therapist spent 3–5 min reading a script of guided imagery to the experimental subject that dealt with identified essential elements of maintaining abstinence. After the guided imagery, the subjects were clearly informed that the objective of the training did not involve explicit rehearsal of the script during the NFB. Subjects reporting previous meditative practices were asked not to use them during the training, because meditation has been observed to override the alpha/theta reinforcement effects (Scott et al. 2005). Following alpha/theta training, the subjects were given the opportunity to process their experience. When it appeared that subjects' delta activity began to increase and that sleep might occur during training, those subjects were told prior to their next session to move a limb if they heard the therapist say for example "left hand." Subsequently, during sessions where delta was increasing toward no responsiveness levels, the feedback sounds were inhibited in order to discourage the sleep transition (Peniston and Saxby 1995; Scott et al. 2005).

Next studies have evaluated the treatment outcomes of Scott–Kaiser NFB protocol in SAD. Burkett et al. (2005) study showed that the addition of this NFB protocol to crack cocaine treatment regimens caused a significant decrease in relapse, depression, and anxiety rates compared to conventional forms of SAD treatment. At follow-up, participants regularly reported no uses, or one through nine uses. Dehghani-Arani et al. (2013) also compared results of 30 sessions of NFB being provided to opioid-dependent patients undergoing outpatient treatment (methadone or buprenorphine maintenance), in comparison with a control group that received outpatient treatment alone. Patients receiving NFB showed significantly more improvements in general health and craving. The next study is the Unterrainer et al. (2014) study in which a mixed substance misuse case received 11 sessions including a 2-month follow-up of NFB protocol combined with short-term psychodynamic psychotherapy. Pre-/post-treatment and follow-up assessment confirmed a significant psychopathology reduction. Furthermore, there was no relapse during the follow-up phase of the study. Rostami and Dehghani-Arani (2015) study is the newest application of Scott–Kaiser NFB protocol, especially for crystal methamphetamine-dependent patients. The study included 100 CMD patients undergoing a medical treatment who were randomly assigned to an experimental or a control group. The results showed the experimental group, who received 30 sessions of NFB, had lower severity of addiction, better psychological health, and better quality of life than the control group.

Other Neurofeedback Approaches in Substance Abuse Disorder

Literature review showed a wide range of research in which different other forms of NFB have been applied. For instance, Horrell and his colleagues used 12 sessions of ADHD-specific NFB protocol (SMR/theta training) and the first part of Scott & Kaiser's modification of Peniston's brainwave training protocol plus at least 2 sessions of motivational interviewing for ten cocaine-abusing/cocaine-dependent subjects. During the SMR/theta NFB protocol, according to its late modifications in Lubar's study (2003, in Horrell et al. 2010), the subjects were trained to enhance the amplitude of SMR within specified frequency band (12–15 Hz at C3 with a monopolar reference on the left mastoid) and/or to suppress the amplitude of theta frequency bands (4–7 Hz at F3 with monopolar reference to the left mastoid). Post-treatment clinical evaluations showed central SMR amplitude increase following with decreased self-reports on depression and stress scores, and urine tests results of decreased use of cocaine and marijuana. On the other hand, effects of NFB resulted in a lower EEG gamma reactivity to drug-related images in a post-NFB cue reactivity test. In particular, evoked gamma showed decreases in power to nontarget and to a lesser extent target drug-related cues, while induced gamma power decreased globally to both target and nontarget drug cues. They finally concluded that gamma-band cue reactivity measures are sufficiently sensitive functional outcomes of NFB treatment. They emphasized the utility of cognitive neuroscience methods based on the EEG gamma-band measures for the assessment of the functional outcomes of NFB-based interventions for cocaine-use disorders (Horrell et al. 2010).

In another innovative works on NFB and SAD, Li et al. (2013) and Hanlon et al. (2013) explored the feasibility of self-regulation of frontal cortical activation using real-time fMRI (rtfMRI) NFB to modify craving in nicotine-dependent cigarette smokers. Actually, this method is a "motivational NFB" approach that uses functional magnetic resonance imaging (fMRI) signals elicited by visual cues (pictures) and related to motivational processes such as craving. The visual feedback subsystem provides simultaneous feedback through these images as their size corresponds to the magnitude of fMRI signal change from a target brain area. During self-regulation of cue-evoked brain responses, decreases and increases in picture size thus provide real motivational consequences in terms of cue approach versus cue avoidance, which increases face validity of the approach in applied settings. Further, the outlined approach comprises of NFB (regulation) and "mirror" runs that allow controlling for non-specific and task-unrelated effects, such as habituation or neural adaptation (Sokunbi et al. 2014). In Li et al. (2013), Hanlon et al. (2013), and Hartwell et al. (2013) studies, to reduce the participant's craving, they were instructed to decrease the anterior cingulate cortex (ACC) activity during four rtfMRI NFB sessions. They were successful in decreasing their ACC activity, and the linear regression analysis results showed a significant correlation between decreased ACC activation and reduced craving ratings. Sokunbi et al. (2014) also, in a pilot study with 10 female volunteers, demonstrated feasibility of this newly developed motivational NFB paradigm to downregulate brain activation in response to appetitive food pictures. They finally mentioned that this newly developed visual feedback subsystem can be integrated into protocols for imaging-based brain–computer interfaces (BCI) and may facilitate NFB research and applications into healthy and dysfunctional motivational processes, such as food craving or addiction. Generally, Li et al. (2013), Hanlon et al. (2013), and Sokunbi et al. (2014) studies suggested that some smokers may be able to use NFB via rtfMRI to regulate ACC activation and to reduce smoking cue-induced craving, although further research is needed to determine the optimal parameters of NFB rtfMRI and whether it might eventually become a therapeutic tool for nicotine dependence.

Low-resolution electromagnetic tomographic (LORETA) neurofeedback (LNFB) in the ACC is another method for SAD treatment that has been started with

Cannon and his colleagues' studies (2006, 2007, 2008). These studies demonstrate relationships between limbic and cortical regions in specific frequencies can be influenced by LNFB in SAD. During LNFB sessions, after a preliminary muscle control session, participant is informed of the inhibitory and reward aspects of the NFB training to increase 14–18 Hz (low-beta) power activity in a seven-voxel cluster of neurons in the right ACC. This protocol provides the opportunity to train SAD patients to influence the electrical activity in regions not likely to be influenced by topographically specific EEG training. Training 14–18 Hz activity in the right anterior cingulate gyrus (rACC) would directly influence activity in cortical and limbic regions of interest (ROI, including the right hippocampus, the right amygdaloid complex, the right orbitofrontal cortex (OFC), the right occipital lobe, the right insular cortex, the right uncus, and two regions in the left prefrontal cortex) shown to be significantly decreased or increased in recovering addicts (Cannon & Lubar 2008; Cannon et al. 2008). In accordance with these studies, Center (2014) also reported a case study which demonstrated the application of LNFB, heart rate variability training, and cognitive restructuring to training a 55-year-old male with a long-term, treatment-resistant, alcohol-use disorder and comorbid mood disorder. The patient demonstrated significant improvements in general cognitive functioning, elevation, and stabilization in mood and sleep, and a significant reduction in alcohol consumption at the conclusion of training and at follow-up 6, 9, and 14 months following the end of training.

Discussion

Altogether, Sokhadze, Stewart, Tasman, Daniels, and Trudeau (2011) have validated the immense potential that NFB protocols have to likely double if not triple the outcome rates in alcoholism and SAD treatment when they are added as an additional component to a comprehensive treatment program. It is because of this method's potential to improve attention, emotion, and behavior self-regulation skills in patients with SAD. Interventions that incorporate NFB techniques are aimed to reeducate patients to control and self-regulate their emotional and motivational states, and to re-establish the normal biological, cognitive, behavioral, and hedonic homeostasis distorted by SAD (Sokhadze et al. 2008; White and Richards 2009; Unterrainer et al. 2014).

According to Rostami and Dehghani-Arani (2015), the most important finding in NFT and SAD studies is that in SAD treatment, a combination of different treatment approaches including pharmachotherapy, psychotherapy, and neurotherapeutic methods such as NFB is highly more effective than using a one-dimensional method. Although pharmacotherapy or psychotherapy approaches alone can lead to some improvement in SAD patients, they come with weak points that include side effects and the high risk of relapse (Simkin et al. 2014; Gossop et al. 2002). Because NFB, on the other hand, deals with the fundamental operational functions of the brain and acts as a mechanism for the brain to self-regulate, it has the ability to correct irregular brain functions and consequently improve psychological abnormalities. Furthermore, researches confirmed the stability of NFB effects and its prevention of negative side effects (Hammond 2011; Unterrainer et al. 2014). Thus, pharmacotherapy can be used to maintain the initial balance between physiological and psychological health in SAD, and then, NFB training can be used to guide the patient toward longer lasting health and balance (Trudeau et al. 2009).

Nowadays, several theoretical opinions exist on the fundamental mechanisms of effectiveness of NFB as a therapeutic method for SAD. Most of these opinions concentrated on the Pension's alpha–theta protocol. McPeak et al. (1991), Rosenfeld (1992), and Taub et al. (1994) introduced this protocol as a kind of meditation technique and suggested that self-induced altered states found in various forms of meditation can sometimes replace the self-destructive pursuit of alcohol and drugs. Cowan (1994) suggested that the effectiveness of such training may be due to the enhanced imprinting of positive temperance suggestions and the feeling of inner empowerment that the alpha/theta state seems to encourage. In a more detailed view, Ochs (1992) has suggested that the most active (and apparently transformational) properties of NFB protocols in SAD treatment may involve teaching the subjects to intentionally increase the amplitude and coherent interaction of both their alpha and theta brainwave frequencies in either of the brain locations. Complementing this finding, Simkin et al. (2014) explained that the alpha–theta NFB protocol trains SAD patients to promote stress reduction and to achieve profoundly relaxed states by increasing alpha and theta brainwaves and decreasing fast beta brainwaves. In Scott et al. (2005) viewpoint, the efficacy of alpha/theta NFB may lie in its ability to allow subjects to better tolerate stress, anxiety, and anxiety-eliciting situations, which are particularly evident during the initial phases of recovery. On the other side, White and Richards (2009) mentioned that alpha–theta protocol can induct higher states of consciousness and insight, helping to alter one's relationship to self and the world as a result of what is seen and understood in those higher states. They concluded that the effectiveness of this protocol may be explained in large part by a neuroplasticity concept known as the malleability of memory, which means that revisiting and re-evaluating early experiences via alpha–theta protocol allow the neurological rewriting of one's memory and consequently modify affective reactions, and alter the nature of memories. Furthermore, in alpha–theta protocol, subconscious (emotional) memories become more available to conscious (episodic) process and traumatic memories are often released and appear as flashbacks from the past. As these flashbacks are relived in the context of current adult resources and perceptions, the subconscious memories may become more readily available for healing and alteration.

On another perspective, explaining effectiveness of NFB protocols in SAD, some neuropsychologists focused on conditional normalization of reinforcement systems in the brain. Blum et al. (2012) were concerned with the reward deprivation syndrome (RDS) as a dysfunction in the brain reward cascade (BRC), which leads to substance craving and being a possible candidate for susceptibility to alcoholism and SAD. Therefore, SAD patients have a neurologically based inability to experience pleasant feelings and calmness from simple stimulation. It has been noticed that dysfunction of this pleasant feeling is the most important factor in forcing patients to feel craving and resort to substance abuse (Kreek et al. 2005). Following this idea, some studies have stated that an apparent neurological "normalization" could be responsible for shifting the trained subject into a physical state of comfortable calmness (Fahrion et al. 1992; Salansky et al. 1998). Studies suggested that NFB training can initiate this neurological normalizing shift (Scott et al. 2005; Sokhadze et al. 2011; Unterrainer et al. 2014).

Recently, mechanisms by which NFB therapy may cause behavioral changes have been suggested by research in neuronal plasticity. A number of investigators (Rosenzweig 2003; VanPraag et al. 2000) are essentially in agreement pointing out that ongoing direct experience that evokes persistent neuronal activation alters brain structure and brain functioning. A possible link is observed between steady-state stimulation, induced neuronal activation, and neuronal plasticity in the increasing body of evidence that the electrical activity of the brain regulates the synthesis, secretion, and actions of neurotrophins (Schindler and Poo 2000), which together promote synaptogenesis. In Sokhadze et al. (2011) explanation, pre- to post-treatment electrical activity changes are considered to positively affect motor control, cortical inhibition function, general arousal, and alertness level. This can mediates the positive effects of proposed NFB protocol on addictive behaviors. The crucial point about NFB is that it directly acts on the brain oscillations, which are altered in SAD. So, NFB-induced modifications could be manifestations of neural plasticity, which is a phenomenon that has been considered a basic mechanism for behavioral modifications.

Finally, while taking into consideration the complexity of the dimensions of this disorder, the worthwhile program must be able to affect various factors while not being prone to the problems of previous methods, such as relapsing, instability, and other side effects (Trudeau 2009). But, as a limitation, although NFT studies attempted to control different factors in the process of NFB training, their use of a new method of technology in NFB and patients' hope and motivation for the new treatment could have had an uncontrollable effect on our research. It is also noticeable about the NFB clinician contact effect. Despite this, the use of a placebo group could have strengthened the design of the NFB studies and created control over other aspects of the program. Furthermore, future studies can include one group of patients who would receive NFB without receiving pharmacotherapy to show the effectiveness of the two methods exclusively.

References

Becerra, J., Fernandez, T., Harmony, T., Caballero, M. I., Garcia, F., Fernandez-Bouzas, A., et al. (2006). Follow-up study of learning-disabled children treated with neurofeedback or placebo. *Clinical EEG & Neuroscience, 37*, 198–203.

Blum, K., Cshen, A. L. C., Giordano, J., Borsten, J., Chen, T. J. H., Hauser, M., et al. (2012). The addictive brain: All roads lead to dopamine. *Journal of Psychoactive Drugs, 44*(2), 134–143.

Bodehnamer, D. E., & Callaway, T. (2004). Extended follow-up of Peniston protocol results with chemical dependency. *Journal of Neurotherapy, 8*(2), 135–148.

Boulay, C. B., Sarnacki, W. A., Wolpaw, J. R., & McFarland, D. J. (2011). Trained modulation of sensorimotor rhythms can affect reaction time. *Clinical Neurophysiology, 122*, 1820–1826.

Breteler, M. H. M., Arns, M., Peters, S., Giepmans, I., & Verhoeven, L. (2010). Improvements in spelling after QEEG-based neurofeedback in dyslexia: A randomized controlled treatment study. *Applied Psychophysiology & Biofeedback, 35*(1), 5–11.

Burkett, V. S., Cummins, J. M., Dickson, R. M., & Skolnick, M. (2005). An open clinical trial utilizing real-time EEG operant conditioning as an adjunctive therapy in the treatment of crack cocaine dependence. *Journal of Neurotherapy, 9*(2), 27–47.

Callaway, T. G., & Bodenhamer-Davis, E. (2008). Long-term follow-up of a clinical replication of the Peniston protocol for chemical dependency. *Journal of Neurotherapy, 12*(4), 243–259.

Cannon, R., & Lubar, J. (2008). EEG spectral power and coherence: Differentiating effects of spatial-specific neuro-operant learning (SSNOL) utilizing LORETA neurofeedback training in the anterior cingulate and bilateral dorsolateral prefrontal cortices. *Journal of Neurotherapy, 11*(3), 25–44.

Cannon, R., Lubar, J., Congedo, M., Thornton, K., Hutchens, T., & Towler, K. (2007). The effects of neurofeedback in the cognitive division of the anterior cingulate gyrus. *The International Journal of Neuroscience, 117*, 337–357.

Cannon, R., Lubar, J., Gerke, A., Thornton, K., Hutchens, T., & McCammon, V. (2006). Topographical coherence and absolute power changes resulting from LORETA neurofeedback in the anterior cingulate gyrus. *Journal of Neurotherapy, 10*, 5–31.

Cannon, R., Lubar, J., Sokhadze, E., & Baldwin, D. (2008). LORETA neurofeedback for addiction and the possible neurophysiology of psychological processes influenced: A case study and region of interest analysis of LORETA neurofeedback in right anterior cingulate cortex. *Journal of Neurotherapy, 12*(4), 227–241.

Center, W. D. (2014). LORETA neurofeedback in alcohol use disorders: A case study. Z score neurofeedback: Clinical applications (pp. 243–272). doi:10.1016/B978-0-12-801291-8.00011-X.

Choi, S. W., Chi, S. E., Chung, S. Y., Kim, J. W., Ahn, C. Y., & Kim, H. T. (2011). Is alpha wave neurofeedback effective with randomized clinical trials in depression? A pilot study. *Neuropsychobiology, 63*, 43–51.

Cortoos, A., De Valck, E., Arns, M., Breteler, M. H., & Cluydts, R. (2010). An exploratory study on the effects of tele-neurofeedback and tele-biofeedback on objective and subjective sleep in patients with primary insomnia. *Applied Psychophysiology & Biofeedback, 35*, 125–134.

Cowan, J. D. (1994). Alpha-theta brain wave biofeedback: The many possible theoretical reasons for its success. Megabrain report. *Journal of Mind Technology, 2*(3), 29–35.

Crocetti, A., Forti, S., & Bo, L. D. (2011). Neurofeedback for subjective tinnitus patients. *Auris Nasus Larnx, 38*, 735–738.

deBeus, R. J., & Kaiser, D. A. (2011). Neurofeedback with children with attention deficit hyperactivity disorder: A randomized doubleblind placebo-controlled study. In R. Coben & J. R. Evans (Eds.), *Neurofeedback and neuromodulation techniques and applications*. New York, NY: Academic Press.

Dehghani-Arani, F., Rostami, R., & Nadali, H. (2013). Neurofeedback training for opiate addiction: Improvement of mental health and craving. *Applied Psychophysiology and Biofeedbck, 38*(2), 133–141.

Dehghani-Arani, F., Rostami, R., & Nosratabadi, M. (2010). Effectiveness of neurofeedback training as a treatment for opioid-dependent patients. *Clinical EEG and Neuroscience, 41*(3), 170–177.

Fahrion, S. L., Walters, E. D., Coyne, L., & Allen, T. (1992). Alteration in EEG amplitude, personality factors and brain electrical mapping after alpha-theta training: A controlled case study of an alcoholic recovery. *Clinical and Experimental Research, 16*(3), 547–552.

Gani, C., Birbaumer, N., & Strehl, U. (2008). Long term effects after feedback of slow cortical potentials and of theta-beta amplitudes in children with attention-deficit/hyperactivity disorder. *International Journal of Bioelectromagnetics, 10*, 209–232.

Gevensleben, H., Holl, B., Albrecht, B., Schlamp, D., Kratz, O., Studer, P., et al. (2010). Neurofeedback training for children with ADHD: 6-month follow-up of a randomised controlled trial. *European Child and Adolescent Psychiatry, 19*, 715–724.

Gevensleben, H., Holl, B., Albrecht, B., Vogel, C., Schlamp, D., Kratz, O., et al. (2009). Is neurofeedback an efficacious treatment for ADHD? A randomized controlled clinical trial. *Journal of Clinical Psychology & Psychiatry, 50*, 780–789.

Goldberg, R. J., Greenwood, J. C., & Taintor, Z. (1976). Alpha conditioning as an adjust treatment for drug dependence. *International Journal of Addiction, 11*, 1085–1089.

Goslinga, J. J. (1975). Biofeedback for chemical problem patients: A developmental process. *Journal of Biofeedback, 2*, 17–27.

Gossop, M., Stewart, D., Browne, N., & Marsden, J. (2002). Factors associated with abstinence, lapse or relapse to heroin use after residential treatment: Protective effect of coping responses. *Addiction, 97*(10), 1259–1267.

Green, E. E., Green, A. M., & Walters, E. D. (1974). Alpha–theta biofeedback training. *Journal of Biofeedback, 2*, 7–13.

Hammer, B. U., Colbert, A. P., Brown, I. A., & Ilioi, E. C. (2011). Neurofeedback for insomnia: A pilot study of Z-score SMR and individualized protocols. *Applied Psychophysiology & Biofeedback, 36*, 251–264.

Hammond, D. C. (2011). What is neurofeedback: An update. *Journal of Neurotherapy, 15*(4), 305–336.

Hanlon, C. A., Hartwell, K. J., Canterberry, M., Li, X., Owens, M., Lematty, T., et al. (2013). Reduction of cue induced craving through real-time neurofeedback in nicotine users: The role of region of interest selection and multiple visits. *Psychiatry Researches, 213*, 79–81.

Hartwell, K. J., Prisciandaro, J. J., Borckardt, J., Li, X., George, M. S., & Brady, K. T. (2013). Real-time fMRI in the treatment of nicotine dependence: A conceptual review and pilot studies. *Psychology of Addictive Behaviors, 27*(2), 501–509.

Horrell, T., El-Baz, A., Baruth, J., Tasman, A., Sokhadze, G., Stewart, C., et al. (2010). Neurofeedback effects on evoked and induced EEG gamma band reactivity to drug-related cues in cocaine addiction. *Journal of Neurotherapy, 14*(3), 195–216.

Ibric, V. L., & Dragomirescu, L. G. (2009). Neurofeedback in pain management. In T. H. Budzyknski, H. K. Budzynski, J. R. Evans, & A. Abarbanel (Eds.), *Introduction to quantitative EEG and neurofeedback: Advanced theory and applications* (2nd ed.). New York, NY: Elsevier.

Johnson, K. A., Hartwell, K., Lematty, T., Borckardt, J., Morgan, P. S., Govindarajan, K., et al. (2012). Intermittent "real-time" fMRI feedback is superior to continuous presentation for a motor imagery task: A pilot study. *Journal of Neuroimaging, 22*, 58–66.

Kaiser, D. A., Othmer, S., & Scott, B. (1999). Effect of neurofeedback on chemical dependency treatment. *Biofeedback & Self-Regulation, 20*(3), 304–305.

Kamiya, J. (2011). The first communications about operant conditioning of the EEG. *Journal of Neurotherapy, 15*(1), 65–73.

Keizer, A. W., Verment, R. S., & Hommel, B. (2010). Enhancing cognitive control through neurofeedback: A role of gamma-band activity in managing episodic retrieval. *Neuroimage, 490*, 3404–3413.

Kelley, M. J. (1997). Native Americans, neurofeedback, and substance abuse theory: Three year outcome of alpha/theta neurofeedback training in the treatment of problem drinking among Dine' (Navajo) people. *Journal of Neurotherapy, 2*(3), 24–60.

Kleber, B., Gruzelier, J., Bensch, M., & Birbaumer, N. (2008). Effects of EEGbiofeedback on professional singing performances. *Revista Espanola Psicologica, 10*, 61–77.

Knezevic, B., Thompson, L., & Thompson, M. (2010). Pilot project to ascertain the utility of Tower of London Test to assess outcomes of neurofeedback in clients with Asperger's syndrome. *Journal of Neurotherapy, 14*(3), 3–19.

Kreek, M. J., Nielsen, D. A., Butelman, E. R., & LaForge, K. S. (2005). Genetic influences on impulsivity, risk taking, stress responsivity and vulnerability to drug abuse and addiction. *Nature Neuroscience, 8*, 1450–1457.

Lansbergen, M. M., van Dongen-Boomsma, M., Buitelaar, J. K., & Slaats-Willemse, D. (2011). ADHD and EEG-neurofeedback: A double-blind randomized placebo-controlled feasibility study. *Journal of Neural Transmission, 118*(2), 275–284.

Leins, U., Goth, G., Hinterberger, T., Klinger, C., Rumpf, N., & Strehl, U. (2007). Neurofeedback for children with ADHD: A comparison of SCP and theta/beta protocols. *Applied Psychophysiology & Biofeedback, 32*, 73–88.

Levesque, J., Beauregard, M., & Mensour, B. (2006). Effect of neurofeedback training on the neural substrates of selective attention in children with attention-deficit/hyperactivity disorder: A functional magnetic resonance imaging study. *Neuroscience Letters, 394*, 216–221.

Li, X., Hartwell, K. J., Borckardt, J., Prisciandaro, J. J., Saladin, M. E., Morgan, P. S., et al. (2013). Volitional reduction of anterior cingulate cortex activity produces decreased cue craving in smoking cessation: A preliminary real-time fMRI study. *Addiction Biology, 18*(4), 739–748.

Lubar, J. F. (1995). Neurofeedback for the management of attention-deficit = hyperactivity disorders. In M. S. Schwartz (Ed.), *Biofeedback: A practitioner's guide*. Guilford: New York, NY.

McPeak, J. D., Kennedy, B. P., & Gordon, S. M. (1991). Altered states of consciousness therapy: A missing component in alcohol and drug rehabilitation treatment. *Journal of Substance Abuse Treatment, 8*, 75–82.

Muller, H. H., Donaldson, C. C. S., Nelson, D. V., & Layman, M. (2001). Treatment of fibromyalgia incorporating EEG-driven stimulation: A clinical study. *Journal of Clinical Psychology, 57*(7), 925–933.

Ochs, L. (1992). EEG biofeedback treatment of addictions. *Applied Psychophysiology and Biofeedback, 20*(1), 8–16.

Passini, F. T., Watson, C. G., Dehnel, L., Herder, J., & Watkins, B. (1977). Alpha wave biofeedback training therapy in alcoholics. *Journal of Clinical Psychology, 33*, 292–299.

Peniston, E. G., & Kulkosky, P. J. (1990). Alcoholic personality and alpha–theta brainwave training. *Medical Psychotherapy, 2*, 37–55.

Peniston, E. G., & Kulkosky, P. J. (1989). Alpha-theta brainwave training and beta-endorphin levels in alcoholics. *Clinical and Experimental Research, 13*, 271–279.

Peniston, E. G., & Saxby, E. (1995). Alpha-theta brainwave neurofeedback training: an effective treatment for male and female alcoholics with depression symptoms. *The Biofeedback Center, 51*(5), 685–693.

Raymond, J., Varney, C., Parkinson, L. A., & Gruzelier, J. H. (2005). The effect of alpha/theta neurofeedback on personality and mood. *Cognitive Brain Research, 23*, 287–292.

Rosenfeld, J. P. (1992). EEG treatment of addictions: Commentary on Ochs, Peniston and Kulkosky. *Applied Psychophysiology and Biofeedback, 20*(2), 12–17.

Rosenzweig, M. R. (2003). Effects of differential experience on the brain and behavior. *Developmental Neuropsychology, 24*(2–3), 523–540.

Rossiter, T. R. (2005). The effectiveness of neurofeedback and stimulant drugs in treating ADHD part II. Replication. *Applied Psychophysiology & Biofeedback, 29*, 233–243.

Rostami, R., & Dehghani-Arani, F. (2015). Neurofeedback training as a new method in treatment of crystal methamphetamine dependent patients: A preliminary study. *Applied Psychophysiology and Biofeedbck, 40*(3), 151–161.

Salansky, N., Fedotchev, A., & Bondar, A. (1998). Responses of the nervous system to low frequency stimulation and EEG rhythms: Clinical implications. *Neuroscience and Biobehavioral Reviews, 22*(3), 395–409.

Saxby, E., & Peniston, E. G. (1995). Alpha-theta brainwave neurofeedback training: An effective treatment for male and female alcoholics with depressive symptoms. *Journal of Clinical Psychology, 51*(5), 685–693.

Schindler, A. F., & Poo, M. (2000). The neurotrophin hypothesis for synaptic plasticity. *Trends in Neuroscience, 23*(12), 639–645.

Scott, W. C., Kaiser, D., Othmer, S., & Sideroff, S. I. (2005). Effects of an EEG biofeedback protocol on a mixed substance abusing population. *The American Journal of Drug and Alcohol Abuse, 3*, 1455–1469.

Simkin, D. R., Thatcher, R. W., & Lubar, J. (2014). Quantitative EEG and neurofeedback in children and adolescents anxiety disorders, depressive disorders, comorbid addiction and attention-deficit/Hyperactivity disorder, and brain injury. *Child and Adolescent Psychiatric Clinics of North America, 23*(3), 427–464.

Sokhadze, T. M., Cannon, R. L., & Trudeau, D. L. (2008). EEG biofeedback as a treatment for substance use disorders: Review, rating of efficacy, and recommendations for further research. *Applied Psychophysiology and Biofeedback, 33*(1), 1–28.

Sokhadze, T. M., Stewart, C. M., & Hollifield, M. (2007). Integrating cognitive neuroscience research and cognitive behavioral treatment with neurofeedback therapy in drug addiction comorbid with posttraumatic stress disorder: A conceptual review. *Journal of Neurotherapy, 11*(2), 13–44.

Sokhadze, E., Stewart, C. M., Tasman, A., Daniels, R., & Trudeau, D. (2011). Review of rationale for neurofeedback application in adolescent substance abusers with comorbid disruptive behavioral disorders. *Journal of Neurotherapy, 15*(3), 232–261.

Sokunbi, M. O., Linden, D. E. J., Habes, I., Johnston, S., & Ihssen, N. (2014). Real-time fMRI brain-computer interface: Development of a "motivational feedback" subsystem for the regulation of visual cue reactivity. *Frontiers in Behavioral Neuroscience.* doi:10.3389/fnbeh. 2014.00392.

Sterman, M. B., LoPresti, R. W., & Fairchild, M. D. (2010). Electroencephalographic and behavioral studies of monomethylhydrazine toxicity in the cat. *Journal of Neurotherapy, 14*, 293–300.

Stokes, D. A., & Lappin, M. S. (2010). Neurofeedback and biofeedback with 37 migraineurs: A clinical outcome study. *Behavior and Brain Functions, 6*, 9–12.

Strehl, U., Leins, U., Gopth, G., Klinger, C., Hinterberger, T., & Birbaumer, N. (2006). Self-regulation of slow cortical potentials: A new treatment for children with attention deficit/hyperactivity disorder. *Pediatrics, 118*, 1530–1540.

Surmeli, T., Ertem, A., Eralp, E., & Kos, I. H. (2011). Obsessive compulsive disorder and the efficacy of qEEG-guided neurofeedback treatment: A case series. *Clinical EEG and Neuroscience, 42*, 195–201.

Taub, E., Steiner, S. S., Smith, R. B., Weingarten, E., & Walton, K. G. (1994). Effectiveness of broad spectrum approaches to relapse prevention in severe alcoholism: A long-term, randomized, controlled trial of transcendental meditation, EMG biofeedback, and electronic neurotherapy. *Alcoholism Treatment Quarterly, 11*, 187–220.

Trudeau, D. L. (2009). Brainwave biofeedback for addictive disorder. *Journal of Neurotherapy, 12* (4), 181–183.

Trudeau, D. L. (2005a). Applicability of brain wave biofeedback to substance use disorder in adolescents. *Child and Adolescent Psychiatric Clinics of North America, 14*(1), 125–136.

Trudeau, D. L. (2005b). EEG Biofeedback for Addictive Disorders—The State of the Art in 2004. *Journal of Adult Development, 12*(2/3), 139–146.

Trudeau, D. L., Sokhadze, T. M., & Cannon, R. L. (2009). Neurofeedback in alcohol and drug dependency. In T. Budzynski, H. Budzynski, J. Evans, & A. Abarbanel (Eds.), *Introduction to quantitative EEG and neurofeedback: Advanced theory and applications series* (2nd ed.). Waltham, MA: Academic Press.

Twemlow, S. W., & Bowen, W. T. (1976). EEG biofeedback induced self-actualization in alcoholics. *Journal of Biofeedback, 3*, 20–25.

Twemlow, S. W., & Bowen, W. T. (1977). Sociocultural predictors of self-actualization in EEG biofeedback-treated alcoholics. *Psychological Reports, 40*, 591–598.

Unterrainer, H. F., Chen, M. J., & Gruzelier, J. H. (2014). EEG-neurofeedback and psychodynamic psychotherapy in a case of adolescent anhedonia with substance misuse: Mood/theta relations. *International Journal of Psychophysiology, 93*(1), 84–95.

VanPraag, H., Kempermann, G., & Gage, F. H. (2000). Neural consequences of environmental enrichment. *Nature Reviews Neuroscience, 1*, 191–198.

Walker, J. E. (2010a). Case report: Dyslexia remediated with QEEG-guided neurofeedback. *NeuroConnections, 28*, 1–5.

Walker, J. E. (2010b). Using QEEG-guided neurofeedback for epilepsy versus standardized protocols: Enhanced effectiveness? *Applied Psychophysiology & Biofeedback, 35*(1), 29–30.

Walker, J. E. (2011). QEEG-guided neurofeedback for recurrent migraine headaches. *Clinical EEG & Neuroscience, 42*(1), 59–61.

White, N. E. (2008). The transformational power of the Peniston protocol: A therapist's experiences. *Journal of Neurotherapy, 12*(4), 261–265.

White, N. E., & Richards, L. M. (2009). Alpha-theta neurotherapy and the neurobehavioral treatment of addictions, mood disorders and trauma. In T. Budzynski, H. Budzynski, J. Evans, & A. Abarbanel (Eds.), *Introduction to quantitative EEG and neurofeedback: Advanced theory and applications series* (2nd ed.). Waltham, MA: Academic Press.

Zoefel, B., Huster, R. J., & Herrmann, C. S. (2010). Neurofeedback training of the upper alpha frequency band in EEG improves cognitive performance. *Neuroimage, 54*, 1427–1431.

Author Biography

Fateme Dehghani-Arani BA in Psychology, University of Tehran; MA in Psychology, University of Tehran; PhD of Health Psychology, University of Tehran; Assistance professor at University of Tehran, Department of Psychology.

Erratum to: Neurobiology of Substance Abuse

André Bedendo, André Luiz Monezi Andrade and Ana Regina Noto

Erratum to:
Chapter 2 in: A.L.M. Andrade and D. De Micheli (eds.), *Innovations in the Treatment of Substance Addiction*, DOI 10.1007/978-3-319-43172-7_2

The names of the authors, respectively, "Denise De Micheli" and "Adriana Scatena" were included incorrectly in the published version of Chapter 2. The erratum chapter and the book have been updated with the changes.

The updated original online version for this chapter can be found at
10.1007/978-3-319-43172-7_2

A. Bedendo (✉) · A.L.M. Andrade · A.R. Noto
Departamento de Psicobiologia, Universidade Federal de São Paulo, Rua Botucatu,
862 – 1o Andar, Edifício de Ciências Biomédicas, São Paulo, SP 04023-062, Brazil
e-mail: andrebedendo@gmail.com

A.L.M. Andrade
e-mail: andremonezi@gmail.com

A.R. Noto
e-mail: anareginanoto@gmail.com; ana.noto@unifesp.br

Index

© Springer International Publishing Switzerland 2016
A.L.M. Andrade and D. De Micheli (eds.), *Innovations in the Treatment
of Substance Addiction*, DOI 10.1007/978-3-319-43172-7

0 1341 1717761 5

CPSIA information can be obtained
at www.ICGtesting.com
Printed in the USA
LVOW13s1548230718
584652LV00003BA/193/P

9 783319 82752